Knee Arthroplasty: Therapeutic and Management Strategies

Knee Arthroplasty: Therapeutic and Management Strategies

Editor

Christian Carulli

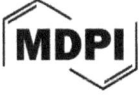

Basel • Beijing • Wuhan • Barcelona • Belgrade • Novi Sad • Cluj • Manchester

Editor
Christian Carulli
University of Florence
Florence
Italy

Editorial Office
MDPI
St. Alban-Anlage 66
4052 Basel, Switzerland

This is a reprint of articles from the Special Issue published online in the open access journal *Journal of Clinical Medicine* (ISSN 2077-0383) (available at: https://www.mdpi.com/journal/jcm/special_issues/E0947N8TM8).

For citation purposes, cite each article independently as indicated on the article page online and as indicated below:

Lastname, A.A.; Lastname, B.B. Article Title. *Journal Name* **Year**, *Volume Number*, Page Range.

ISBN 978-3-7258-0889-2 (Hbk)
ISBN 978-3-7258-0890-8 (PDF)
doi.org/10.3390/books978-3-7258-0890-8

© 2024 by the authors. Articles in this book are Open Access and distributed under the Creative Commons Attribution (CC BY) license. The book as a whole is distributed by MDPI under the terms and conditions of the Creative Commons Attribution-NonCommercial-NoDerivs (CC BY-NC-ND) license.

Contents

About the Editor vii

Preface ix

Caspar W. J. Hulleman, Tommy S. de Windt, Karin Veerman, Jon H. M. Goosen,
Frank-Christiaan B. M. Wagenaar and Gijs G. van Hellemondt
Debridement, Antibiotics and Implant Retention: A Systematic Review of Strategies for
Treatment of Early Infections after Revision Total Knee Arthroplasty
Reprinted from: *J. Clin. Med.* **2023**, *12*, 5026, doi:10.3390/jcm12155026 1

Jung-Wee Park, Tae Woo Kim, Chong Bum Chang, Minji Han, Jong Jin Go,
Byung Kyu Park, et al.
Effects of Thrombin-Based Hemostatic Agent in Total Knee Arthroplasty: Meta-Analysis
Reprinted from: *J. Clin. Med.* **2023**, *12*, 6656, doi:10.3390/jcm12206656 12

Emerito Carlos Rodriguez-Merchan and Alberto D. Delgado-Martinez
Risk Factors for Periprosthetic Joint Infection after Primary Total Knee Arthroplasty
Reprinted from: *J. Clin. Med.* **2022**, *11*, 6128, doi:10.3390/jcm11206128 23

Emerito Carlos Rodriguez-Merchan, Hortensia De la Corte-Rodriguez, Teresa Alvarez-Roman,
Primitivo Gomez-Cardero, Carlos A. Encinas-Ullan and Victor Jimenez-Yuste
Complications and Implant Survival of Total Knee Arthroplasty in People with Hemophilia
Reprinted from: *J. Clin. Med.* **2022**, *11*, 6244, doi:10.3390/jcm11216244 41

Giuseppe Polizzotti, Alfredo Lamberti, Fabio Mancino and Andrea Baldini
New Horizons of Cementless Total Knee Arthroplasty
Reprinted from: *J. Clin. Med.* **2024**, *13*, 233, doi:10.3390/jcm13010233 55

Melanie Schindler, Stephanie Schmitz, Jan Reinhard, Petra Jansen, Joachim Grifka
and Achim Benditz
Pain Course after Total Knee Arthroplasty within a Standardized Pain Management Concept: A
Prospective Observational Study
Reprinted from: *J. Clin. Med.* **2022**, *11*, 7204, doi:10.3390/jcm11237204 66

Krystian Kazubski, Łukasz Tomczyk, Andrzej Bobiński and Piotr Morasiewicz
Prognostic Factors in Staged Bilateral Total Knee Arthroplasty—A Retrospective Case
Series Analysis
Reprinted from: *J. Clin. Med.* **2023**, *12*, 3547, doi:10.3390/jcm12103547 77

Christian Carulli, Matteo Innocenti, Rinaldo Tambasco, Alessandro Perrone
and Roberto Civinini
Total Knee Arthroplasty in Haemophilia: Long-Term Results and Survival Rate of a Modern
Knee Implant with an Oxidized Zirconium Femoral Component
Reprinted from: *J. Clin. Med.* **2023**, *12*, 4356, doi:10.3390/jcm12134356 86

Jong Hwa Lee, Ho Jung Jung, Byung Sun Choi, Du Hyun Ro and Joong Il Kim
Effectiveness of Robotic Arm-Assisted Total Knee Arthroplasty on Transfusion Rate in Staged
Bilateral Surgery
Reprinted from: *J. Clin. Med.* **2023**, *12*, 4570, doi:10.3390/jcm12144570 97

Yoshinori Ishii, Hideo Noguchi, Junko Sato, Ikuko Takahashi, Hana Ishii, Ryo Ishii, et al.
Characteristics of Preoperative Arteriosclerosis Evaluated by Cardio-Ankle Vascular Index in
Patients with Osteoarthritis before Total Knee Arthroplasty
Reprinted from: *J. Clin. Med.* **2023**, *12*, 4685, doi:10.3390/jcm12144685 106

Jong Hwa Lee, Ho Jung Jung, Joon Kyu Lee, Ji Hyo Hwang and Joong Il Kim
Large Osteophytes over 10 mm at Posterior Medial Femoral Condyle Can Lead to Asymmetric
Extension Gap Following Bony Resection in Robotic Arm–Assisted Total Knee Arthroplasty with
Pre-Resection Gap Balancing
Reprinted from: *J. Clin. Med.* **2023**, *12*, 5980, doi:10.3390/jcm12185980 115

Stefano Campi, Rocco Papalia, Carlo Esposito, Vincenzo Candela, Andrea Gambineri and Umile Giuseppe Longo
The Correlation between Objective Ligament Laxity and the Clinical Outcome of Mechanically Aligned TKA
Reprinted from: *J. Clin. Med.* **2023**, *12*, 6007, doi:10.3390/jcm12186007 . . . . **122**

Luboš Nachtnebl, Vasileios Apostolopoulos, Michal Mahdal, Lukáš Pazourek, Pavel Brančík, Tomáš Valoušek, et al.
Implant Preference and Clinical Outcomes of Patients with Staged Bilateral Total Knee Arthroplasty: All-Polyethylene and Contralateral Metal-Backed Tibial Components
Reprinted from: *J. Clin. Med.* **2023**, *12*, 7438, doi:10.3390/jcm12237438 . . . . **135**

Ulrike Wittig, Amir Koutp, Patrick Reinbacher, Konstanze Hütter, Andreas Leithner and Patrick Sadoghi
Enhancing Precision and Efficiency in Knee Arthroplasty: A Comparative Analysis of Computer-Assisted Measurements with a Novel Software Tool versus Manual Measurements for Lower Leg Geometry
Reprinted from: *J. Clin. Med.* **2023**, *12*, 7581, doi:10.3390/jcm12247581 . . . . **144**

About the Editor

Christian Carulli

Christian Carulli is an Associate Professor and Deputy Chief of the Orthopaedic Clinic at the University of Florence, Italy. He is specialist in Orthopaedics and Traumatology and in Hand Surgery, and completed a fellowship at Hospital for Special Surgery and a Master in Bone Metabolism. He performed more than 2000 major surgeries, and 3000 minor procedures.

His member of several national (SIOT, AICE, SIAGASCOT, ORTOMED, AIR, AUOT, SICM) and international societies (WFH, ESSKA, EKA, ISHA) and co-founding member of the EHPA. He is also Associate Editor for prestigious scientific journals (JOOT, JCM) and editorial member of many other high-impact journals. He is author and co-author of more than 100 papers and books, with a current IF of more than 130. He wrote also a book in Haemophilia in 2017 and a new book on this topic is currently under writing.

His clinical and scientific fields of interest are: rare diseases (Haemophilia, Multiple Sclerosis, Rheumatic conditions); joint replacement of the lower limbs; traumatology in fragile patients; hip, knee, and ankle arthroscopy.

Preface

In recent decades, knee arthroplasty has been one of the most evolving branches of orthopaedic surgery. Very few historical surgical techniques, biomaterials, implantation philosophies, and postoperative approaches are maintained; however, most have been fully implemented, and clinical outcomes, such as patients' postoperative perceptions, have been associated with new paradigms. Nowadays, knee arthroplasty may be considered an "ultra-specialty on specialty" due to the many brand-new aspects arising from its clinical and surgical issues.

Thus, this Special Issue on "Knee Arthroplasty: Therapeutic and Management Strategies" includes several modern aspects representing a new vision of this simple but complex surgery.

The articles included in this Special Issue propose specific preoperative evaluations and risk factor analyses, the adoption of peculiar surgical techniques or computerized/robotic devices, the use of modern implants and biomaterials, the innovative management of postoperative infections, postoperative strategies, and the evaluation of long-term results.

Well-known authors from various countries have contributed to this collection with their expertise and leadership, sharing the highly technical capacity while also providing a clear exposition of these modern aspects that have made and will continue to make knee arthroplasty a highly dynamic sector of orthopaedic art.

We are sure that readers will find a treasure of information and technical sparks to improve their clinical and surgical practice and even think about further implementations of knee arthroplasty; so much has indeed been achieved, but improving the analysis of clinical cases and management is also mandatory.

Christian Carulli
Editor

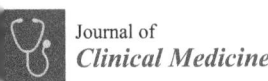

Systematic Review

Debridement, Antibiotics and Implant Retention: A Systematic Review of Strategies for Treatment of Early Infections after Revision Total Knee Arthroplasty

Caspar W. J. Hulleman [1], Tommy S. de Windt [2], Karin Veerman [1], Jon H. M. Goosen [1], Frank-Christiaan B. M. Wagenaar [2] and Gijs G. van Hellemondt [1,*]

1. Sint Maartenskliniek, Orthopedic Surgery, 6574 NA Nijmegen, The Netherlands; casparhulleman96@gmail.com (C.W.J.H.)
2. Orthopedisch Centrum Oost Nederland, Orthopedic Center, 7555 DL Hengelo, The Netherlands
* Correspondence: g.vanhellemondt@maartenskliniek.nl

Abstract: Goal: The purpose of this review is to provide a systematic and comprehensive overview of the available literature on the treatment of an early prosthetic joint infection (PJI) after revision total knee arthroplasty (TKA) and provide treatment guidelines. Methods: This systematic review was performed in accordance with the Preferred Reporting Items for Systematic Reviews and Meta-Analysis (PRISMA) guidelines. The search was conducted using the electronic databases of PubMed, Trip, Cochrane, Embase, LILACS and SciElo. After the inclusion of the relevant articles, we extracted the data and results to compose a treatment algorithm for early and acute PJI after revision TKA. Results: After applying the in- and exclusion criteria, seven articles were included in this systematic review focusing on debridement, antibiotics and implant retention (DAIR) for PJI following revision TKA, of which one was prospective and six were retrospective. All studies were qualified as level IV evidence. Conclusions: The current literature suggests that DAIR is a valid treatment option for early infections after revision TKA with success rates of 50–70%. Repeat DAIR shows success rates of around 50%. Further research should be aimed at predicting successful (repeat/two-stage) DAIRs in larger study populations, antibiotic regimes and the cost effectiveness of a second DAIR after revision TKA.

Keywords: debridement; antibiotics and implant retention; revision knee arthroplasty; periprosthetic joint infection

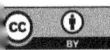

1. Introduction

The ongoing growth of the elderly population increases demand for joint arthroplasty. In fact, the incidence of total knee arthroplasty (TKA) for osteoarthritis (OA) is estimated to rise by 276% by 2030 [1]. This will inevitably lead to an increase in the number of revision arthroplasties. One of the most feared complications after total knee arthroplasty is a periprosthetic joint infection (PJI). With an incidence of 1–2%, this complication is relatively uncommon after primary TKA. For revision TKA, however, the infection rate is higher, at 2 to 5% [2]. A recent systematic review showed a significantly higher incidence of PJIs after revision TKA with a pooled reinfection rate (95% CI) of 12.7% (7.0–19.7%) after one-stage revision TKA and 16.2% (13.7–19.0%) after two-stage revision (Goud et al.) [3]. Additionally, a PJI after revision TKA has a significantly reduced percentage of successful eradication, leading to even more reoperations, longer hospitalization and a higher prevalence of multidrug-resistant organisms [4]. A PJI is one of the most significant and potentially lethal complications following TKA and is physically and mentally disastrous for the patient. In addition, it is a known burden to society due to the high costs. It is estimated that in the US the projected cost of PJI treatment is USD 1.62 billion [5]. Parvizi et al. [6] found significant differences in mortality rates in patients undergoing revision for a PJI compared to aseptic loosening at 30–90 days (3.7% vs. 0.8%) and 90 days to 1 year (10.6% vs. 2%), respectively. The mortality rates for PJIs have been shown to be comparable to breast cancer and higher than those for colorectal and lung cancer, again stressing their burden on society [7]. There are different types of PJIs, with different treatment strategies for each type. The most common types are classified by Tsukayama et al. as type IIb, early deep postoperative infection (within 4 weeks after surgery), and type III, acute hematogenous infection [8].

Historically, debridement, antibiotics and implant retention (DAIR) is considered a reasonable treatment option for an early PJI (i.e., a PJI occurring in the first 3 months after surgery) if the duration of clinical signs and symptoms is less than three weeks, the implant is stable and the soft tissue is in good condition [9]. DAIR aims to eliminate the infection and prevent recurrence. It is a well-established treatment for PJI after primary arthroplasty, with an overall success rate of 60 to 80% [10–13]. While treating an early PJI after revision TKA is more challenging, our group found an overall success rate of DAIR (with success defined as retention of components and absence of infection) of 62% after two years [14]. Currently, a treatment algorithm for early PJIs after knee revision arthroplasty is lacking. The purpose of this review is to provide a systematic and comprehensive overview of the available literature on the treatment of early PJIs after revision TKA with DAIR and provide early treatment guidelines.

2. Methods

2.1. Data Source and Search

We have not registered this systematic review in the public registry of Prospero, as this is a UK-based registry. However, this systematic review was performed in accordance with the Preferred Reporting Items for Systematic Reviews and Meta-Analysis (PRISMA) statement [15]. The search was conducted in July 2023 using the following electronic databases: PubMed, Cochrane Library, Embase, Trip Medical Database, SciElo and LILACS. We used a combination and variation of the terms 'revision arthroplasty', 're-revision', 'aseptic revision', 'total knee arthroplasty', 'infection', 'periprosthetic joint infection', 'positive cultures' and 'debridement, antibiotics, implant retention'. For each database, a specific search was generated and converted accordingly. The full search strategies can be found in Supplementary Materials.

2.2. Study Selection

After the search was conducted, the articles were screened by title and abstract and the following steps were selected as described in Figure 1. Articles on early and acute PJI (Tsukayama type IIb and III) after revision TKA treated with DAIR were included in this review. The exclusion criteria were defined as PJI after primary TKA, joints other than the knee, articles not written in English and systematic reviews. After applying the exclusion criteria, duplicate articles were removed. Finally, two more articles were removed because they reported insufficient outcome data. The following data were extracted: patient demographics (study population and mean age), reason of revision, type of infection that occurred after revision, prophylactic antibiotic regime, postoperative antibiotic strategy, mean follow-up period and rate of success.

2.3. Definitions of Infection

Different definitions of PJI were used in the included studies. Early PJI was defined as a deep infection occurring within three months after surgery (Zimmerli et al. [9]) or within four weeks after surgery (Tsykayama et al. type IIb [8]), and acute hematogenous PJI was defined as occurring more than four weeks after surgery following a symptom-free postoperative period, but with symptoms for three weeks or less (Tsukayama et al. type III [8]). Based on clinical applicability, the classification system of Tsukayama was primarily used in this review.

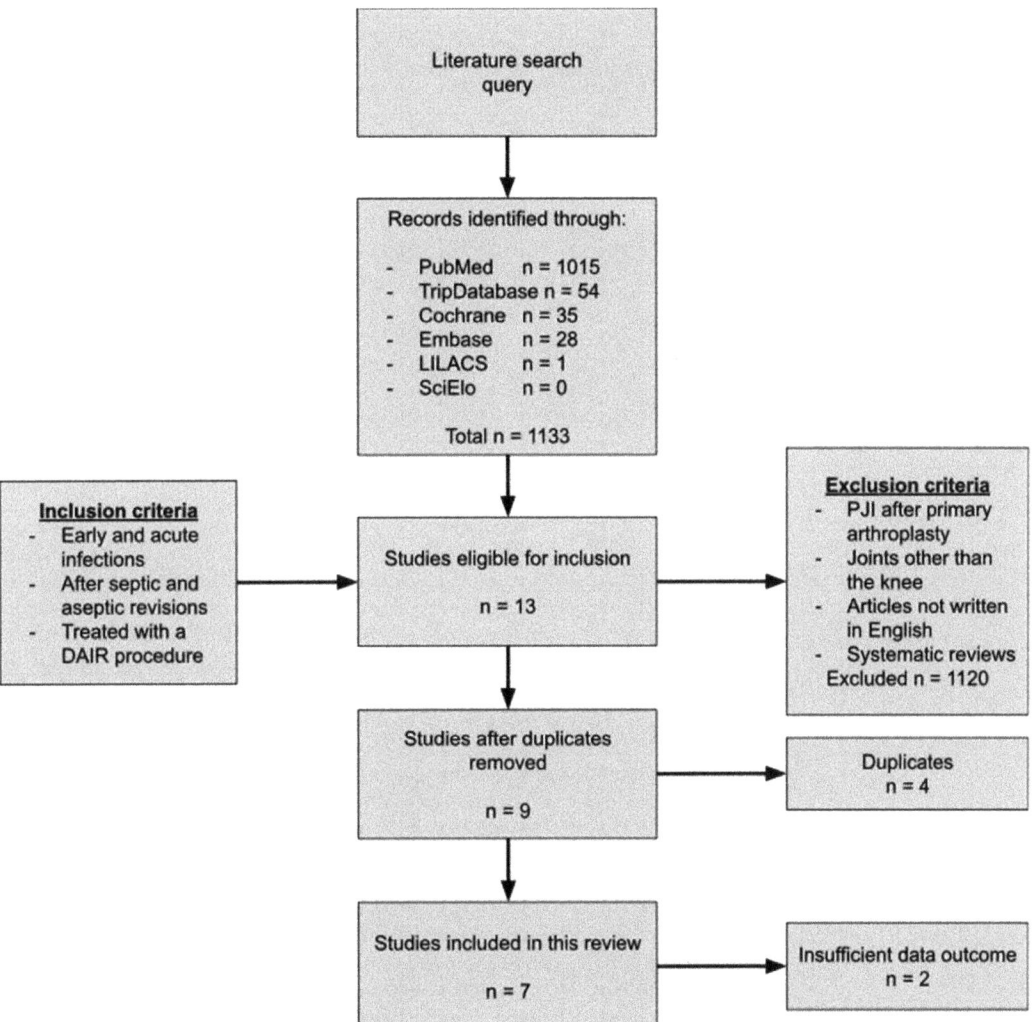

Figure 1. Flowchart of study selection. DAIR: debridement, antibiotics and implant retention. PJI: prosthetic joint infection.

3. Results

3.1. The DAIR Procedure

The DAIR procedures described in these articles are highly comparable regarding the technique of incision, removal of modular components, collection of tissue samples and debridement and irrigation. An overview is shown in Table 1. The study of Faschingbauer et al. [16] specifically describes cleaning of the surgical field, new instruments and new gloves for the surgeon following irrigation. If they were not able to close the wound properly, a vacuum-assisted closure system (VAC) was used. Only Veerman et al. [14] mention how many cultures were taken during the DAIR ($n = 6$) and how they were processed afterwards. Salomons et al. [17] is the only study reporting the use of a planned two-stage DAIR procedure for selected cases in their population.

Table 1. DAIR procedure.

Surgical Procedure	Chiu et al. [18]	Faschingbauer et al. [16]	Vahedi et al. [19]	Bongers et al. [20]	Cochrane et al. [21]	Veerman et al. [14]	Salomons et al. [17]
Opening via pre-existing incision	Yes	Yes	Did not mention	Yes	Did not mention	Yes	Did not mention
Synovectomy (taking cultures)	Yes	Yes	Did not mention	Yes	Did not mention	Yes	Did not mention
Debridement of infected soft tissue (taking cultures)	Yes	Yes	Yes	Did not mention	Did not mention	Yes	Yes
Replacement of modular parts	Yes	Yes	Yes	Yes	Yes	Yes	Did not mention
Irrigation of implants	Antibiotic solution using pulsed lavage	10 L of anti-infectious irrigation	Did not mention	3 L betadine saline solution and 3 L saline	Did not mention	6 L of saline using pulsed lavage	6–9 L of saline, in some cases along with antibiotic and/or betadine solution

3.2. DAIR as Treatment for Early and Acute Infections after Revision Total Knee Arthroplasty

The literature search yielded 1133 titles that were screened for title and abstract. After applying the in- and exclusion criteria, seven articles focusing on DAIR for early PJIs following revision TKA were included in this systematic review, of which one was a prospective study and six were retrospective studies. The extracted data is shown in Table 2. All studies were qualified as level IV evidence.

Chiu et al. [18] analyzed 40 early and late PJIs after revision TKA. They defined failure of DAIR as failure to control the infection after one DAIR and recurrence of infection during the follow-up period which necessitated removal of the implant, arthrodesis, or above the knee amputation. They used a culture-directed parenteral antibiotic therapy of at least six weeks and no oral antibiotics were given after this period. Success was defined as implant salvage with clinical eradication of the infection at the latest follow-up. The overall success rate was 30%. However, the success rate between the different types of infection differed. They used the classification system as proposed by Tsukayama et al. which was previously mentioned [8]. For the type IIb infections ($n = 10$) DAIR was successful in 70% of cases, while for the type IV ($\leq$4 weeks) infections ($n = 20$) 0% of cases were successful. For these failed DAIRs, the infection was managed after a two-stage revision ($n = 9$), arthrodesis ($n = 6$), resection arthroplasty ($n = 3$) and above the knee amputation ($n = 2$). From the patients with a type III infection (acute hematogenous) ($n = 10$), 50% were successful ($n = 5$) and the infection was eradicated after two-stage revision ($n = 3$) and after arthrodesis ($n = 2$).

Table 2. Study specifications and patient characteristics.

Autor	Study Design	Study Size	Mean Age (Years)	Reason for Index Revision	Type of (Re-)Infection	Causative Pathogen	Prophylactic/Preoperative Antibiotic Regime	Postoperative Culture-Directed Antibiotic Therapy	Mean Follow-Up (Months)	Overall Success Rate (%)
Chiu 2007 [18]	Prospective	40 knees	72.7 (range 59–85)	Aseptic loosening 70% Wear 30%	25% Early 50% Late (>4 weeks) 25% Acute hematogenous	13 MRSA 12 CoNS 5 Multiple organisms 2 GBS 2 GGS 1 E. coli	1 S. epidermidis 1 S. aureus 1 C. parapsilosis 1 C. glabrata 1 P. aeruginosa	Did not mention	Parenteral for 6 weeks	79 (range 36–143)	30
Faschingbauer 2018 [16]	Retrospective	7 knees	67.3 (range 45–84)	PJI 100%	Early or acute hematogenous	7 MRSE 3 E. coli 2 S. aureus 2 Multiple organisms	1 S. intermedius 1 Enterococcus 1 Enterobacter 1 Culture negative	Successful cases 7 Le, Ri 3 no antibiotics 1 Va, Ti, Ri 1 Fl, Ri	Failed cases 2 no antibiotics 2 Le, Ri 1 Cl, Ri 1 Me	Parenteral, oral or both for 2 weeks	39 (range 24–90)	57.1
Vahedi 2019 [19]	Retrospective matched cohort study	24 knees	64 (range 43–77)	PJI 100%	Acute	7 S. aureus 4 S. epidermidis 4 Gram negative	2 MRSA 2 Multiple organisms 5 Culture negative	Did not mention	Parenteral for 6 weeks + oral for 6 months	46 (range 29–86)	71 (50 for second DAIR)
Bongers 2020 [20]	Retrospective	11 knees	67 (range 46–86)	PJI 100%	Early (<6 weeks) or acute hematogenous	Did not mention	Before 2-stage revision: 3 g Ce daily until culture results, Va in case of resistance of allergy or antibiotics based on previously cultivated susceptibility	Not specifically given for DAIR	94 (range 24–172)	50
Cochrane 2021 [21]	Retrospective	11 knees	65 (SD 7.3)	Mechanical failure 100%	Early or acute hematogenous	4 MRSA 2 CoNS 2 Enterobac.	1 S. aureus 1 Enterococcus 1 P. acnes	Before 2-stage revision: 2 or 3 g of Ce before incision	Not specifically given for DAIR	46 (SD 34)	64
Veerman 2022 [14]	Retrospective	35 knees	66 (SD 11)	Mechanical failure 100%	Early or acute hematogenous	37 Staphylococcus species 18 Gram negative bacilli 17 Multiple organisms 33 Culture negative	One dose of 2 g Ce followed by 3 × 1 g for 5 days or until culture samples are available; Ri was added for susceptible Staphylococcus species	Parenteral for 5 days + oral or iv for 3 months	24	62 (50 for second DAIR)
Salomons 2023 [17]	Retrospective	12 knees	71 (range 41–90)	Aseptic loosening 42% Instability 25% Periprosthetic fracture 17% Arthrofibrosis 17%	Early (8%) or acute hematogenous (92%)	3 S. aureus 3 S. mitis, S. viridans, S. agalactiae 1 S. aureus + Enterococcus 1 CoNS 4 Culture negative	Did not mention	Parenteral for 3–6 weeks followed by culture directed suppressive antibiotics for the life of the implant	84 (range 24–180)	92

MRSA: methicillin-resistant staphylococcus aureus, S. aureus: methicillin-sensitive staphylococcus aureus, MRSE: methicillin-resistant staphylococcus epidermidis, CoNS: coagulase-negative staphylococcus, P. acnes: propionibacterium acnes, S. epidermidis: staphylococcus epidermidis, S. intermedius: streptococcus intermedius, S. mitis: streptococcus mitis, S. viridans: streptococcus viridans, S. aglactiae: streptococcus agalactiae, E. coli: escheria coli, P. aeruginosa: pseudomonas aeruginosa, Le: levofloxacin, Ri: rifampicin, Va: vancomycin, Ti: tigecycline, Fl: flucloxacillin, Cl: clindamycin, Me: meropenem, Ce: cefazolin.

In the study of Faschingbauer et al. [16], the incidence of re-infection after 440 two-stage septic revision total hip and knee arthroplasties was reported. The overall re-infection-rate was 11.6% ($n = 51$). Of these 51 patients, 19 were subjected to DAIR therapy. DAIR was performed when a re-infection occurred within 30 days after the two-stage revision or in patients with an acute re-infection with symptoms occurring within less than three weeks. A repeated DAIR, after three to six days, was performed if a persistent micro-organism was found intra-operatively, persistent wound drainage occurred or no decrease in C-reactive protein (CRP) with concomitant clinical signs was observed. This was repeated up to 11 times. Culture-directed oral or parenteral antibiotic therapy was continued for two weeks after the last surgery and no suppression therapy was used. Failure of DAIR was defined as any additional surgery due to infection after discharge. The success rate was 57.1% ($n = 4$) after revision TKA. The management of the six patients with a persistent infection was not specified.

The study of Vahedi et al. [19] evaluated 24 patients undergoing DAIR for a PJI after a two-stage revision total knee arthroplasty. The indication for DAIR was early infection (defined in the study as symptoms less than three weeks before DAIR) without signs of implant loosening or malposition. Antibiotic therapy was culture directed and involved parenteral antibiotics for six weeks followed by oral antibiotics for six months. Success (defined as no recurrence of infection and implant survival after two years of follow-up) occurred in 71% of patients ($n = 17$). Three patients underwent a second DAIR, of which two were successful. The one patient with a recurrent infection after the second DAIR and four other patients underwent a second two-stage revision. The matched control group ($n = 48$) that underwent two-stage revision for chronic PJIs after primary TKA and did not receive DAIR showed a success rate of 73% ($n = 35$).

Bongers et al. [20] analyzed 113 two-stage revisions for infected TKA; 99 patients completed the five-year follow-up. From these 99 patients, 23% ($n = 23$) had a reinfection, of which 14% ($n = 14$) had new pathogens and 9% ($n = 9$) were relapses. The 14 new infections were treated with a second revision ($n = 5$), DAIR ($n = 8$) or conservative treatment ($n = 1$), and the 9 relapse infections were treated with a second revision ($n = 6$) and DAIR ($n = 3$). DAIR was performed in recurrent early postoperative infections within 6 weeks after revision surgery or within two weeks of onset of an acute hematogenous infection. In 50% ($n = 11$) of the patients with a reinfection, (repeated) DAIR eradicated the infection and implant removal was not needed.

The study of Cochrane et al. [21] investigated the incidence of early infections after one year of aseptic revision TKA. The reasons for revision were component loosening, component malrotation, polyethylene wear, failed unicompartmental knee arthroplasty, arthrofibrosis, extensor mechanism failure, periprosthetic fracture and anterior knee pain. After the 157 aseptic TKA revisions were analyzed, an infection rate of 9% ($n = 14$) was observed. Treatment of these 14 PJIs was a DAIR (or repeat DAIRs) procedure in 11 patients and a two-stage re-revision in the other 3 patients. Seven patients treated with DAIR had a successful outcome (infection free at most recent follow-up), two patients underwent an above the knee amputation and two patients underwent a two-stage re-revision.

The team of Veerman et al. [14] analyzed the outcome of 88 DAIRs performed within 90 days after the revision arthroplasty (35 TKAs). Success was defined as no need for further surgery of any kind (revision, explantation or amputation), no persistent or recurrent PJI, no need for suppressive antibiotic therapy and patient survival after a follow-up of two years. For the interval between the revision and the DAIR, a cut-off point was used: DAIRs performed <30 days and DAIRs performed >30 days after the index revision. This cut-off was based on the current recommendation of the 2018 Philadelphia consensus meeting to perform DAIR within 30 days after the index revision when a PJI is suspected [22].

If needed, a second DAIR was performed to control the infection during the initial antimicrobial treatment. Directly after the DAIR, empirical parenteral antibiotic therapy was started and modified according to the culture results when they became available. Antibiotic therapy was continued for three months after the last surgical procedure. The success rate of the DAIR after revision TKA was 62% ($n = 22$). In 10 cases, a second DAIR was necessary, with a success rate of 50% ($n = 5$). An interval of >30 days between the index revision and the first DAIR was associated with a reduced success rate (OR 0.24, 95% CI 0.08–0.72, $p = 0.008$). A second DAIR procedure within 90 days also reduced the success rate significantly (OR 0.37, 95% CI 0.14–0.97, $p = 0.040$).

Finally, Salomons et al. [17] examined the results of DAIR combined with suppressive antibiotic therapy (SAT) for acute infection after aseptic revision TKA. The PJIs after revision TKA ($n = 12$) included in this study were classified as early postoperative and acute hematogenous following the same definition as used by Tsukayama et al. In four cases, antibiotic beats or an antibiotic impregnated spacer was placed on the spot of the arthroplasty insert, followed by a second planned DAIR. Why these patients were selected for a planned second DAIR is not mentioned. SAT started after 3–6 weeks of parenteral antibiotic therapy, in some cases combined with oral antibiotics, for the life of the implant. The outcomes were defined as survival of the implant free from reoperation for infection or free from re-revision for infection. Reoperation for infections included revisions for infection, unplanned additional DAIR procedures and debridement of superficial wound infections. The survivorship free from reoperation and re-revision for infection after 5 years is 67% (95% CI 37–100) and 92% (95% CI 72–100), respectively. A planned double DAIR procedure as described above had a success rate of 75%. They also mentioned that a single prior aseptic revision and acute hematogenous PJI performed better compared to multiple revised joints and early postoperative PJI.

3.3. Proposed Treatment Algorithm

One could argue that the level IV data from several small retrospective cohorts is insufficient to support a comprehensive treatment algorithm. Moreover, it remains difficult to determine which success rate is acceptable to consider DAIR to be a reasonable treatment option for early and acute infections after revision TKA. Nevertheless, according to the literature reviewed in this article, a first treatment algorithm can be proposed, albeit with a weak recommendation. A flowchart of this algorithm is shown in Figure 2.

The types of PJI are based on the classification system by Tsukayama et al. [8].

DAIR is a good treatment option for early (Tsukayama type IIb, within one month after revision) and acute hematogenous (Tsukayama type III) PJIs following revision TKA. At least five or six intraoperative periprosthetic tissue samples should be routinely obtained with separate clean instruments from the synovium, capsule and interfaces. Subsequent debridement, complete synovial resection (synovectomy) and exchange of the mobile parts should be performed. The joint and wound should be thoroughly irrigated with six liters of saline using pulsed lavage. One DAIR might not be enough to control the infection and depending on the virulence of the micro-organism or relapse of the infection a second DAIR might be necessary. It is important to stress that the success rate of a second DAIR decreases significantly to less than 50%, which warrants adequate information to be given to the patient.

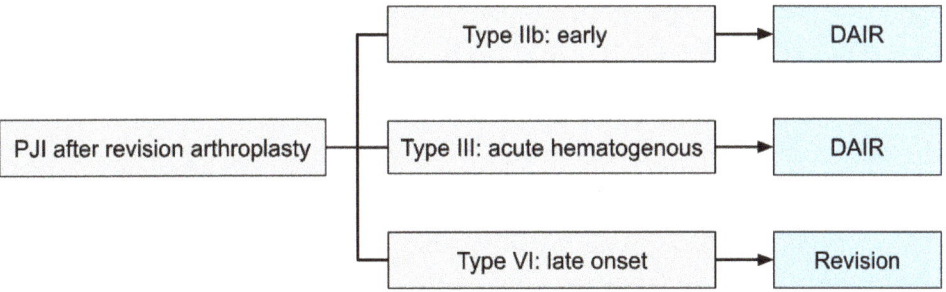

Figure 2. Flowchart of treatment algorithm. PJI types based on the classification described by Tsukayama et al. [8].

Late (Tsukayama type IV) infections (more than one month after revision) are associated with lower success rates after DAIR and warrant a two-stage revision. Reasons for DAIR could be bacterial load reduction or patient and/or surgeon preference in selected cases.

Empiric antibiotic treatment should be started immediately after taking the tissue cultures, followed by a 6-to-12-week course of culture-directed antibiotics.

Empiric intravenous antibiotic treatment should be started and given for at least seven days. Adjustments should be made based on the culture results. The empiric treatment is dependent on local etiology and resistance patterns and should be discussed in a multidisciplinary approach.

4. Discussion

This is the first systematic review on DAIR after revision TKA. Despite the heterogeneous treatment approaches and relatively small study populations presented, pooled together they provide tools to take the first step in composing treatment guidelines for infections after knee revision arthroplasty. DAIR is a good treatment option for PJIs occurring after revision TKA, with success rates up to 71%. However, a high variation in success rates was seen in the included studies, ranging from 30–92%. One reason is the variation in inclusion criteria in the study of Chiu et al. [18], as they also included late chronic PJIs and therefore reported a low success rate. Moreover, there was variation in the definition of a failure, as several studies considered repeat DAIR as a failure. There are relatively small variations in surgical procedures and the antibiotic regimes used in the different studies vary, possibly contributing to the alternating success rates. Notably, the high success rate reported by the article of Salomons et al. [17] is remarkable. Unlike the other articles they use SAT and, in some cases, a planned second DAIR procedure. Weston et al. [23] reported a 5-year survival rate of 66% for a PJI after TKA treated with DAIR followed by SAT. The study of Chung et al. [24] investigated the effect of a planned two-stage DAIR procedure for a PJI after TKA and reported a success rate of 89%. Taking this into account, the high success rate in the study of Salomons seems to be mainly attributed to the implementation of a two-stage DAIR procedure.

The success rate of DAIR after revision TKA is comparable to that after primary TKA. Gerritsen et al. [13] conducted a large systematic review including 3559 PJIs after primary TKA treated with DAIR, reporting a success rate of 63%. In contrast with our findings, Wouthuyzen-Bakker et al. [25] reported very good success rates (73%) of a second DAIR. However, their report remains unclear as to whether the index surgery was a primary or revision arthroplasty. Vilchez et al. [26] state that a second DAIR is associated with higher rates of failure in PJIs after primary arthroplasty, especially those caused by staphylococcus aureus. A cost-effectiveness analysis of Antonios et al. [27] states that a second DAIR for a PJI after primary TKA improves health utility and saves costs. Determining whether the same is applicable for a second DAIR after revision arthroplasty remains difficult based on current literature.

Previously, guidelines for the treatment of PJIs as introduced by Osmon et al. [28] recommend a DAIR for patients with an acute PJI, no implant loosening and without the presence of a sinus tract. However, only Faschingbauer et al. [16] excluded patients with the presence of a sinus tract. This is in contrast with the articles of Veerman et al. [14] and Bongers et al. [20], who specifically mention a sinus tract as an indication for DAIR or its resection as part of the DAIR procedure. Other more recent articles show that the presence of a sinus tract is not associated with a significantly lower success rate after DAIR. [29,30].

A DAIR procedure is followed by antibiotic treatment. The duration of antibiotic treatment differs between the studies included in this review, ranging from two weeks to chronic suppressive treatment. The study of Putho et al. [31] reported no difference between a total antibiotic course of three or six months after DAIR for a PJI following primary TKA. Bernard et al. [32] suggested that antibiotic therapy for a primary PJI can be limited to a 6-week course, with 1 week of intravenous administration. Another study showed no association between the duration of intravenous antibiotics (median 42 days;

IQR 38–42) and treatment failure [33]. Importantly, a recent review supports the use of oral antibiotics after seven days of intravenous antibiotics for the treatment of a PJI. Although these findings should be considered with care, this can have a considerable impact on patient and caregiver burden with potentially fewer complications [34].

Another important issue is the increase in culture-negative PJIs seen after primary TKA. In these cases, DAIR has shown similar or even slightly better outcomes compared to culture-positive cases [35,36]. Indeed, a recent meta-analysis demonstrated a culture-negative PJI to have similar or better survival rates when compared with a culture-positive PJI group for patients who underwent DAIR, one-stage or two-stage revision. A negative perioperative culture was not a worse prognostic factor for PJIs [37]. Given these results, it is assumed that culture-negative PJIs after revision arthroplasty will not be contraindicated when considering DAIR.

5. Conclusions

The current literature suggests that DAIR is a valid treatment option for early (Tsukayama type IIb) and acute hematogenous (Tsukayama type III) PJIs after revision TKA with success rates of 50–70%. A second DAIR shows success rates of around 50%. These success rates may vary between hospitals due to varying DAIR techniques and antibiotic regimes. The described standard treatment protocol for DAIR after revision TKA may be of added value. Further research should be aimed at predicting successful (repeat/two-stage) DAIRs in larger study populations, antibiotic regimes and the cost effectiveness of a second DAIR after revision TKA.

Supplementary Materials: The following supporting information can be downloaded at: https://www.mdpi.com/article/10.3390/jcm12155026/s1, Systematic search strategy.

Author Contributions: Writing—original draft preparation, C.W.J.H. and T.S.d.W. Review and editing, K.V., J.H.M.G., F-C.B.M.W. and G.G.v.H. Supervision, G.G.v.H. All authors have read and agreed to the published version of the manuscript.

Funding: This research received no external funding.

Institutional Review Board Statement: Not applicable.

Informed Consent Statement: Not applicable.

Data Availability Statement: Not applicable.

Conflicts of Interest: The authors declare no conflict of interest.

References

1. Ackerman, I.N.; Bohensky, M.A.; Zomer, E.; Tacey, M.; Gorelik, A.; Brand, C.A.; de Steiger, R. The projected burden of primary total knee and hip replacement for osteoarthritis in Australia to the year 2030. *BMC Musculoskelet. Disord.* **2019**, *20*, 90. [CrossRef]
2. Lenguerrand, E.; Whitehouse, M.; Beswick, A.; Toms, A.D.; Porter, M.L.; Blom, A.W.; National Joint Registry for England, Wales, Northern Ireland and the Isle of Man. Description of the rates, trends and surgical burden associated with revision for prosthetic joint infection following primary and revision knee replacements in England and Wales: An analysis of the National Joint Registry for England, Wales, Northern Ireland and the Isle of Man. *BMJ Open* **2017**, *7*, e014056. [CrossRef]
3. Goud, A.L.; Harlianto, N.I.; Ezzafzafi, S.; Veltman, E.S.; Bekkers, J.E.J.; van der Wal, B.C.H. Reinfection rates after one- and two-stage revision surgery for hip and knee arthroplasty: A systematic review and meta-analysis. *Arch. Orthop. Trauma Surg.* **2023**, *143*, 829–838. [CrossRef]
4. Rajgor, H.; Dong, H.; Nandra, R.; Parry, M.; Stevenson, J.; Jeys, L. Repeat revision TKR for failed management of peri-prosthetic infection has long-term success but often require multiple operations: A case control study. *Arch. Orthop. Trauma Surg.* **2023**, *143*, 987–994. [CrossRef]
5. Haddad, F.S.; Ngu, A.; Negus, J.J. Prosthetic Joint Infections and Cost Analysis? *Adv. Exp. Med. Biol.* **2017**, *971*, 93–100. [CrossRef]
6. Pravizi, J.; Zmistowski, B. A Quarter of Patients Treated for PJI Dead within 5 Years. December 2012. Available online: https://www.healio.com/news/orthopedics/20130104/a-quarter-of-patients-treated-for-pji-dead-within-5-years (accessed on 7 March 2023).
7. Sandifrod, N.; Frencescini, M.; Kendoff, D. The Burden of Prosthetic Joint Infection (PJI). July 2021. Available online: https://aoj.amegroups.com/article/view/6209/html#B5 (accessed on 7 March 2023).

8. Tsukayama, D.T.; Goldberg, V.M.; Kyle, R. Diagnosis and management of infection after total knee arthroplasty. *J. Bone Jt. Surg* **2003**, *85* (Suppl. 1), S75–S80. [CrossRef]
9. Zimmerli, W.; Trampuz, A.; Ochsner, P.E. Prosthetic-Joint Infections. *N. Engl. J. Med.* **2004**, *351*, 1645–1654. [CrossRef]
10. de Vries, L.; van der Weegen, W.; Neve, W.; Das, H.; Ridwan, B.; Steens, J. The Effectiveness of Debridement, Antibiotics and Irrigation for Periprosthetic Joint Infections after Primary Hip and Knee Arthroplasty. A 15 Years Retrospective Study in Two Community Hospitals in the Netherlands. *J. Bone Jt. Infect.* **2016**, *1*, 20–24. [CrossRef]
11. Barros, L.H.; Barbosa, T.A.; Esteves, J.; Abreu, M.A.; Soares, D.; Sousa, R. Early Debridement, antibiotics and implant retention (DAIR) in patients with suspected acute infection after hip or knee arthroplasty—Safe, effective and without negative functional impact. *J. Bone Jt. Infect.* **2019**, *4*, 300–305. [CrossRef]
12. Iza, K.; Foruria, X.; Moreta, J.; Uriarte, I.; Loroño, A.; Aguirre, U.; Mozos, J.L.M.d.L. DAIR (Debridement, Antibiotics and Implant Retention) less effective in hematogenous total knee arthroplasty infections. *J. Orthop. Surg. Res.* **2019**, *14*, 278. [CrossRef]
13. Gerritsen, M.; Khawar, A.; Scheper, H.; van der Wal, R.; Schoones, J.; de Boer, M.; Nelissen, R.; Pijls, B. Modular component exchange and outcome of DAIR for hip and knee periprosthetic joint infection: A systematic review and meta-regression analysis *Bone Jt. Open* **2021**, *2*, 806–812. [CrossRef]
14. Veerman, K.; Raessens, J.; Telgt, D.; Smulders, K.; Goosen, J.H.M. Debridement, antibiotics, and implant retention after revision arthroplasty: Antibiotic mismatch, timing, and repeated DAIR associated with poor outcome. *Bone Jt. J.* **2022**, *104-B*, 464–471 [CrossRef]
15. Moher, D.; Liberati, A.; PRISMA Group. Preferred reporting items for systematic reviews and meta-analyses: The PRISMA statement. *PLoS Med.* **2009**, *6*, e1000097. [CrossRef]
16. Faschingbauer, M.; Boettner, F.; Bieger, R.; Weiner, C.; Reichel, H.; Kappe, T. Outcome of Irrigation and Debridement after Failed Two-Stage Reimplantation for Periprosthetic Joint Infection. *BioMed Res. Int.* **2018**, *2018*, 2875018. [CrossRef]
17. Salmons, H.I.; Bettencourt, J.W.; Wyles, C.C.; Osmon, D.R.; Berry, D.J.; Abdel, M.P. Irrigation and Debridement with Chronic Antibiotic Suppression for the Management of Acutely Infected Aseptic Revision Total Joint Arthroplasties. *J. Arthroplast.* **2023** [CrossRef]
18. Chiu, F.-Y.; Chen, C.-M. Surgical Débridement and Parenteral Antibiotics in Infected Revision Total Knee Arthroplasty. *Clin. Orthop. Relat. Res.* **2007**, *461*, 130–135. [CrossRef]
19. Vahedi, H.; Aali-Rezaie, A.; Shahi, A.; Conway, J.D. Irrigation, Débridement, and Implant Retention for Recurrence of Periprosthetic Joint Infection Following Two-Stage Revision Total Knee Arthroplasty: A Matched Cohort Study. *J. Arthroplast.* **2019**, *34*, 1772–1775. [CrossRef]
20. Bongers, J.; Jacobs, A.M.; Smulders, K.; Van Hellemondt, G.G.; Goosen, J.H. Reinfection and re-revision rates of 113 two-stage revisions in infected TKA. *J. Bone Jt. Infect.* **2020**, *5*, 137–144. [CrossRef]
21. Cochrane, N.H.; Wellman, S.S.; Lachiewicz, P.F. Early Infection After Aseptic Revision Knee Arthroplasty: Prevalence and Predisposing Risk Factors. *J. Arthroplast.* **2022**, *37*, S281–S285. [CrossRef]
22. Argenson, J.N.; Arndt, M.; Babis, G.; Battenberg, A.; Budhiparama, N.; Catani, F.; Chen, F.; de Beaubien, B.; Ebied, A.; Esposito, S.; et al. Hip and Knee Section, Treatment, Debridement and Retention of Implant: Proceedings of International Consensus on Orthopedic Infections. *J. Arthroplast.* **2019**, *34*, S399–S419. [CrossRef]
23. Weston, J.T.; Watts, C.D.; Mabry, T.M.; Hanssen, A.D.; Berry, D.J.; Abdel, M.P. Irrigation and debridement with chronic antibiotic suppression for the management of infected total knee arthroplasty: A Contemporary Analysis. *Bone Jt. J.* **2018**, *100-B*, 1471–1476. [CrossRef]
24. Chung, A.S.; Niesen, M.C.; Graber, T.J.; Schwartz, A.J.; Beauchamp, C.P.; Clarke, H.D.; Spangehl, M.J. Two-Stage Debridement With Prosthesis Retention for Acute Periprosthetic Joint Infections. *J. Arthroplast.* **2019**, *34*, 1207–1213. [CrossRef]
25. Wouthuyzen-Bakker, M.; Löwik, C.A.; Ploegmakers, J.J.; Knobben, B.A.; Dijkstra, B.; de Vries, A.J.; Mithoe, G.; Kampinga, G.; Zijlstra, W.P.; Jutte, P.C.; et al. A Second Surgical Debridement for Acute Periprosthetic Joint Infections Should Not Be Discarded. *J. Arthroplast.* **2020**, *35*, 2204–2209. [CrossRef]
26. Vilchez, F.; Martínez-Pastor, J.; García-Ramiro, S.; Bori, G.; Maculé, F.; Sierra, J.; Font, L.; Mensa, J.; Soriano, A. Outcome and predictors of treatment failure in early post-surgical prosthetic joint infections due to Staphylococcus aureus treated with debridement. *Clin. Microbiol. Infect.* **2011**, *17*, 439–444. [CrossRef]
27. Antonios, J.K.; Bozic, K.J.; Clarke, H.D.; Spangehl, M.J.; Bingham, J.S.; Schwartz, A.J. Cost-effectiveness of Single vs Double Debridement and Implant Retention for Acute Periprosthetic Joint Infections in Total Knee Arthroplasty: A Markov Model. *Arthroplast. Today* **2021**, *11*, 187–195. [CrossRef]
28. Osmon, D.R.; Berbari, E.F.; Berendt, A.R.; Lew, D.; Zimmerli, W.; Steckelberg, J.M.; Rao, N.; Hanssen, A.; Wilson, W.R.; Infectious Diseases Society of America. Diagnosis and management of prosthetic joint infection: Clinical practice guidelines by the Infectious Diseases Society of America. *Clin. Infect. Dis.* **2013**, *56*, e1–e25. [CrossRef]
29. Deng, W.; Li, R.; Shao, H.; Yu, B.; Chen, J.; Zhou, Y. Comparison of the success rate after debridement, antibiotics and implant retention (DAIR) for periprosthetic joint infection among patients with or without a sinus tract. *BMC Musculoskelet. Disord.* **2021**, *22*, 895. [CrossRef]
30. Xu, Y.; Wang, L.; Xu, W. Risk factors affect success rate of debridement, antibiotics and implant retention (DAIR) in periprosthetic joint infection. *Arthroplasty* **2020**, *2*, 37. [CrossRef]

31. Puhto, A.-P.; Puhto, T.; Syrjala, H. Short-course antibiotics for prosthetic joint infections treated with prosthesis retention. *Clin. Microbiol. Infect.* **2012**, *18*, 1143–1148. [CrossRef]
32. Bernard, L.; Legout, L.; Zürcher-Pfund, L.; Stern, R.; Rohner, P.; Peter, R.; Assal, M.; Lew, D.; Hoffmeyer, P.; Uçkay, I. Six weeks of antibiotic treatment is sufficient following surgery for septic arthroplasty. *J. Infect.* **2010**, *61*, 125–132. [CrossRef]
33. Tai, D.B.G.; Berbari, E.F.; Suh, G.A.; Lahr, B.D.; Abdel, M.P.; Tande, A.J. Truth in DAIR: Duration of Therapy and the Use of Quinolone/Rifampin-Based Regimens after Debridement and Implant Retention for Periprosthetic Joint Infections. *Open Forum Infect. Dis.* **2022**, *9*, ofac363. [CrossRef]
34. Miller, R.; Higuera, C.A.; Wu, J.; Klika, A.; Babic, M.; Piuzzi, N.S. Periprosthetic Joint Infection: A Review of Antibiotic Treatment. *JBJS Rev.* **2020**, *8*, e19.00224. [CrossRef]
35. Tirumala, V.; Smith, E.; Box, H.; Kieboom, J.v.D.; Klemt, C.; Kwon, Y.-M. Outcome of Debridement, Antibiotics, and Implant Retention with Modular Component Exchange in Acute Culture-Negative Periprosthetic Joint Infections. *J. Arthroplast.* **2021**, *36*, 1087–1093. [CrossRef]
36. van Eck, J.; Liu, W.-Y.; Goosen, J.H.M.; Rijnen, W.H.C.; van der Zwaard, B.C.; Heesterbeek, P.; van der Weegen, W.; The Further Members of Regional Prosthetic Joint Infection Group. Higher 1-year risk of implant removal for culture-positive than for culture-negative DAIR patients following 359 primary hip or knee arthroplasties. *J. Bone Jt. Infect.* **2022**, *7*, 143–149. [CrossRef]
37. Li, F.; Qiao, Y.; Zhang, H.; Cao, G.; Zhou, S. Comparable clinical outcomes of culture-negative and culture-positive periprosthetic joint infections: A systematic review and meta-analysis. *J. Orthop. Surg. Res.* **2023**, *18*, 210. [CrossRef]

Disclaimer/Publisher's Note: The statements, opinions and data contained in all publications are solely those of the individual author(s) and contributor(s) and not of MDPI and/or the editor(s). MDPI and/or the editor(s) disclaim responsibility for any injury to people or property resulting from any ideas, methods, instructions or products referred to in the content.

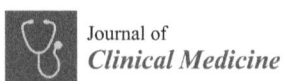

Systematic Review

Effects of Thrombin-Based Hemostatic Agent in Total Knee Arthroplasty: Meta-Analysis

Jung-Wee Park [1,2,†], Tae Woo Kim [2,3,†], Chong Bum Chang [1,2], Minji Han [4], Jong Jin Go [1], Byung Kyu Park [1], Woo-Lam Jo [5,*,‡] and Young-Kyun Lee [1,2,*,‡]

[1] Department of Orthopaedic Surgery, Seoul National University Bundang Hospital, Seongnam 13620, Republic of Korea; jwepark@gmail.com (J.-W.P.); ccbknee@gmail.com (C.B.C.); gjjjl@naver.com (J.J.G.); hellowbk@gmail.com (B.K.P.)
[2] Department of Orthopaedic Surgery, Seoul National University College of Medicine, Seoul 03080, Republic of Korea; orthopassion@naver.com
[3] Department of Orthopaedic Surgery, SMG-SNU Boramae Medical Center, Seoul 07061, Republic of Korea
[4] Department of Health Science and Technology, Graduate School of Convergence Science and Technology, Seoul National University, Seoul 08826, Republic of Korea; mj830@snu.ac.kr
[5] Department of Orthopaedic Surgery, Seoul St. Mary's Hospital, College of Medicine, The Catholic University of Korea, Seoul 06591, Republic of Korea
* Correspondence: jis25@naver.com (W.-L.J.); ykleemd@gmail.com (Y.-K.L.); Tel.: +82-2-2258-2838 (W.-L.J.); +82-31-787-7204 (Y.-K.L.)
† These authors contributed equally to this work.
‡ These authors contributed equally to this work.

Abstract: The effectiveness of Floseal, a thrombin-based hemostatic matrix, in total knee arthroplasty (TKA) in minimizing blood loss and transfusion requirements remains a topic of debate. This meta-analysis aims to evaluate the up-to-date randomized controlled trials (RCTs) on the efficacy and safety of Floseal in TKA. A comprehensive search was conducted in electronic databases to identify relevant RCTs. The methodological quality of the included studies was assessed, and data extraction was performed. The pooled effect sizes were calculated using standardized mean difference (SMD) or odds ratios (OR) with 95% confidence intervals (CIs). Eight studies involving 904 patients were included in the meta-analysis. The use of a thrombin-based hemostatic agent significantly reduced hemoglobin decline (SMD = −0.49, 95% CI: −0.92 to −0.07) and the risk of allogenic transfusion (OR = 0.45, 95% CI: 0.25 to 0.81) but showed no significant difference in the volume of drainage or total blood loss. Funnel plots showed no evidence of publication bias. This meta-analysis provides robust evidence supporting the effectiveness of Floseal in reducing hemoglobin decline and transfusion in TKA. Further well-designed RCTs with longer follow-up periods are warranted to assess long-term efficacy and safety.

Keywords: total knee arthroplasty; thrombin-based hemostatic agent; hemostatic matrix; blood loss; transfusion; meta-analysis

Citation: Park, J.-W.; Kim, T.W.; Chang, C.B.; Han, M.; Go, J.J.; Park, B.K.; Jo, W.-L.; Lee, Y.-K. Effects of Thrombin-Based Hemostatic Agent in Total Knee Arthroplasty: Meta-Analysis. *J. Clin. Med.* **2023**, *12*, 6656. https://doi.org/10.3390/jcm12206656

Academic Editor: Christian Carulli

Received: 12 September 2023
Revised: 13 October 2023
Accepted: 18 October 2023
Published: 20 October 2023

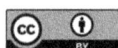

Copyright: © 2023 by the authors. Licensee MDPI, Basel, Switzerland. This article is an open access article distributed under the terms and conditions of the Creative Commons Attribution (CC BY) license (https://creativecommons.org/licenses/by/4.0/).

1. Introduction

Total knee arthroplasty (TKA) is a satisfactory surgical option in elderly patients with intractable symptoms and advanced osteoarthritis of the knee joint [1,2]. However, TKA is usually associated with significant perioperative blood loss and an increased need for allogenic blood transfusion because it requires soft tissue exposure, extensive bony resection, and a lengthy operation time [3,4]. The acute anemia and the allogeneic blood transfusion used to treat the anemia could lead to perioperative comorbidities and increase medical costs [5,6]. Therefore, surgeons prioritize minimizing perioperative blood loss and have employed various methods to achieve this goal and reduce the need for blood transfusion following TKA. These methods include the use of erythropoietic agents, autologous blood transfusion from pre-donated blood, cell salvage, hemostatic agents, and antifibrinolytic agents [7].

One of the widely used methods is the administration of Floseal (Baxter, Deerfield, IL, USA), a hemostatic matrix composed of thrombin and bovine gelatin, which can promote blood coagulation [8]. This thrombin-saturated gelatin plays a role in the initial hemostasis process where the vessel injury due to surgery occurs. Aggregation of platelets and activating the coagulation pathway leads to the conversion of prothrombin to thrombin and the subsequent formation of insoluble fibrin composites [9]. When the thrombin-rich gelatin is applied to the bleeding site, it affects the coagulation process by not only creating a fibrin clot, activating and inducing the platelet aggregation but also triggering a tamponade effect that mechanically stops the bleeding by swelling the gelatin granules by 10% to 20% [10]. The function of gelatin in this composite is the excellent absorbent feature, which enables it to absorb and carry 200% of its volume in liquid [11]; this enhances the coagulation process by maximizing the local platelet concentration in the bleeding site and the efficient release of prothrombin kinase that is required in the coagulation cascade [12]. Thrombin-based hemostatic agents have been traditionally adopted in various fields, including general, cardiac, gynecologic, neurovascular, and orthopedic surgeries [8,13–16], and now are expanding their indication to otorhinolaryngologic, dental, and urologic surgeries [17–21].

In the scope of TKA, some clinical studies have shown the prominent effect of Floseal in terms of a decrease in perioperative bleeding or hemoglobin drop [22–28]. However, these studies suffer from methodological flaws, such as poor study design, small sample sizes, and inconsistent outcomes. Due to these flaws, the use of thrombin-based hemostatic agents in TKA is still a topic of debate, and there is a need for more reliable and convincing data to assess its efficacy and safety. There are two previous meta-analyses that incorporated the outcomes of thrombin-based hemostatic matrix use in TKA [29,30]. However, these studies were published in 2014 and 2017, and only four randomized clinical trials (RCTs) were included. Therefore, the aim of this study was to evaluate up-to-date RCTs on the effectiveness and safety of thrombin-based hemostatic agents in TKA.

2. Materials and Methods

2.1. Search Strategy

This study was conducted following the PRISMA (Preferred Reporting Items for Systematic Reviews and Meta-Analyses) guidelines but not registered in the International Prospective Register of Systematic Reviews (PROSPERO). Electronic databases, including PubMed, Embase Cochrane Library, and Web of Science, were searched. The systematic search was carried out in January 2023. There was no restriction on the publication date or the language. The search process was conducted as illustrated in Figure 1.

Search terms were generated using the Boolean operators (AND or OR) and the keywords "thrombin" OR "Floseal" OR "hemostatic matrix" and "knee replacement" in combination. The search process was conducted by two reviewers separately, and in case of any disagreement, a third reviewer was consulted. To assess the methodological quality of the included literature, the risk of bias outlined in the Cochrane Handbook for Systematic Reviews of Interventions version 6.3 was used [31].

2.2. Selection Criteria

The inclusion criteria were as follows: (1) the studies on patients who received TKA; (2) the studies that used Floseal with comparison to the control group (control groups could be treated with other intervention or no intervention); (3) the studies that included outcomes relevant to patient blood management; and (4) the studies that were published RCTs. The studies were excluded if hemostatic agents other than Floseal were used in the experimental group.

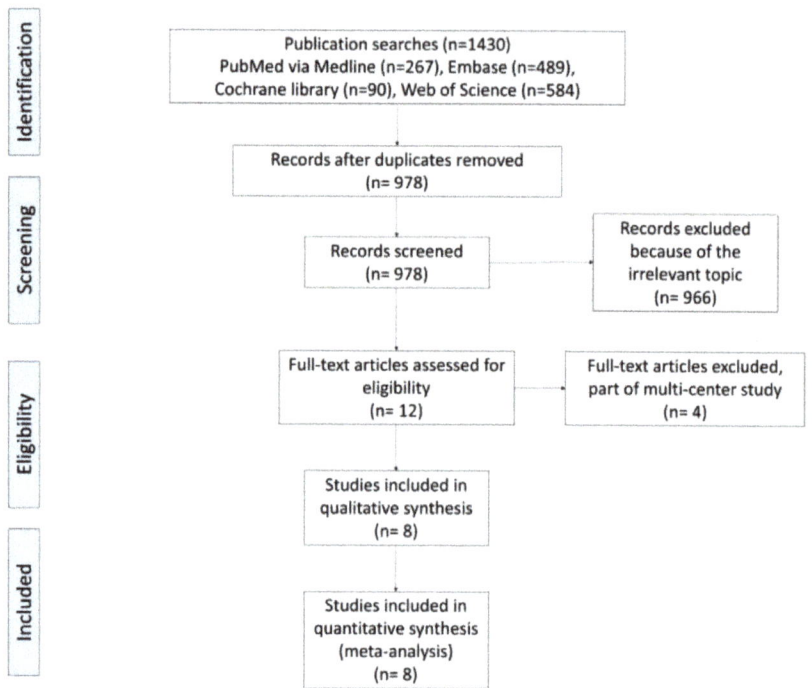

Figure 1. PRISMA flowchart of the systematic search. PRISMA, Preferred Reporting Items for Systematic Reviews and Meta-Analyses.

2.3. Data Extraction

The data extraction process was conducted independently by two researchers. They extracted various types of data from the included literature, such as the name of the first author, publication year, details of the interventions, demographics, number of included patients, and outcome measures. Additionally, other relevant parameters from individual studies were also extracted.

2.4. Data Analysis and Statistical Methods

Effect sizes were calculated based on the type of data: the standardized mean difference (SMD) was used for continuous data, calculated by dividing the mean difference (MD) by the common standard deviation (SD). For binary data, odds ratios (OR) were used. The pooled standard deviation (SD) was calculated by applying the following formula $SD = \sqrt{\frac{(n_1-1) \times s_1^2 + (n_2-1) \times s_2^2}{(n_1+n_2-2)}}$, where n_1 and n_2 represent the sample sizes of the treatment and control groups, respectively, and s_1 and s_2 denote the standard deviations of the mean difference before and after treatment in the treatment and control groups, respectively [32].

Heterogeneity was estimated depending on the value of p and I^2 using the standard chi-square test. When $I^2 > 50\%$, $p < 0.1$ was considered to be significant heterogeneity [33]. Therefore, a random-effect model was applied for data analysis. A fixed-effect model was used when no significant heterogeneity was found. To evaluate biases related to publication, we utilized funnel plots, which visually depict the characteristics and results of individual studies. We conducted a meta-analysis using Excel, a Microsoft application, and R (version 4.2.2). The data pooling process was performed in Excel, while the meta-analysis was conducted in R using the 'meta' and 'metafor' packages.

3. Results

3.1. Literature Search

A total of 1430 potential studies were identified with the first search strategy. Additionally, 452 duplicated articles were deleted, leaving 978 records. After screening, in total, 12 full-text articles were assessed for eligibility. Out of twelve, four reports were excluded according to the eligibility criteria. No additional studies were obtained after the reference review. Finally, eight independent comparison studies were eligible for data extraction and meta-analysis, as indicated by the flowchart in Figure 1 [22,24–28,34,35]. These studies involved a total of 485 patients in the Floseal group and 418 patients in the control group.

3.2. Study Characteristics

The main characteristics of the included studies are reported in Table 1. All the studies evaluated primary TKA. Statistically similar baseline characteristics were observed between the Floseal and control groups, including age, sex, body mass index, preoperative hemoglobin, comorbidities, and anesthesia. In each study, thrombin-based hemostatic matrix was administered intra-articularly before suturing, though the dosages varied (5–10 mL).

Table 1. Demographic features of the included studies.

Author	Year	Number (F/C)	Age (Years) (F/C)	Male (F/C)	BMI (kg/m^2) (F/C)	Antithrombotic Agent	Transfusion Criteria (g/dL)	Dosage (mL)
Kim HJ [27]	2012	97/99	72.7/70.1	N/S	N/S	Aspirin or warfarin	N/S	10
Helito CP [26]	2013	10/10	67.8/66.6	N/S	N/S	Enoxaparin	V/S change [a]	10
Di Francesco A [24]	2013	51/42	67.9/70.2	24/17	26.0/26.2	Enoxaparin	Hb 8.5	10
Suarez JC [28]	2014	56/52	65.9/65.1	20/21	29.8/33.7	Enoxaparin	Hb 8.0	5
Bae KC [22]	2014	50/50	68.8/69.0	4/8	26.4/24.8	N/S	Hb 8.5	10
Velyvis JH [34]	2015	157/100	72.5/73.0	71/47	N/S	N/S	Hb 8 or 9 and associated symptoms [b]	10 or 5
Helito CP [25]	2019	30/30	N/S	N/S	N/S	Enoxaparin	N/S	10
Yen SH [31]	2021	34/35	69.7/69.7	6/3	29.4/28.6	Enoxaparin	N/S	10

F/C, Floseal group/control group; BMI, body mass index; N/S, not stated; Hb, hemoglobin; V/S, vital sign. V/S change [a]: heart rate >120 with mean arterial blood pressure < 80 mmHg or blood pressure < 100 mmHg (systolic) and 60 mmHg (diastolic), pulse oximetry < 90%, and tachypnea. Associated symptoms [b]: weakness, dizziness, fainting, slow capillary refill, shortness of breath, or hypotension.

3.3. Risk of Bias Assessment

The included trials had small sample sizes, ranging from 10 to 157 patients; however, they were relatively well-designed and well-implemented. The quality of the included studies, according to the Cochrane Handbook for Systematic Reviews of Interventions, is reported in Table 2.

Table 2. Risk of bias of the included studies.

Author	Year	D1	D2	D3	D4	D5	Overall
Kim HJ [27]	2012	Low risk	Low risk	Low risk	Low risk	Low risk	Low risk
Helito CP [26]	2013	Low risk	Low risk	Low risk	Low risk	Low risk	Low risk
Di Francesco A [24]	2013	Some concerns	Low risk	Low risk	Some concerns	Low risk	Some concerns
Suarez JC [28]	2014	Low risk	Low risk	Low risk	Low risk	Some concerns	Some concerns
Bae KC [22]	2014	Some concerns	Low risk	Low risk	Low risk	Some concerns	Some concerns
Velyvis JH [34]	2015	Low risk	Low risk	Low risk	Low risk	Low risk	Low risk
Helito CP [25]	2019	Some concerns	Low risk	Low risk	Some concerns	Some concerns	Some concerns
Yen SH [35]	2021	Some concerns	Low risk	Low risk	Low risk	Low risk	Some concerns

D1: Randomization process; D2: deviations from intended interventions; D3: missing outcome data; D4: measurement of the outcome; D5: selection of the reported result.

In four studies [24,27,28,35], random numbers generated by a computer and proper concealment of allocation were used, and two studies [27,28] implemented a double-blind approach involving blinding of participants and personnel.

All the included studies did not have an unclear bias due to incomplete outcome data or selective outcome reporting.

3.4. Outcomes for Meta-Analysis

3.4.1. Hemoglobin Decline

Details regarding hemoglobin decline after TKA were available in all eight studies [22,24–28,34,35]. Two studies demonstrated a significant difference between the groups [24,25]. There was significant heterogeneity ($I^2 = 83\%$, $p < 0.01$); therefore, a random-effect model was performed. The pooled results showed that hemoglobin decline in the Floseal group was significantly lower than that in the control group (SMD = −0.49, 95% CI: −0.92 to −0.07) (Figure 2).

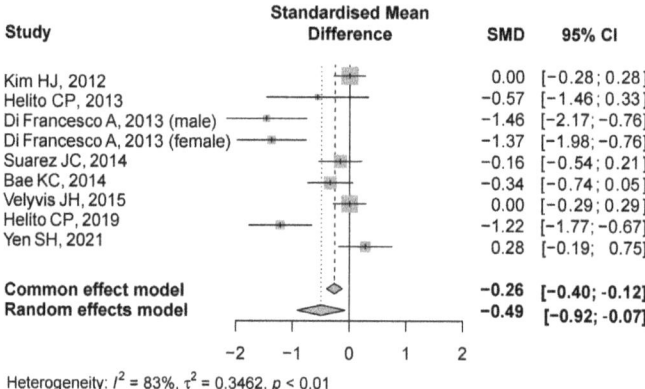

Figure 2. The forest plot of hemoglobin decline from the included studies [22,24–28,34,35].

3.4.2. Volume of Drainage

Details regarding the volume of drainage after TKA were available in all studies [22,24–28,34,35]. Five studies demonstrated a significant difference between the groups [22,24,25,28,34]. There was significant heterogeneity ($I^2 = 99\%$, $p < 0.01$); therefore, a random effect model was performed. The pooled results showed that there was no significant difference in drainage between the two groups (SMD = −2.11, 95% CI: −4.77 to 0.54) (Figure 3).

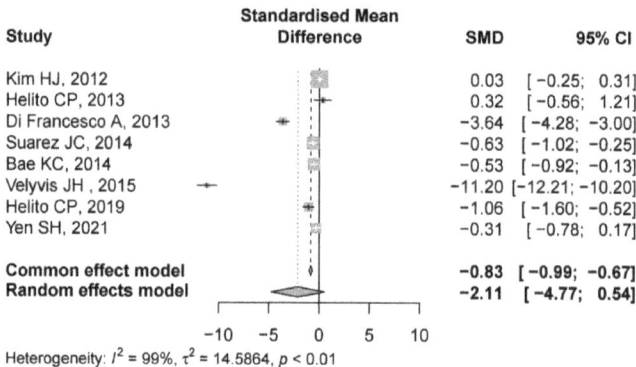

Figure 3. The forest plot of the volume of drainage from the included studies [22,24–28,34,35].

3.4.3. Total Blood Loss

Details regarding total blood loss after TKA were available in five studies [22,24,25,28,35]. Three studies demonstrated a significant difference between the groups [22,24,28]. There was significant heterogeneity ($I^2 = 96\%$, $p < 0.01$); therefore, a random-effect model was performed. There was no significant difference in total blood loss between the two groups (SMD = −0.90, 95% CI: −2.17 to 0.38) (Figure 4).

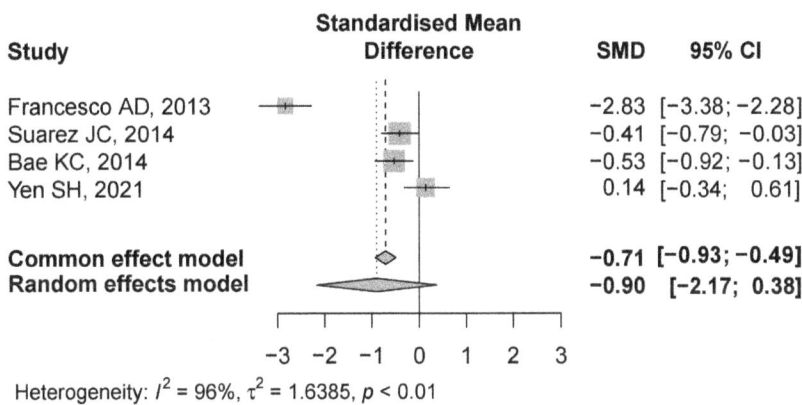

Figure 4. The forest plot of total blood loss from the included studies [22,24,25,28,35].

3.4.4. Risk of Allogenic Transfusion

Details regarding transfusion rate after TKA were available in six studies [22,24,25,28,34,35]. One study demonstrated a significant difference between the groups [22]. There was no significant heterogeneity ($I^2 = 0\%$, $p = 0.53$); therefore, a common effect model was performed. The pooled results showed that the transfusion rate in the Floseal group was significantly lower than that in the control group (OR = 0.45, 95% CI: 0.25 to 0.81) (Figure 5).

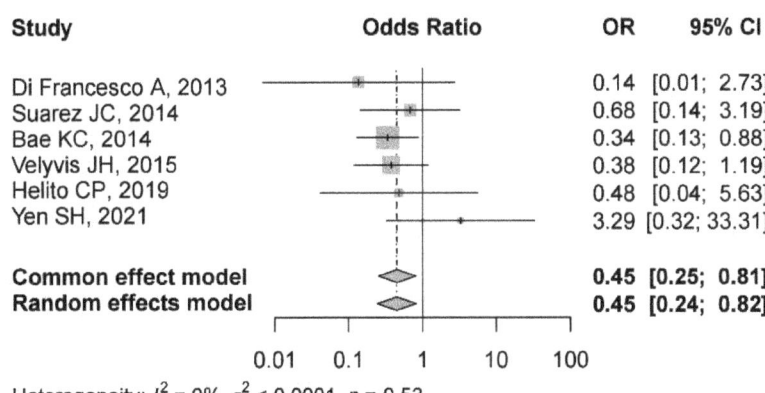

Figure 5. The forest plot of allogenic blood transfusion from the included studies [22,24,25,28,34,35].

3.5. Publication Bias

Funnel plots showed that there was no publication bias (Figure 6).

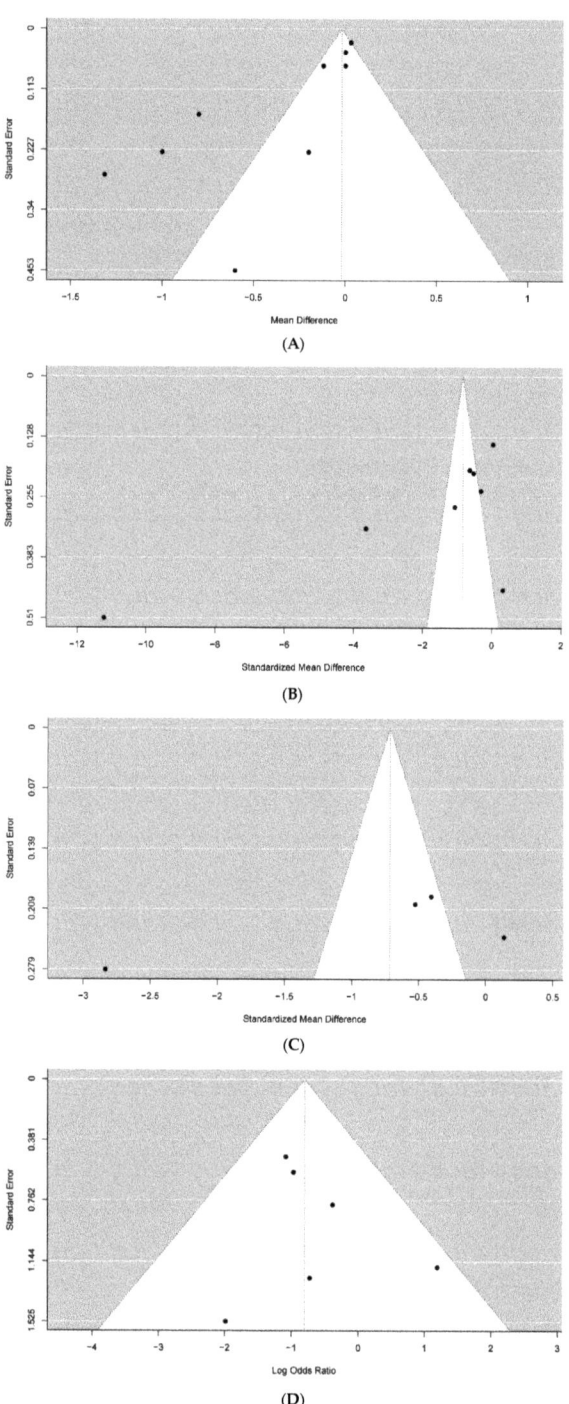

Figure 6. Funnel plots of the meta-analysis. Hemoglobin decline (**A**), volume of drainage (**B**), total blood loss (**C**), allogenic blood transfusion (**D**).

3.6. Complications

Complications, including superficial infection, deep infection, and venous thromboembolism (VTE), were investigated in five studies. In Kim et al.'s study [27], two superficial infections were reported in each of the Floseal and control groups. In Bae et al.'s study [22], VTE occurred in seven and nine cases in groups of thrombin-based hemostatic matrix and control, respectively. However, there was no case of deep infection that could be related to the use of a thrombin-based hemostatic matrix in any of the studies.

4. Discussion

This meta-analysis aimed to evaluate the effectiveness and safety of a thrombin-based hemostatic matrix in TKA based on up-to-date RCTs. The analysis focused on several key outcomes, including hemoglobin decline, the volume of drainage, total blood loss, and the risk of allogeneic transfusion. The results of the meta-analysis indicate that the use of a thrombin-based hemostatic matrix in TKA has a significant impact on reducing hemoglobin decline and the need for allogenic transfusion.

There has been a debate on the effectiveness of the application of topical hemostatic agents in TKA. Two previous meta-analyses have shown promising results regarding the effectiveness of thrombin-based hemostatic matrix in TKA. In 2014, Wang C. et al. reported that there was a significant advantage in hemoglobin decline and calculated total blood loss but no difference in postoperative drainage volume and rate of transfusion in TKA when using a thrombin-based hemostatic matrix [30]. In contrast, Fu X. et al. found that there was a significant difference in hemoglobin decline, total blood loss, drainage volume, and transfusion rate in the Floseal group compared to the control group [29]. Although there is no other previous meta-analysis on the use of Floseal in TKA, in two retrospective studies, Schwab PE demonstrated that there were no differences in hemoglobin and transfusion rate in patients who received minimal invasive TKA with or without aspirin [36,37]. Among the eight studies evaluated in this meta-analysis, RCTs by Yen SH et al. and Kim HJ et al. showed no advantage of Floseal in terms of hemoglobin level, transfusion rate, drainage volume, and total blood loss [27,35]. In contrast, studies by Bae KC et al. and Di Francesco A. et al. favored the use of Floseal in TKA [24,34]. Through this meta-analysis, we found advantages in using a thrombin-based hemostatic matrix in reducing hemoglobin decline and allogenic transfusion. With current meta-analyses, we added to the collective evidence in favor of the use of thrombin-based hemostatic matrix in TKA, along with other studies that support its use as a part of patient blood management.

In this meta-analysis, three studies [22,24,28] reported the effectiveness of a thrombin-based hemostatic matrix in reducing blood loss, while two other studies showed no significant effect. The conflicting results can be explained by different surgical and blood management protocols. In Yen et al.'s study, minimal invasive TKA that minimizes soft-tissue injury and subsequent bleeding was performed, and it can be related to a reduced difference between Floseal and control groups [35]. However, in other studies, conventional TKAs were performed, or TKA types were not described. Different blood drainage protocols also can affect the results of the study. Kim et al.'s study that placed a drain with low pressure for 24 h [27], and Yen et al.'s study that maintained a vacuum bag for 12 h with no full compression, followed by full compression until removal showed no difference between thrombin-based hemostatic matrix and control groups [35]. However, Di Francesco et al.'s study that placed a drain with high vacuum pressure for 24 h showed reduced blood drainage and transfusion rate in the Floseal group [24]. The use of tranexamic acid (TXA) also influences the postoperative bleeding and the study results. However, only two recent studies reported that the Floseal group did not use TXA [25,35], and it is not clear whether TXA was used perioperatively in the other six studies [22,24,26–28,34]. The amount of the Floseal used can also affect the results. However, the amount of Floseal was almost similar among studies (seven studies: 10 mL Floseal; one study: 5 ml Floseal), and therefore, its effect is likely to be minimal. Also, funding may become an issue that affects study results. However, among the three studies with funding [24,27,34], Kim et al.'s study showed no difference in hemoglobin drop between the thrombin-based hemostatic matrix and control groups [27]. On the contrary, among the five studies without funding [22,25,26,28,35], Bae et al.'s study [22] and Helito et al.'s study [25] reported reduced blood drainage and hemoglobin drop in the thrombin-based hemostatic matrix group compared to the control group. From these results, it is difficult to say that funding had an effect on the results of this study.

Comparing our findings with previous studies, our meta-analysis provides more recent and comprehensive evidence regarding the effectiveness of thrombin-based hemostatic matrix in TKA. Previous meta-analyses by Smith et al. and Li et al. also explored the outcomes of the use of a thrombin-based hemostatic matrix in TKA but included fewer RCTs and were published in 2018 and 2017, respectively [22,29,30]. Our study incorporates additional RCTs published since then, thereby strengthening the overall evidence base.

One of the reasons that the thrombin-based hemostatic matrix was effective in hemoglobin decrease and transfusion but not in drainage and total blood loss might be because the latter indices do not include hidden blood loss in the interstitial area. In contrast, hemoglobin decreases, and the risk of allogeneic blood transfusion represents perioperative blood loss from a more systemic point of view. Applying the thrombin-based hemostatic matrix in TKA might not show a significant difference in the amount of drainage or measured total blood loss, but it could be effective in occult bleeding [30].

Although our study demonstrates the potential benefits of the thrombin-based hemostatic matrix in TKA, certain limitations should be acknowledged. First, the included studies varied in terms of patient characteristics, surgical techniques, and outcome measures, which may introduce heterogeneity and affect the generalizability of the results. Second, the follow-up durations in the included studies were relatively short, limiting the assessment of long-term outcomes. Third, limited statistical significance was observed in a few studies included in the meta-analysis: hemoglobin reduction was significant in two studies, total weight loss in three studies, and transfusion rate in one study. Integrating the findings from individual studies in a meta-analysis, especially when there are only a few studies with statistically significant results, can lead to greater heterogeneity in the results and exacerbate the influence of publication bias. We used a random-effect model rather than a common-effect model when the $I^2 > 50\%$, indicating severe heterogeneity. Future studies with larger sample sizes and standardized protocols are needed to further validate the findings of this meta-analysis.

5. Conclusions

In conclusion, our meta-analysis suggests that thrombin-based hemostatic matrix is an effective hemostatic agent in TKA, leading to reduced hemoglobin decline, lower transfusion requirements, and improved postoperative outcomes. These findings provide valuable insights for orthopedic surgeons and enhance the existing evidence base. Further well-designed RCTs with longer follow-up periods are warranted to assess the long-term efficacy and safety of thrombin-based hemostatic matrix in TKA.

Author Contributions: Conceptualization, C.B.C.; methodology, Y.-K.L.; validation, T.W.K.; formal analysis, M.H.; investigation, T.W.K.; data curation, J.-W.P., J.J.G. and B.K.P.; writing—original draft preparation, J.-W.P.; writing—review and editing, Y.-K.L. and W.-L.J.; funding acquisition, C.B.C. All authors have read and agreed to the published version of the manuscript.

Funding: This research was supported by grant No. HI22C1879 from the Korea Health Industry Development Institution.

Institutional Review Board Statement: Ethical review and approval were waived for this study due to its design as a meta-analysis not involving any individual data (IRB exemption from SNUBH IRB No. Z-2023-103, date: 28 June 2023).

Data Availability Statement: The data presented in this study are available on reasonable request from the corresponding author.

Conflicts of Interest: The authors declare no conflict of interest.

References

1. Goh, G.S.; Fillingham, Y.A.; Ong, C.B.; Krueger, C.A.; Courtney, P.M.; Hozack, W.J. Redefining Indications for Modern Cementless Total Knee Arthroplasty: Clinical Outcomes and Survivorship in Patients >75 Years Old. *J. Arthroplast.* **2022**, *37*, 476–481.e1. [CrossRef]
2. Kurtz, S.; Ong, K.; Lau, E.; Mowat, F.; Halpern, M. Projections of primary and revision hip and knee arthroplasty in the United States from 2005 to 2030. *J. Bone Jt. Surg. Am.* **2007**, *89*, 780–785. [CrossRef]
3. Hu, Y.; Li, Q.; Wei, B.G.; Zhang, X.S.; Torsha, T.T.; Xiao, J.; Shi, Z.J. Blood loss of total knee arthroplasty in osteoarthritis: An analysis of influential factors. *J. Orthop. Surg. Res.* **2018**, *13*, 325. [CrossRef]
4. Liu, W.; Yang, C.; Huang, X.; Liu, R. Tranexamic Acid Reduces Occult Blood Loss, Blood Transfusion, and Improves Recovery of Knee Function after Total Knee Arthroplasty: A Comparative Study. *J. Knee Surg.* **2018**, *31*, 239–246. [CrossRef]
5. Klika, A.K.; Small, T.J.; Saleh, A.; Szubski, C.R.; Chandran Pillai, A.L.; Barsoum, W.K. Primary total knee arthroplasty allogenic transfusion trends, length of stay, and complications: Nationwide inpatient sample 2000-2009. *J. Arthroplast.* **2014**, *29*, 2070–2077. [CrossRef]
6. Suh, Y.S.; Choi, H.S.; Lee, J.S.; Jang, B.W.; Hwang, J.; Song, M.G.; Joo, J.; Chung, H.; Lee, J.J.; Nho, J.H. Transfusion Trends of Knee Arthroplasty in Korea: A Nationwide Study Using the Korean National Health Insurance Service Sample Data. *Int. J. Environ. Res. Public Health* **2022**, *19*, 5982. [CrossRef]
7. Liu, D.; Dan, M.; Martinez Martos, S.; Beller, E. Blood Management Strategies in Total Knee Arthroplasty. *Knee Surg. Relat. Res.* **2016**, *28*, 179–187. [CrossRef]
8. Echave, M.; Oyaguez, I.; Casado, M.A. Use of Floseal(R), a human gelatine-thrombin matrix sealant, in surgery: A systematic review. *BMC Surg.* **2014**, *14*, 111. [CrossRef]
9. Gale, A.J. Continuing education course #2: Current understanding of hemostasis. *Toxicol. Pathol.* **2011**, *39*, 273–280. [CrossRef] [PubMed]
10. Chiara, O.; Cimbanassi, S.; Bellanova, G.; Chiarugi, M.; Mingoli, A.; Olivero, G.; Ribaldi, S.; Tugnoli, G.; Basilico, S.; Bindi, F.; et al. A systematic review on the use of topical hemostats in trauma and emergency surgery. *BMC Surg.* **2018**, *18*, 68. [CrossRef]
11. Sae-Jung, S.; Apiwatanakul, P. Chitosan Pad, Cellulose Membrane, or Gelatin Sponge for Peridural Bleeding: An Efficacy Study on a Lumbar Laminectomized Rat Model. *Asian Spine J.* **2018**, *12*, 195–201. [CrossRef] [PubMed]
12. Schreiber, M.A.; Neveleff, D.J. Achieving hemostasis with topical hemostats: Making clinically and economically appropriate decisions in the surgical and trauma settings. *AORN J.* **2011**, *94*, S1–S20. [CrossRef] [PubMed]
13. Lemmer, R.; Albrech, M.; Bauer, G. Use of FloSeal hemostatic matrix in a patient with severe postpartum hemorrhage. *J. Obstet. Gynaecol. Res.* **2012**, *38*, 435–437. [CrossRef]
14. Nasso, G.; Piancone, F.; Bonifazi, R.; Romano, V.; Visicchio, G.; De Filippo, C.M.; Impiombato, B.; Fiore, F.; Bartolomucci, F.; Alessandrini, F.; et al. Prospective, randomized clinical trial of the FloSeal matrix sealant in cardiac surgery. *Ann. Thorac. Surg.* **2009**, *88*, 1520–1526. [CrossRef] [PubMed]
15. Nomura, K.; Yoshida, M.; Okada, M.; Nakamura, Y.; Yawatari, K.; Nakayama, E. Effectiveness of a Gelatin-Thrombin Matrix Sealant (Floseal(R)) for Reducing Blood Loss During Microendoscopic Decompression Surgery for Lumbar Spinal Canal Stenosis: A Retrospective Cohort Study. *Glob. Spine J.* **2021**, *13*, 764–770. [CrossRef]
16. Waldert, M.; Remzi, M.; Klatte, T.; Klingler, H.C. FloSeal reduces the incidence of lymphoceles after lymphadenectomies in laparoscopic and robot-assisted extraperitoneal radical prostatectomy. *J. Endourol.* **2011**, *25*, 969–973. [CrossRef] [PubMed]
17. Ali, T.; Keenan, J.; Mason, J.; Hseih, J.T.; Batstone, M. Prospective study examining the use of thrombin-gelatin matrix (Floseal) to prevent post dental extraction haemorrhage in patients with inherited bleeding disorders. *Int. J. Oral. Maxillofac. Surg.* **2022**, *51*, 426–430. [CrossRef]
18. Bonduelle, Q.; Biggs, T.C.; Sipaul, F. Floseal: A novel application technique for the treatment of challenging epistaxis. *Clin. Otolaryngol.* **2020**, *45*, 960–962. [CrossRef]
19. Brand, Y.; Narayanan, V.; Prepageran, N.; Waran, V. A Cost-Effective Delivery System for FloSeal During Endoscopic and Microscopic Brain Surgery. *World Neurosurg.* **2016**, *90*, 492–495. [CrossRef]
20. Gazzeri, R.; Galarza, M.; Alfier, A. Safety biocompatibility of gelatin hemostatic matrix (Floseal and Surgiflo) in neurosurgical procedures. *Surg. Technol. Int.* **2012**, *22*, 49–54.
21. Ujam, A.; Awad, Z.; Wong, G.; Tatla, T.; Farrell, R. Safety trial of Floseal((R)) haemostatic agent in head and neck surgery. *Ann. R. Coll. Surg. Engl.* **2012**, *94*, 336–339. [CrossRef]
22. Bae, K.C.; Cho, C.H.; Lee, K.J.; Son, E.S.; Lee, S.W.; Lee, S.J.; Lim, K.H. Efficacy of intra-articular injection of thrombin-based hemostatic agent in the control of bleeding after primary total knee arthroplasty. *Knee Surg. Relat. Res.* **2014**, *26*, 236–240. [CrossRef]
23. Comadoll, J.L.; Comadoll, S.; Hutchcraft, A.; Krishnan, S.; Farrell, K.; Kreuwel, H.T.; Bechter, M. Comparison of hemostatic matrix and standard hemostasis in patients undergoing primary TKA. *Orthopedics* **2012**, *35*, e785–e793. [CrossRef]
24. Di Francesco, A.; Flamini, S.; Fiori, F.; Mastri, F. Hemostatic matrix effects on blood loss after total knee arthroplasty: A randomized controlled trial. *Indian. J. Orthop.* **2013**, *47*, 474–481. [CrossRef]

25. Helito, C.P.; Bonadio, M.B.; Sobrado, M.F.; Giglio, P.N.; Pecora, J.R.; Camanho, G.L.; Demange, M.K. Comparison of Floseal(R) and Tranexamic Acid for Bleeding Control after Total Knee Arthroplasty: A Prospective Randomized Study. *Clinics* **2019**, *74*, e1186 [CrossRef]
26. Helito, C.P.; Gobbi, R.G.; Castrillon, L.M.; Hinkel, B.B.; Pecora, J.R.; Camanho, G.L. Comparison of Floseal(r) and electrocautery in hemostasis after total knee arthroplasty. *Acta Ortop. Bras.* **2013**, *21*, 320–322. [CrossRef]
27. Kim, H.J.; Fraser, M.R.; Kahn, B.; Lyman, S.; Figgie, M.P. The efficacy of a thrombin-based hemostatic agent in unilateral total knee arthroplasty: A randomized controlled trial. *J. Bone Jt. Surg. Am.* **2012**, *94*, 1160–1165. [CrossRef]
28. Suarez, J.C.; Slotkin, E.M.; Alvarez, A.M.; Szubski, C.R.; Barsoum, W.K.; Patel, P.D. Prospective, randomized trial to evaluate efficacy of a thrombin-based hemostatic agent in total knee arthroplasty. *J. Arthroplast.* **2014**, *29*, 1950–1955. [CrossRef]
29. Fu, X.; Tian, P.; Xu, G.J.; Sun, X.L.; Ma, X.L. Thrombin-Based Hemostatic Agent in Primary Total Knee Arthroplasty. *J. Knee Surg.* **2017**, *30*, 121–127. [CrossRef]
30. Wang, C.; Han, Z.; Zhang, T.; Ma, J.X.; Jiang, X.; Wang, Y.; Ma, X.L. The efficacy of a thrombin-based hemostatic agent in primary total knee arthroplasty: A meta-analysis. *J. Orthop. Surg. Res.* **2014**, *9*, 90. [CrossRef]
31. Higgins, J.P.; Savović, J.; Page, M.J.; Elbers, R.G.; Sterne, J.A. Chapter 8: Assessing Risk of Bias in a Randomized Trial. In *Cochrane Handbook for Systematic Reviews of Interventions*; John & Wiley & Sons: Hoboken, NJ, USA, 2022.
32. Shim, S.R.; Kim, S.J. Intervention meta-analysis: Application and practice using R software. *Epidemiol. Health* **2019**, *41*, e2019008. [CrossRef]
33. Higgins, J.P.; Thompson, S.G. Quantifying heterogeneity in a meta-analysis. *Stat. Med.* **2002**, *21*, 1539–1558. [CrossRef]
34. Velyvis, J.H. Gelatin matrix use reduces postoperative bleeding after total knee arthroplasty. *Orthopedics* **2015**, *38*, e118–e123. [CrossRef]
35. Yen, S.H.; Lin, P.C.; Wu, C.T.; Wang, J.W. Comparison of Effects of a Thrombin-Based Hemostatic Agent and Topical Tranexamic Acid on Blood Loss in Patients with Preexisting Thromboembolic Risk Undergoing a Minimally Invasive Total Knee Arthroplasty. A Prospective Randomized Controlled Trial. *Biomed. Res. Int.* **2021**, *2021*, 2549521. [CrossRef]
36. Schwab, P.E.; Thienpont, E. Use of a haemostatic matrix does not reduce blood loss in minimally invasive total knee arthroplasty. *Blood Transfus.* **2015**, *13*, 435–441. [CrossRef]
37. Schwab, P.E.; Thienpont, E. Use of a haemostatic matrix (Floseal(R)) does not reduce blood loss in minimally invasive total knee arthroplasty performed under continued aspirin. *Blood Transfus.* **2016**, *14*, 134–139. [CrossRef]

Disclaimer/Publisher's Note: The statements, opinions and data contained in all publications are solely those of the individual author(s) and contributor(s) and not of MDPI and/or the editor(s). MDPI and/or the editor(s) disclaim responsibility for any injury to people or property resulting from any ideas, methods, instructions or products referred to in the content.

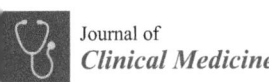

Review

Risk Factors for Periprosthetic Joint Infection after Primary Total Knee Arthroplasty

Emerito Carlos Rodriguez-Merchan [1,2,*] and Alberto D. Delgado-Martinez [3,4]

1. Department of Orthopedic Surgery, La Paz University Hospital, Paseo de la Castellana 261, 28046 Madrid, Spain
2. Osteoarticular Surgery Research, Hospital La Paz Institute for Health Research—IdiPAZ (La Paz University Hospital—Autonomous University of Madrid), 28046 Madrid, Spain
3. Department of Orthopedic Surgery, Hospital Universitario de Jaen, 23007 Jaen, Spain
4. Department of Surgery, University of Jaen, 23071 Jaen, Spain
* Correspondence: ecrmerchan@hotmail.com

Abstract: Periprosthetic joint infection (PJI) is a major adverse event of primary total knee arthroplasty (TKA) from the patient's perspective, and it is also costly for health care systems. In 2010, the reported incidence of PJI in the first 2 years after TKA was 1.55%, with an incidence of 0.46% between the second and tenth year. In 2022, it has been published that 1.41% of individuals require revision TKA for PJI. The following risk factors have been related to an increased risk of PJI: male sex, younger age, type II diabetes, obesity class II, hypertension, hypoalbuminemia, preoperative nutritional status as indicated by prognostic nutritional index (PNI) and body mass index, rheumatoid arthritis, post-traumatic osteoarthritis, intra-articular injections prior to TKA, previous multi-ligament knee surgery, previous steroid therapy, current tobacco use, procedure type (bilateral), length of stay over 35 days, patellar resurfacing, prolonged operative time, use of blood transfusions, higher glucose variability in the postoperative phase, and discharge to convalescent care. Other reported independent risk factors for PJI (in diminishing order of importance) are congestive heart failure, chronic pulmonary illness, preoperative anemia, depression, renal illness, pulmonary circulation disorders, psychoses, metastatic tumor, peripheral vascular illness, and valvular illness. Preoperative intravenous tranexamic acid has been reported to diminish the risk of delayed PJI. Knowing the risk factors for PJI after TKA, especially those that are avoidable or controllable, is critical to minimizing (ideally preventing) this complication. These risk factors are outlined in this article.

Keywords: periprosthetic joint infection; risk factors; total knee arthroplasty

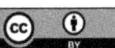

1. Introduction

According to Carulli et al., total knee arthroplasty (TKA) is one of the most successful surgical techniques in orthopedic surgery, with good clinical outcomes and a high survival percentage of more than 90% of cases at long-term follow-up. The increasing mean population age, worsening of joint degenerative disorders, and joint sequelae related to previous fractures have caused a continuous rise in the number of TKAs in every country annually, along with an expected increase in adverse events [1]. A frequent cause of revision TKA following primary TKA is periprosthetic joint infection (PJI) [2–6]. PJI was published by the Musculoskeletal Infection Society (MSIS) in 2011 [7] (Table 1).

Table 1. MSIS definition of PJI [7].

	PJI Exists When
1	There is a sinus tract communicating with the implant; or
2	A bacterium is isolated by culture from 2 or more separate tissue or fluid samples attained from the affected knee; or

Table 1. Cont.

	PJI Exists When
3	When 4 of the following 6 criteria exist: a. Raised serum erythrocyte sedimentation rate and serum C-reactive protein concentration b. Raised synovial white blood cell count c. Raised synovial polymorphonuclear percentage d. Existence of purulence in the affected joint e. Isolation of a microorganism in one culture of periprosthetic tissue or fluid f. Greater than 5 neutrophils per high-power field in 5 high-power fields noticed from histologic analysis of periprosthetic tissue at ×400 magnification

In 2018, Parvizi et al. reported an evidence-based definition for knee PJI that has demonstrated very good performance on formal external validation [8]. Two positive cultures or the existence of a sinus tract were deemed primary factors and diagnostic of PJI. The estimated weights of increased serum C-reactive protein (CRP) (>1 mg/dL), D-dimer (>860 ng/mL), and erythrocyte sedimentation rate (ESR) (>30 mm/h) were 2, 2, and 1 point, respectively. Moreover, increased synovial fluid white blood cell count (>3000 cells/µL), alpha-defensin (signal-to-cutoff ratio > 1), leukocyte esterase (++), polymorphonuclear percentage (>80%), and synovial CRP (>6.9 mg/L) were given 3, 3, 3, 2, and 1 point, respectively. Individuals with a total score of greater than or equal to 6 were deemed infected, whereas a score between 2 and 5 needed the addition of intraoperative findings for proving or disproving the diagnosis. Intraoperative findings of positive histology, purulence, and single positive culture were given 3, 3, and 2 points, respectively. Put together with the preoperative score, an aggregate of greater than or equal to 6 was deemed infected, a score between 4 and 5 was uncertain, and a score of 3 or less was not infected. These standards showed a greater sensitivity of 97.7% compared with the MSIS (79.3%) and the International Consensus Meeting definition (86.9%), with an akin specificity of 99.5% [8].

In 2021, McNally et al. reported the result of a plan created by the European Bone and Joint Infection Society (EBJIS) and endorsed by the MSIS and the European Society of Clinical Microbiology and Infectious Diseases Study Group for Implant-Associated Infections (ESGIAI). McNally et al. defined PJI using a three-degree method to the diagnostic sequence, leading to a definition set and guidance that was fully backed by the EBJIS, MSIS, and ESGIAI [9]. There are three possibilities: infection unlikely, infection likely, and infection established based on the following data: clinical and blood workup (clinical features, CRP); synovial fluid cytological analysis (leukocyte count (cells/µL); polymorphonuclear percentage); synovial fluid biomarkers (alpha-defensin); microbiology (aspiration fluid, intraoperative fluid and tissue, sonication (CFU/mL); and histology (high-power field, 400× magnification). This new EBJIS definition can now be used worldwide [9].

PJI is a severe complication of primary TKA from the patient's perspective, and it is also very costly for health care systems [10]. In fact, PJI is one of the most overwhelming adverse events of TKA [11].

Although one-stage revision TKA is performed in certain situations and centers, a PJI usually requires a two-stage revision TKA, which involves a double surgical intervention. First, the removal of the infected implant (septic loosening) is required. Following this procedure, a period of several weeks of antibiotic treatment is needed until the infection is considered cured (normalization of the ESR and CRP and healing of the surgical wound). The second intervention is the insertion of a new implant, using a model that is stable for proper functioning of the knee [11]. Figure 1 shows a case of PJI (septic loosening) that was solved by a two-stage revision TKA.

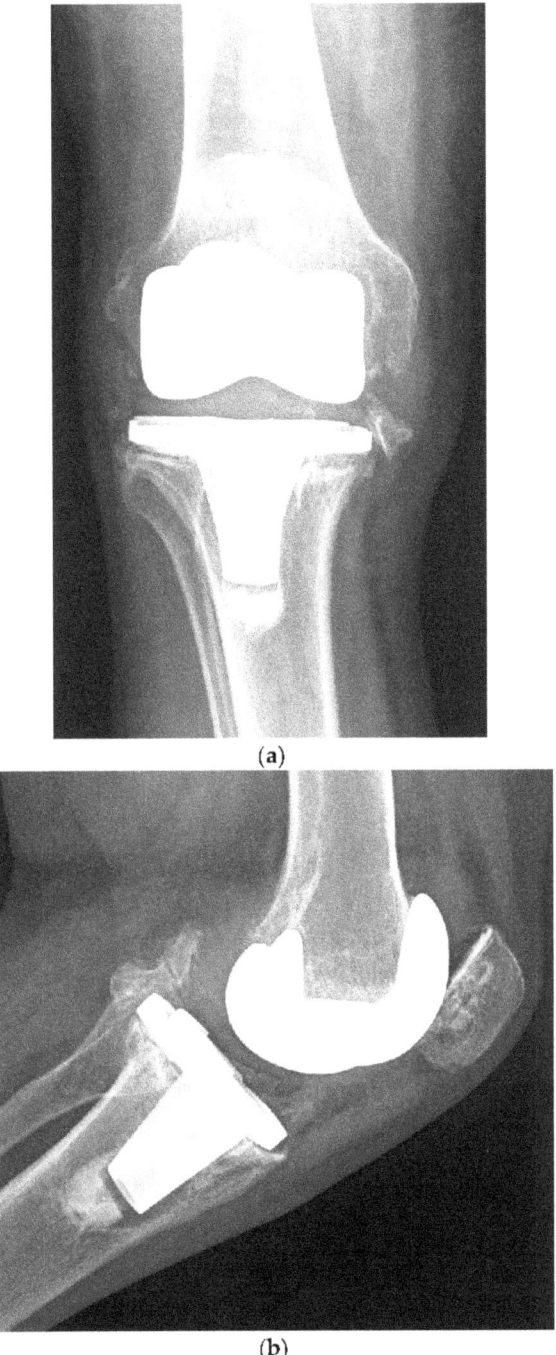

Figure 1. Cont.

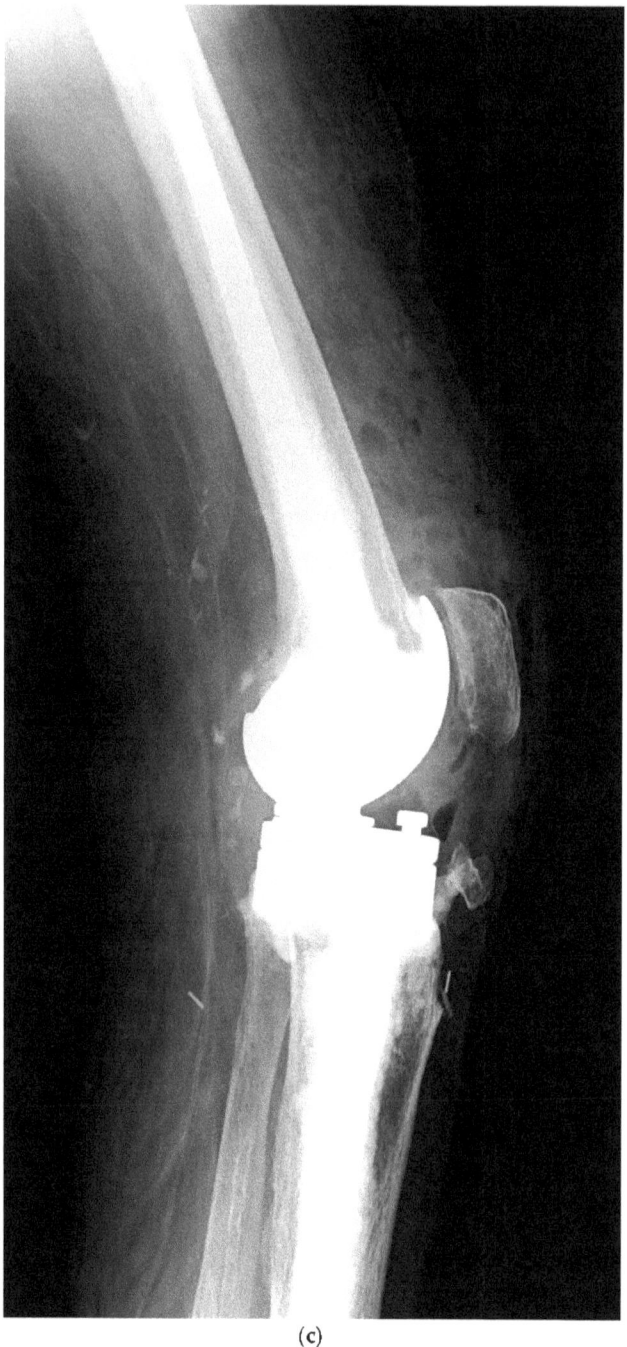

(c)

Figure 1. *Cont.*

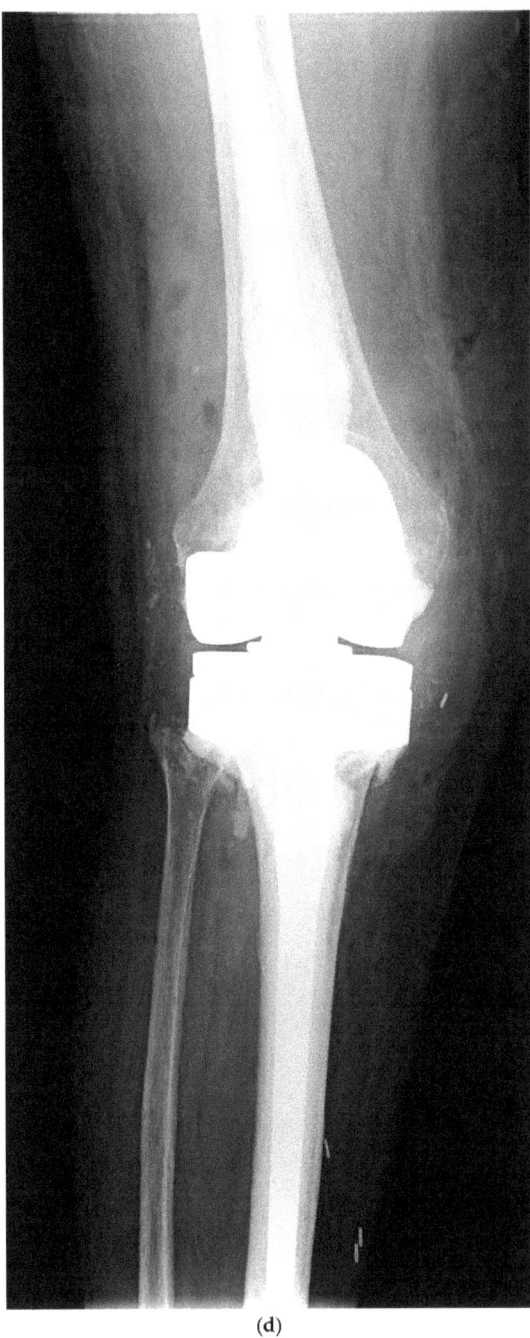

(d)

Figure 1. (a–d). Periprosthetic joint infection of a primary total knee arthroplasty (TKA) that was resolved by a two-stage revision TKA: (**a**) preoperative anteroposterior (AP) radiograph; (**b**) preoperative lateral image; (**c**) postoperative AP radiograph showing the prosthesis implanted in the second-stage revision (rotational hinge design); (**d**) lateral image of the aforementioned prosthesis.

It is important to emphasize that debridement, antibiotics, and implant retention (DAIR) is today a frequently utilized procedure in early infections [12–16]. Toh et al. reported that DAIR is the procedure of preference for individuals with acute postoperative and acute hematogenous PJI [15]. They stated that DAIR failure was related to premature mortality. Repeated DAIRs, increased ESR > 107.5, and *S. aureus* PJI were related to treatment failure, and two-stage revision TKA was advised. It is also relevant to remark that the likelihood of PJI after primary TKA can be reduced by decreasing the patient's weight, which will also minimize the risk of implant failure [17].

The aim of this narrative review is to present an overview of the risk factors for PJI after primary TKA. To this end, we have outlined the most important points to facilitate further investigation into specific aspects of the topic. This article seeks to explain the risk factors for PJI after primary TKA, with the aim of controlling or preventing this complication whenever possible.

A PubMed (MEDLINE), Cochrane Library, Web of Science, and Scopus search of reports on PJI in TKA was conducted. The key words utilized were "PJI TKA risk factors". The inclusion criterion was reports focused on the risk factors for PJI in TKA. Studies not focused on such risk factors were disregarded. The searches were dated from the creation of the search engines until 30 September 2022. From the 13,304 articles (10,300 in the Web of Science, 2860 in Scopus, 136 in PubMed, 8 in The Cochrane Library), we chose those that seemed most directly related to the title of this article (66 articles).

2. Incidence of PJI after TKA

Several authors have reported infection rates of 2–5% after TKA [4–7,18,19]. However, in a level 2 evidence study (prognostic study) published in 2010, among 69,663 patients operated on for TKA, Kurtz et al. identified 1400 infections. The incidence of infection in the first 2 years was 1.55%. The incidence between the second and tenth year was 0.46%. PJI was observed to occur at a fairly elevated percentage in Medicare individuals, with the highest risk in the first 2 years following TKA; roughly a quarter of PJIs occur after 2 years [20].

In 2022, the McMaster Arthroplasty Collaborative (MAC) found that 1.41% of individuals experienced revision TKA for PJI [11]. Figure 2 shows a comparison between the rates of PJI after TKA reported in 2010 and 2022.

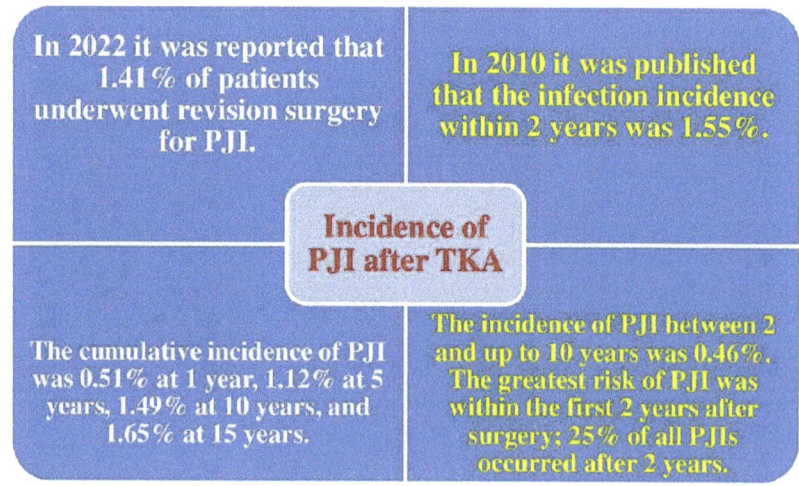

Figure 2. Rates of periprosthetic joint infection (PJI) after primary total knee arthroplasty (TKA) published in 2010 [20] and 2022 [11].

3. Risk Factors for Periprosthetic Joint Infection following Primary TKA

3.1. Patient-Related Risk Factors

3.1.1. Male Gender, Procedure Type (bilateral), Length of Stay over 35 Days, and Usage of Transfusions Have Been Shown to Be Risk Factors for Postoperative PJI

In 2021, Ko et al. found that male sex, low family earnings, surgical technique type (bilateral), length of stay (LOS) ≥ 35 days, and transfusions were risk factors for postoperative adverse events after TKA in individuals with idiopathic knee osteoarthritis. The aforementioned authors analyzed 560,954 individuals older than 50 years. The risk of PJI was evaluated with 8 independent parameters: sex, age, place of residence, family earnings, hospital bed size, type of surgical technique (unilateral or bilateral, primary or revision TKA), LOS, and the use of transfusions [21].

3.1.2. Male Gender, Younger Age, Type II Diabetes, Posttraumatic Osteoarthritis, Patellar Resurfacing, and Discharge to Nursing Home Were Related to an Increased Risk of PJI

In 2022, the MAC carried a population-based cohort investigation utilizing linked administrative databases. The multivariable analysis showed that male gender, younger age, type II diabetes, posttraumatic osteoarthritis, patellar resurfacing, and discharge to convalescent care were related to an increased risk of PJI [11].

In an article with level 2 evidence (prognostic study), the independent risk factors for PJI (in diminishing order of importance) were congestive heart failure, chronic pulmonary illness, preoperative anemia, diabetes, depression, renal illness, pulmonary circulation disorders, obesity, rheumatologic illness, psychoses, metastatic tumor, peripheral vascular illness, and valvular illness [22].

In 2013, Chen et al. showed that the principal factors associated with PJI following TKA were body mass index (BMI), diabetes mellitus, hypertension, steroid treatment, and rheumatoid arthritis. The study had insufficient evidence to demonstrate that the male sex was associated with PJI after TKA. A statistical analysis showed no correlations between urinary tract infection, fixation technique, American Society of Anesthesiology (ASA) score, bilateral procedure, age, transfusion, antibiotics, bone graft, and PJI [23].

A study with level 2 evidence (prognostic study) reported by Kurtz et al. in 2010 showed that women had a lower risk of PJI than men. Comorbidities also increased TKA infection risk. Individuals receiving public assistance for Medicare premiums were at increased risk for PJI. Hospital factors did not contribute to an increased risk of infection. PJI occurred at a fairly elevated percentage in Medicare individuals, with the greatest risk of PJI within the first 2 years following TKA; nonetheless, around 25% of all PJIs occurred after 2 years [20].

Cordtz et al. observed that individuals with rheumatoid arthritis had a diminished 10-year risk of revision TKA, whereas the risk of PJI was increased compared with individuals with osteoarthritis after TKA. Previous treatment with biological disease-modifying antirheumatic drugs was not related to an increased risk of PJI [24].

In an investigation with level 3 evidence (therapeutic study), Pancio et al. found that a higher proportion of individuals who had undergone multi-ligament knee surgery experienced infections compared with matched controls (7% vs. 1%), respectively. Previous multi-ligament surgery was associated with a greater risk of PJI [25].

3.1.3. Previous Septic Arthritis Has Been Shown to Be a Risk Factor for Postoperative PJI

Previous septic arthritis has also been recognized as a PJI risk factor [25]. Pooled data from more than 1300 arthroplasties in published papers revealed a PJI rate of 5.96% when a previous infection occurred in the same articulation. The risk of infection was lower because the TKA surgery was delayed from the resolution of the previous infection.

3.1.4. Smoking Is related to Higher Percentages of PJI

In 2015, Singh et al. found that smoking was related to an elevated risk of PJI after primary TKA. Tobacco use status was accessible for 7926 (95%) individuals and was not accessible for 446 (5%); 565 (7%) currently smoked tobacco. The hazard ratios for PJI were higher in current tobacco users than in nonusers [26]. Cessation of smoking before TKA is strongly recommended.

3.1.5. Hypoalbuminemia and Obesity Class II Are Dependable Predictors of PJI

According to Man et al., malnutrition is a relevant but changeable risk factor for postoperative adverse events and unfavorable results in orthopedic surgery [27]. They sought to detect biomarkers of malnutrition in individuals undergoing TKA that could be predictive of adverse postoperative complications in the hospital, to identify patients at risk and optimize their nutritional status prior to TKA. These authors analyzed 624 patients in whom possible biomarkers of pre-operative malnutrition, including hypoalbuminemia (serum albumin < 3.5 g/dL), total lymphocyte count (TLC) (<1500 cells/mm^3), and BMI, were evaluated for associations with in-hospital postoperative adverse events. The frequencies of hypoalbuminemia, low TLC, overweight, obesity class I, and obesity class II were 2.72%, 33.4%, 14.8%, 44.5%, and 26.9%, respectively. There were significant relationships between hypoalbuminemia and type II obesity (BMI $\geq$ 30.0 kg/m^2) and PJI percentages and no significant relationships between these adverse events and low TLC, overweight, or type I obesity. It was also found that individuals with hypoalbuminemia or type II obesity with gouty arthritis were more prone to experience PJI. The authors concluded that hypoalbuminemia and type II obesity together were dependable biomarkers of preoperative malnutrition that could predict PJI following TKA; however, low TLC, overweight, and type I obesity were not significantly related to an increased risk of PJI [27].

3.1.6. Intra-Articular Injections Prior to TKA Are Related to a Higher Risk of PJI

In a level 3 evidence study (therapeutic study) published in 2017, Bedard et al. observed that intra-articular knee injections with corticosteroids, hyaluronic acid, or other drugs prior to TKA were related to an increased risk of PJI, and this association appeared to be time dependent: the shorter the delay between injection and TKA, the greater the likelihood of PJI [28]. The proportion of patients undergoing TKAs who developed PJI was greater in those who were given an injection prior to TKA than in those who were not (4.4% vs. 3.6%). Similarly, the proportion of patients undergoing TKAs who developed PJI requiring surgical reintervention was also greater among those who received an injection prior to TKA than in those who did not (1.49% vs. 1.04%). An analysis of the months between injection and TKA showed that the odds of PJI were greater for patients injected up to 6 months between injection and TKA, as were the odds of surgical intervention for TKA infection when the injection was within 7 months of TKA. When the time span between injection and TKA was longer than 6–7 months, the ORs were no longer raised [28].

3.1.7. Greater Glucose Variability in the Postoperative Period Is Related to Higher Percentages of PJI

In 2018, Shohat et al. investigated the relationship between glucose variability and postoperative adverse events after TKA (level 4 of evidence study) [29]. They analyzed data on 2698 individuals who had experienced TKA at a single center. Individuals with a minimum of two postoperative glucose values per day or more than three values overall were included in the research. Glucose variability was evaluated utilizing a coefficient of variation. The MSIS criteria were utilized to establish PJI. Some 19.9% of the patients had diabetes. Greater glycemic variability was related to increased LOS, 90-day mortality, PJI, and SSI. Adjusted analyses showed that for every 10-percentage-point rise in the coefficient of variation, the LOS increased by 6.1%, and the risks of PJI and SSI increased by 20% and 14%, respectively. These associations were independent of the year of the surgical procedure, age, BMI, Elixhauser comorbidity index, diagnosis of diabetes, in-hospital utilization of insulin or steroids, or mean glucose values throughout hospitalization. They concluded that greater glucose variability in the postoperative period was related to increased percentages of SSI and PJI after TKA. According to Shohat et al., it is paramount to control glucose variability in the early postoperative phase [29].

3.1.8. Reduction of Patient's Weight Diminishes the Probability of PJI and Minimizes Implant Failure

It has been published that the likelihood of PJI following primary TKA can be reduced by decreasing the patient's weight, which will also minimize the risk of implant failure [17].

4. Surgical Risk Factors

4.1. Prolonged Surgical Time Correlates with Increased Infection Risk

In 2006, Peersman et al. stated that the time span of the surgical procedure had a definite impact on infection rates, especially regarding postoperative infection after TKA. The study confirmed the significance of the time span of TKA as a risk factor for SSI and subsequent PJI. Therefore, the time span of the surgical intervention can be a predictor of PJI [30].

4.2. Unilateral versus Bilateral TKA

In 2021, Ko et al. reported that the procedure type (bilateral TKA versus unilateral TKA), was a risk factor for postoperative adverse events following TKA [21]. Some reports have shown that when bilateral TKA is carried out, the LOS, anesthesia duration and rehabilitation period can be reduced and that there are advantages to individuals and hospitals in terms of cost [31,32].

Despite these benefits, there were issues over the safety of bilateral TKA. According to Odum et al., concurrent bilateral TKA had greater percentages of adverse events compared with unilateral TKA [31]. Memtsoudis et al. stated that staging bilateral TKA had either a greater or similar frequency of adverse events compared with simultaneous bilateral TKA [33]. The study by Ko et al. proved the outcomes of those studies, given that the complication hazard ratios for bilateral TKA were consistently higher than those for unilateral TKA [21].

4.3. Patellar Resurfacing

A multivariable model reported by the MAC showed that patellar resurfacing was related to an increased risk of PJI. However, patellar resurfacing was the weakest of all significant predictors ($p = 0.04$) [11]. In contrast, a meta-analysis of randomized controlled trials (RCTs) encountered no difference in infection percentages between patellar resurfacing and non-resurfacing [34]. Clearly, future studies should examine the association between patellar resurfacing and PJI after primary TKA.

4.4. Risk Factors in the Postoperative Phase

It has been reported that the use of blood transfusions [21], LOS over 35 days [20], higher glucose variability [28], and discharge to convalescent care [11] are important risk factors for PJI following TKA. Ko et al. found that the risk was increased in the longer LOS cohort and in the transfusion cohort [21]. The Cox proportional hazards model reported by the MAC showed that discharge to a nursing home was related to an increased risk of developing PJI after primary TKA [10]. Table 2 summarizes the patient-related and surgical risk factors for PJI after primary TKA as well as risk factors in the postoperative period.

Table 2. Patient-related and surgical risk factors for PJI after primary TKA, as well as risk factors in the postoperative period.

	Risk Factors
Patient-related risk factors	<ul><li>Male gender</li><li>Younger age</li><li>Type II diabetes</li><li>Obesity class II</li><li>Hypertension</li><li>Hypoalbuminemia</li><li>Poor preoperative nutritional status</li><li>Rheumatoid arthritis</li><li>Post-traumatic osteoarthritis</li><li>Intraarticular injections before TKA</li><li>Previous multi-ligament knee surgery</li><li>Previous septic arthritis</li><li>Previous steroid therapy</li><li>Current tobacco use</li><li>Congestive heart failure</li><li>Chronic pulmonary disease</li><li>Preoperative anemia</li><li>Depression</li><li>Renal illness</li><li>Pulmonary circulation disorders</li><li>Psychoses</li><li>Metastatic tumor</li><li>Peripheral vascular illness</li><li>Valvular illness</li></ul>
Surgical risk factors	<ul><li>Prolonged operative time</li><li>Procedure type (bilateral)</li><li>Patellar resurfacing</li></ul>
Risk factors in the postoperative period	<ul><li>Use of blood transfusion</li><li>Higher glucose variability</li><li>Length of stay over 35 days</li><li>Discharge to convalescent care</li></ul>

5. Other Topics of Interest Related to the Risk of PJI following TKA

5.1. Tranexamic Acid Diminishes the Risk of Revision TKA for Acute and Late PJI

In 2020, Lacko et al. analyzed the impact of intravenous usage of tranexamic acid (TXA) on the risk of revision TKA for acute and late PJI following primary TKA [35]. This study included 1529 TKAs (396 men, 1133 women; mean age 67.8 years). Lacko et al. analyzed the revision percentage for acute and late PJI in a cohort of 787 TKAs with preoperative intravenously used TXA (TXA cohort) compared with a cohort of 742 TKAs without TXA (non-TXA cohort). A multiple logistic regression analysis was conducted to assess significant predictors of TKA revision for acute and late PJI. Revision TKA due to PJI was observed in one individual in the TXA cohort and one individuals in the non-TXA cohort. The cumulative revision percentage of TKA was significantly lower in the TXA group (0.13% vs. 1.08%). A multivariate logistic regression analysis detected 2 predictors of revision TKA: being older than 75 years at the time of primary TKA and male sex. The utilization of TXA was demonstrated to be a significant protective factor. These authors identified a lower cumulative revision percentage of TKA for acute and late PJI when TXA was utilized. Lacko et al. concluded that the pre-operative intravenous utilization of TXA could be an efficacious, safe, and inexpensive approach to preventing PJI [35].

In 2021, Hong et al. found that use of TXA on the day of surgery in TKA was associated with significantly diminished odds of PJI in the first 3 months. Some 46% received TXA on the day of surgery, and 0.13% developed PJI within 3 months. After adjusting for individual and hospital-related covariates, TXA administration was related to significantly lower odds of PJI within 3 months of surgery. They concluded that TXA might play a significant role in decreasing PJI after TKA [36]. Figure 3 summarizes the role of TXA for the prevention of PJI following TKA. Table 2 summarizes patient-related and surgical risk factors for PJI after primary TKA.

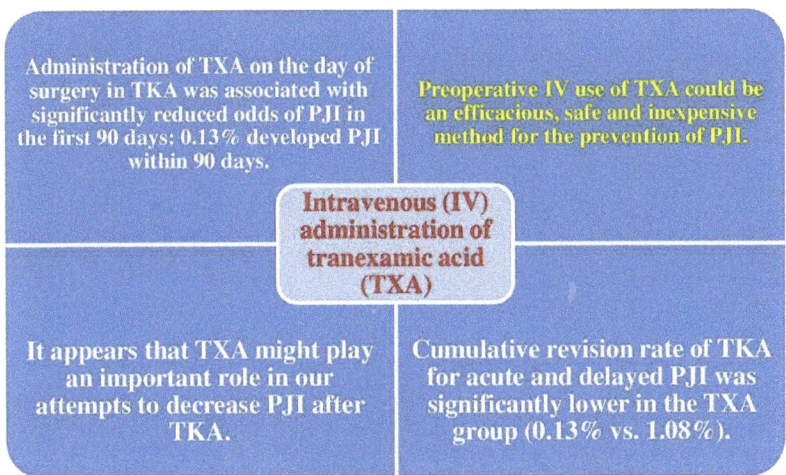

Figure 3. Intravenous administration of tranexamic acid appears to play an important role in the prevention of periprosthetic joint infection (PJI) after primary total knee arthroplasty (TKA) [35,36].

5.2. Prognostic Nutritional Index as a Predictor of Postoperative PJI

According to Hanada et al., individuals with malnutrition have an elevated risk of postoperative adverse events after TKA. In addition, serum albumin and total lymphocyte count are deemed preoperative nutritional evaluation parameters. The prognostic nutritional index (PNI) is estimated by combining serum albumin and total lymphocyte counts. The objective of this investigation was to detect risk factors for postoperative adverse events after TKA, including preoperative nutritional evaluation, and to evaluate preoperative PNI as a predictor of postoperative adverse events [37]. A total of 160 individuals (234 knees) undergoing primary TKA were analyzed. The serum albumin (g/dL) and total lymphocyte count (/mm^3) were studied within 90 days prior to TKA; then, the PNI was estimated. Postoperative aseptic wound complications were studied, such as skin erosion and dehiscence within 14 days and PJI following TKA. PJIs occurred in 14 (6%) knees. Postoperative aseptic wound complications within 14 days were significant risk factors for PJI. No significant dissimilarities in individual demographics, such as age, gender, BMI, or comorbidities were observed between patients with and without PJI except for the percentage of aseptic surgical wound complications. In addition, postoperative aseptic wound problems were affected by elevated BMI and low PNI. They concluded that pre-operative nutritional status, as shown by PNI and BMI, was related to postoperative wound complications within 14 days. PJI following TKA was related to early postoperative aseptic wound complications [37].

5.3. BMI Is a Superior Predictor of PJI Risk Than Local Quantities of Adipose Tissue

According to Shearer et al., both BMI and local quantities of adiposity at the surgical area have been found to be independent risk factors for PJI after TKA [38]. They evaluated previously utilized means of determining knee adiposity and found the best measure for forecasting both surgical time span and PJI after TKA, reviewing 4745 individuals who experienced primary TKA. Individual demographic data, surgical time span, and postoperative infection status within 12 months were obtained. Preoperative weight-bearing anteroposterior (AP) and lateral X-rays were studied to detect the thickness of the prepatellar adipose tissue, the width of the tibial plateau, and the total soft tissue knee width. The knee adipose index (KAI) was estimated from the ratio of bone to total knee width. They found considerable variability in both local parameters of adiposity compared with BMI. Neither parameter of local knee adipose tissue demonstrated a substantial correlation with PJI risk. By contrast, there was a significant correlation between PJI risk and BMI > 35. The surgical time span correlated with both BMI and parameters of local adipose tissue (KAI and prepatellar fat thickness). They concluded that BMI was a superior predictor of PJI after TKA compared with local parameters of the adipose tissue of the knee joint [38].

5.4. American College of Surgeons National Surgical Quality Improvement Program SSI Calculator

In a study with level 3 evidence published in 2016, Wingert et al. assessed the reliability of the American College of Surgeons National Surgical Quality Improvement Program (ACS NSQIP) SSI Calculator in forecasting 30-day and 90-day postoperative infection. The minimum follow-up was 90 days [10]. Individuals who experienced a repeat surgical intervention within 90 days of the TKA and in whom at least 1 positive intraoperative culture was obtained at the time of re-intervention were deemed to have PJI. Individual-specific risk possibilities for PJI based on demographics and comorbidities were obtained from the ACS NSQIP Surgical Risk Calculator website. The ACS NSQIP Surgical Risk Calculator demonstrated only moderate reliability in forecasting 30-day PJI. For 90-day PJI, the risk calculator was also only moderate in reliability. They concluded that the ACS NSQIP Surgical Risk Calculator was only a moderate predictor of acute PJI at the 30- and 90-day intervals following primary TKA. Therefore, orthopedic surgeons should be cautious when employing this instrument as a predictive tool for PJI [10].

6. Discussion

A recent study confirmed a relevant agreement among European orthopedic surgeons regarding prevention of PJI after TKA, and Table 3 shows the measures recommended by these authors to decrease the risk of PJI. However, the authors also noted that there is still room for improvement [39].

Table 3. Measures recommended to minimize the risk of periprosthetic joint infection (PJI) following TKA [38].

Measures
Changeable Risk Factors Should Be Optimized before TKA
Patient education should involve skin cleaning methods with a remnant antiseptic solution
Alcoholic chlorhexidine provides better protection than alcoholic povidone-iodine against PJI
Alcohol-based solutions should be utilized in surgical hand preparation
A standardized method to the utilize of antiseptics should be in place, with special attention to the incision area
Antibiotic prophylaxis should be given before surgery and not routinely prolonged
Traffic and number of personnel in the operating room should be maintained to a minimum
Tranexamic acid and hemostatic drug utilization should be optimized to diminish the need for a surgical drain
Structured monitoring and reporting protocols for PJI should be in place
Specific instructions for PJI should be created and executed; these should be tailored to individual patient risk factors
Instructions based on level 1 or 2 of evidence should be deemed compulsory
Infections that appear 30 days after surgery can still be deemed to be PJI

Even though a number of deterrent actions during surgeries including prophylactic IV utilization of antibiotics; preoperative disinfection of the skin; and intrawound lavage with a great quantity of saline have been carried out pre-, intra- and postoperatively, the risk of infection persists [11].

Given the high individual and societal influence of PJI and revision TKA, it is encouraging to note that the percentages of PJI are decreasing over time. However, with increasing percentages of osteoarthritis and TKA worldwide, it is likely that the absolute burden of PJI will continue to grow. Therefore, there is still a need to diminish the percentages of PJI after TKA. One approach is the use of antibiotic cement, although there are still conflicting data in the literature [40–43]. An RCT showed an 87% relative risk decrease in PJI after revision TKA utilizing a dilute povidone-iodine lavage compared with saline [44]. Both procedures deserve further analysis in the context of primary TKA through large RCTs, given that they are low-cost and potentially effective interventions. Preoperative risk factors for PJI must be addressed; for example, reducing body weight [45], controlling diabetes mellitus [46], improving malnutrition [47], and stopping smoking [48]. Individuals with malnutrition have an elevated risk of postoperative infection [47,49,50], and the frequency of malnutrition in individuals experiencing TKA has been revealed to be as high as 40% [51]. Therefore, it is important to assess nutritional status among preoperative patients.

PNI has been employed to assess nutrition in individuals with heart failure [52] and who experienced gastrointestinal surgery [53]. PNI can be easily estimated with serum albumin and total lymphocyte counts and is helpful for the nutritional assessment of individuals prior to TKA [50]. In fact, PNI has been shown as a predictor of 5-year overall survival following colorectal cancer surgical procedures and postoperative delirium [54,55].

It is important to mention the Swedish nationwide plan called Prosthesis Related Infections Shall be Stopped (PRISS), which was recently reported by Thompson et al. [18]. They calculated the incidence percentage of PJI after primary TKA prior to and after PRISS. These authors observed a 2-year incidence rate of 1.45%. The incidence rate was 1.44% prior to PRISS and 1.46% after. Diagnoses were confirmed within 30 days of primary TKA in 52%, and within 90 days in 73% of cases. A similar incidence prior to and after the PRISS plan was found. In addition, the time span to diagnosis was similar throughout both time intervals [19]. The likelihood of PJI after primary TKA can also be reduced by decreasing the patient's weight, which will likewise minimize the risk of implant failure [17].

Kirschbaum et al. observed that the likelihood of survival of primary TKA is substantially diminished with each consecutive revision and also that PJI is the principal source of multiple revisions [56]. Muwanis et al. found that dilute povidone-iodine (Betadine, Avrio Health L.P, Stamford, CT, USA) compared with normal saline irrigation is an economical and simple technique to reduce PJI and more specifically SSI in TKA [57]. According to Buchalter et al., in spite of the utilization of topical irrigation solutions and addition of local antimicrobial agents, the use of a non-cephalosporin perioperative antibiotic (either vancomycin or clindamycin) is related to a higher risk of TKA PJI compared with cefazolin [58]. An increased frequency of PJI in individuals experiencing mobilization under anesthesia (MUA) was reported by Parkulo et al. [59].

Kurz et al. determined that intra-articular injections of hyaluronic acid or corticosteroid given within the 4-month period before TKA were not related to a high PJI risk within the elderly Medicare patient population [60]. According to Avila et al., individuals receiving intra-articular injections should wait at least 3 months prior to experiencing TKA to lessen infection risk [61]. Yang et al. reported that intra-articular injections of corticosteroid or hyaluronic acid prior to TKA increased the risk of postoperative infection. Injections given more than 3 months prior to TKA did not substantially augment the risk of infection [62].

Colonoscopy has been related to an increased PJI risk in TKA recipients [63]. The utilization of the Surgical Helmet Systems was related to a lower percentage of PJI following primary TKA than with conventional surgical gowning [64]. According to Blanchard et al., individuals with preoperative urinary tract infection within 1 week of TKA have an increased risk of postoperative PJI. Moreover, antibiotics do not seem to lessen the risk [65]. Individuals with a higher number of reported allergies could be at a higher risk of PJI after TKA [66].

The main limitation of this article is that the selection of studies that were finally analyzed was subjective, i.e., those that we considered most directly related to the title of the article were chosen. Therefore, it is possible that some important articles were not included. This article is not a systematic review of the literature, but a narrative review of the articles we found most interesting.

7. Conclusions

PJI is a serious adverse event following primary TKA. It has been found that 1.41% of patients experience revision TKA for PJI. The reported cumulative frequency for PJI is 0.51% at 1 year, 1.12% at 5 years, 1.49% at 10 years, and 1.65% at 15 years. The infection frequency within 2 years is 1.55%, and the frequency between 2 and up to 10 years is 0.46%.

Male gender, younger age, type II diabetes, posttraumatic arthritis, patellar resurfacing, discharge to a nursing home, obesity class II, hypertension, prior steroid therapy, rheumatoid arthritis, procedure type (bilateral), LOS longer than 35 days, prolonged operative time, current tobacco use, intra-articular injections before TKA, previous knee infections, previous multi-ligament knee surgery and utilization of blood transfusions have all been related to an increased risk of PJI. Other independent risk factors for PJI (in diminishing order of importance) are congestive heart failure, chronic pulmonary illness, pre-operative anemia, depression, renal illness, pulmonary circulation disorders, psychoses, metastatic tumor, peripheral vascular illness, and valvular illness.

Greater glucose variability in the postoperative phase has also been related to higher percentages of PJI, with hypoalbuminemia a reliable predictor. Preoperative nutritional status, as shown by PNI and BMI, is related to postoperative wound complications within 14 days. PJI following TKA has been related to early postoperative aseptic wound complications. Pre-operatively intravenously administered tranexamic acid decreases the risk of delayed PJI.

The likelihood of PJI after primary TKA can be reduced by decreasing the patient's weight, which will also minimize the risk of implant failure. The likelihood of survival of primary TKA is substantially diminished with each consecutive revision, and PJI is the principal source of multiple revisions. Dilute povidone-iodine compared with normal saline irrigation is an economical and easy technique to reduce any PJI and more especially SSI. The utilization of a non-cephalosporin perioperative antibiotic (either vancomycin or clindamycin) is related to a higher risk of TKA PJI compared with cefazolin. An increased frequency of PJI in individuals experiencing MUA has been reported.

Intra-articular injections of hyaluronic acid or corticosteroid given within the 4-month period before TKA are not associated with higher PJI risk within the elderly Medicare patient population. Individuals receiving intra-articular injections should wait at least 3 months prior to undergoing TKA to mitigate the infection risk. Intra-articular injections of corticosteroid or hyaluronic acid prior to TKA augment the risk of postoperative infection. Injections given more than 3 months prior to TKA do not significantly augment the risk of infection.

Colonoscopy has been associated with an increased PJI risk in TKA recipients. The utilization of the Surgical Helmet Systems has been associated with an inferior percentage of PJI following primary TKA than conventional surgical gowning. Individuals with pre-operative urinary tract infection within 1 week of TKA have an increased risk of postoperative PJI. Moreover, antibiotics do not appear to mitigate this risk. Individuals with a higher number of reported allergies might be at increased risk of PJI after TKA.

The main limitation of this article is that the selection of articles that were ultimately analyzed was subjective, i.e., those that we considered most directly related to the title of the article. Therefore, it is possible that some important articles were not included in the end. This article is not a systematic review of the literature but a narrative review of the articles we found most relevant.

Of all the aforementioned risk factors, some are modifiable, and others are not. To minimize the risk of PJI, modifiable factors must be reversed or controlled (Table 4). The risk of PJI after TKA has diminished in small but uniform amounts over the past 15 years. The majority of PJIs are diagnosed within the first 2 years postoperatively, although a slight percentage continues to happen after a decade. The frequency of PJI has diminished barely over the past 15 years, it endures as one of the most disturbing adverse events of TKA, and continuous research to reduce its occurrence is needed. It is essential to be conscious of the risk factors for PJI after primary TKA, as discussed in this article, and to manage them as well as possible before surgery. It is also important for patients undergoing TKA to know to some extent their risk of developing PJI.

Table 4. Main modifiable risk factors of periprosthetic joint infection (PJI) before surgery.

Risk Factor	Control Needed
Hyperglycemia	Control preoperatively
Obesity	Try to control
Hypertension	Control preoperatively
Previous intra-articular injections	Avoid 6 months before
Hypoalbuminemia	Unknown if control decreases risk
Tobacco use	Cessation of smoking at least 1 month before
Previous infection	Wait at least 3 months after infection is resolved
Nutritional status	Unknown if control decreases risk
Preoperative anemia	Correct preoperatively
Steroid therapy	Avoid for 1 month before, if possible

Author Contributions: Both authors participated equally in all tasks: Conceptualization; methodology; writing—original draft preparation; writing—review and editing. All authors have read and agreed to the published version of the manuscript.

Funding: This research received no external funding.

Institutional Review Board Statement: Not applicable.

Informed Consent Statement: Not applicable.

Conflicts of Interest: The authors declare no conflict of interest.

References

1. Carulli, C.; Villano, M.; Bucciarelli, G.; Martini, C.; Innocenti, M. Painful knee arthroplasty: Definition and overview. *Clin. Cases Miner. Bone Metab.* **2011**, *8*, 23–25. [PubMed]
2. Bengtson, S.; Knutson, K. The infected knee arthroplasty. A 6-year follow-up of 357 cases. *Acta Orthop. Scand.* **1991**, *62*, 301–311. [CrossRef] [PubMed]
3. Kapadia, B.H.; Berg, R.A.; Daley, J.A.; Fritz, J.; Bhave, A.; Mont, M.A. Periprosthetic joint infection. *Lancet* **2016**, *387*, 386–394. [CrossRef]
4. Kurtz, S.M.; Lau, E.; Schmier, J.; Ong, K.L.; Zhao, K.; Parvizi, J. Infection Burden for Hip and Knee Arthroplasty in the United States. *J. Arthroplast.* **2008**, *23*, 984–991. [CrossRef] [PubMed]
5. Petrie, R.S.; Hanssen, A.D.; Osmon, D.R.; Ilstrup, D. Metal-backed patellar component failure in total knee arthroplasty: A possible risk for late infection. *Am. J. Orthop.* **1998**, *27*, 172–176. [PubMed]
6. Zmistowski, B.; Restrepo, C.; Hess, J.; Adibi, D.; Cangoz, S.; Parvizi, J. Unplanned readmission after total joint arthroplasty: Rates, reasons, and risk factors. *J. Bone Joint Surg. Am.* **2013**, *95*, 1869–1876. [CrossRef] [PubMed]
7. Parvizi, J.; Zmistowski, B.; Berbari, E.F.; Bauer, T.W.; Springer, B.D.; Della Valle, C.J.; Garvin, K.L.; Mont, M.A.; Wongworawat, M.D.; Zalavras, C.G. New Definition for Periprosthetic Joint Infection: From the Workgroup of the Musculoskeletal Infection Society. *Clin. Orthop. Relat. Res.* **2011**, *469*, 2992–2994. [CrossRef]
8. Parvizi, J.; Tan, T.L.; Goswami, K.; Higuera, C.; Della Valle, C.; Chen, A.F.; Shohat, N. The 2018 Definition of Periprosthetic Hip and Knee Infection: An Evidence-Based and Validated Criteria. *J. Arthroplast.* **2018**, *33*, 1309–1314.e2. [CrossRef]
9. McNally, M.; Sousa, R.; Wouthuyzen-Bakker, M.; Chen, A.F.; Soriano, A.; Vogely, H.C.; Clauss, M.; Higuera, C.A.; Trebše, R. The EBJIS definition of periprosthetic joint infection. *Bone Joint J.* **2021**, *103*, 18–25. [CrossRef]
10. Wingert, N.C.; Gotoff, J.; Parrilla, E.; Gotoff, R.; Hou, L.; Ghanem, E. The ACS NSQIP Risk Calculator Is a Fair Predictor of Acute Periprosthetic Joint Infection. *Clin. Orthop. Relat. Res.* **2016**, *474*, 1643–1648. [CrossRef]
11. McMaster Arthroplasty Collaborative (MAC). Incidence and predictors of prosthetic joint infection following primary total knee arthroplasty: A 15-year population-based cohort study. *J Arthroplast.* **2022**, *37*, 367–372.e1. [CrossRef]

12. Leonard, H.A.C.; Liddle, A.D.; Burke, O.; Murray, D.W.; Pandit, H. Single- or Two-stage Revision for Infected Total Hip Arthroplasty? A Systematic Review of the Literature. *Clin. Orthop. Relat. Res.* **2014**, *472*, 1036–1042. [CrossRef] [PubMed]
13. Urish, K.L.; Bullock, A.G.; Kreger, A.M.; Shah, N.B.; Jeong, K.; Rothenberger, S.D.; the Infected Implant Consortium. A Multicenter Study of Irrigation and Debridement in Total Knee Arthroplasty Periprosthetic Joint Infection: Treatment Failure Is High. *J. Arthroplast.* **2018**, *33*, 1154–1159. [CrossRef] [PubMed]
14. Zhu, M.F.; Kim, K.; Cavadino, A.; Coleman, B.; Munro, J.T.; Young, S.W. Success Rates of Debridement, Antibiotics, and Implant Retention in 230 Infected Total Knee Arthroplasties: Implications for Classification of Periprosthetic Joint Infection. *J. Arthroplast.* **2021**, *36*, 305–310.e1. [CrossRef] [PubMed]
15. Toh, R.X.; Yeo, Z.N.; Liow, M.H.L.; Yeo, S.J.; Lo, N.N.; Chen, J.Y. Debridement, antibiotics, and implant retention in periprosthetic joint infection: What predicts success or failure? *J. Arthroplast.* **2021**, *36*, 3562–3569. [CrossRef]
16. Walkay, S.; Wallace, D.T.; Balasubramaniam, V.S.C.; Maheshwari, R.; Changulani, M.; Sarungi, M. Outcomes of Debridement, Antibiotics and Implant Retention (DAIR) for Periprosthetic Joint Infection in a High-Volume Arthroplasty Centre. *Indian J. Orthop.* **2022**, *56*, 1449–1456. [CrossRef]
17. Ammarullah, M.I.; Santoso, G.; Sugiharto, S.; Supriyono, T.; Kurdi, O.; Tauviqirrahman, M.; Winarni, T.I.; Jamari, J. Tresca stress study of CoCrMo-on-CoCrMo bearings based on body mass index using 2D computational Mmdel. *J. Tribol.* **2022**, *33*, 31–38. Available online: https://jurnaltribologi.mytribos.org/v33/JT-33-31-38.pdf (accessed on 12 October 2022).
18. Shahi, A.; Parvizi, J. Prevention of Periprosthetic Joint Infection. *Arch. Bone Jt. Surg.* **2015**, *3*, 72–81. [CrossRef]
19. Thompson, O.; W-Dahl, A.; Lindgren, V.; Gordon, M.; Robertsson, O.; Stefánsdóttir, A. Similar periprosthetic joint infection rates after and before a national infection control program: A study of 45,438 primary total knee arthroplasties. *Acta Orthop.* **2022**, *93*, 3–10. [CrossRef]
20. Kurtz, S.M.; Ong, K.L.; Lau, E.; Bozic, K.J.; Berry, D.; Parvizi, J. Prosthetic Joint Infection Risk after TKA in the Medicare Population. *Clin. Orthop. Relat. Res.* **2010**, *468*, 52–56. [CrossRef]
21. Ko, M.S.; Choi, C.H.; Yoon, H.K.; Yoo, J.H.; Oh, H.C.; Lee, J.H.; Park, S.H. Risk factors of postoperative complications following total knee arthroplasty in Korea: A nationwide retrospective cohort study. *Medicine* **2021**, *100*, e28052. [CrossRef] [PubMed]
22. Bozic, K.J.; Lau, E.; Kurtz, S.; Ong, K.; Berry, D.J. Patient-related Risk Factors for Postoperative Mortality and Periprosthetic Joint Infection in Medicare Patients Undergoing TKA. *Clin. Orthop. Relat. Res.* **2012**, *470*, 130–137. [CrossRef]
23. Chen, J.; Cui, Y.; Li, X.; Miao, X.; Wen, Z.; Xue, Y.; Tian, J. Risk factors for deep infection after total knee arthroplasty: A meta-analysis. *Arch. Orthop. Trauma. Surg.* **2013**, *133*, 675–687. [CrossRef] [PubMed]
24. Cordtz, R.L.; Zobbe, K.; Højgaard, P.; Kristensen, L.E.; Overgaard, S.; Odgaard, A.; Lindegaard, H.; Dreyer, L. Predictors of revision, prosthetic joint infection and mortality following total hip or total knee arthroplasty in patients with rheumatoid arthritis: A nationwide cohort study using Danish healthcare registers. *Ann. Rheum. Dis.* **2018**, *77*, 281–288. [CrossRef]
25. Pancio, S.I.; Sousa, P.L.; Krych, A.J.; Abdel, M.P.; Levy, B.A.; Dahm, D.L.; Stuart, M.J. Increased Risk of Revision, Reoperation, and Implant Constraint in TKA After Multiligament Knee Surgery. *Clin. Orthop. Relat. Res.* **2017**, *475*, 1618–1626. [CrossRef] [PubMed]
26. Singh, J.A.; Schleck, C.; Harmsen, W.S.; Jacob, A.K.; Warner, D.O.; Lewallen, D.G. Current tobacco use is associated with higher rates of implant revision and deep infection after total hip or knee arthroplasty: A prospective cohort study. *BMC Med.* **2015**, *13*, 283. [CrossRef] [PubMed]
27. Man, S.L.-C.; Chau, W.-W.; Chung, K.-Y.; Ho, K.K.W. Hypoalbuminemia and obesity class II are reliable predictors of periprosthetic joint infection in patient undergoing elective total knee arthroplasty. *Knee Surg. Relat. Res.* **2020**, *32*, 21. [CrossRef]
28. Bedard, N.A.; Pugely, A.J.; Elkins, J.M.; Duchman, K.R.; Westermann, R.W.; Liu, S.S.; Gao, Y.; Callaghan, J.J. Do intraarticular injections increase the risk of infection after TKA? *Clin. Orthop. Relat. Res.* **2017**, *475*, 45–52. [CrossRef]
29. Shohat, N.; Restrepo, C.; Allierezaie, A.; Tarabichi, M.; Goel, R.; Parvizi, J. Increased Postoperative Glucose Variability Is Associated with Adverse Outcomes Following Total Joint Arthroplasty. *J. Bone Jt. Surg.* **2018**, *100*, 1110–1117. [CrossRef]
30. Peersman, G.; Laskin, R.; Davis, J.; Peterson, M.G.E.; Richart, T. Prolonged Operative Time Correlates with Increased Infection Rate After Total Knee Arthroplasty. *HSSJ* **2006**, *2*, 70–72. [CrossRef]
31. Odum, S.M.; Springer, B.D. In-Hospital Complication Rates and Associated Factors After Simultaneous Bilateral Versus Unilateral Total Knee Arthroplasty. *J. Bone Jt. Surg. Am.* **2014**, *96*, 1058–1065. [CrossRef] [PubMed]
32. Stubbs, G.; Pryke, S.E.R.; Tewari, S.; Rogers, J.; Crowe, B.; Bridgfoot, L.; Smith, N. Safety and cost benefits of bilateral total knee replacement in an acute hospital. *ANZ J. Surg.* **2005**, *75*, 739–746. [CrossRef] [PubMed]
33. Memtsoudis, S.G.; Ma, Y.; González Della Valle, A.; Mazumdar, M.; Gaber-Baylis, L.K.; MacKenzie, C.R.; Sculco, T.P. Perioperative outcomes after unilateral and bilateral total knee arthroplasty. *J. Am. Soc. Anesthesiol.* **2009**, *111*, 1206–1216. [CrossRef] [PubMed]
34. Pilling, R.W.; Moulder, E.; Allgar, V.; Messner, J.; Sun, Z.; Mohsen, A. Patellar resurfacing in primary total knee replacement: A meta-analysis. *J. Bone Jt. Surg. Am.* **2012**, *94*, 2270–2278. [CrossRef]
35. Lacko, M.; Jarčuška, P.; Schreierova, D.; Lacková, A.; Gharaibeh, A. Tranexamic acid decreases the risk of revision for acute and delayed periprosthetic joint infection after total knee replacement. *Jt. Dis. Relat. Surg.* **2020**, *31*, 8–13. [CrossRef]
36. Hong, G.J.; Wilson, L.A.; Liu, J.; Memtsoudis, S.G. Tranexamic Acid Administration is Associated with a Decreased Odds of Prosthetic Joint Infection Following Primary Total Hip and Primary Total Knee Arthroplasty: A National Database Analysis. *J. Arthroplast.* **2020**, *36*, 1109–1113. [CrossRef]
37. Hanada, M.; Hotta, K.; Matsuyama, Y. Prognostic nutritional index as a risk factor for aseptic wound complications after total knee arthroplasty. *J. Orthop. Sci.* **2021**, *26*, 827–830. [CrossRef]

38. Shearer, J.; Agius, L.; Burke, N.; Rahardja, R.; Young, S.W. BMI is a Better Predictor of Periprosthetic Joint Infection Risk Than Local Measures of Adipose Tissue After TKA. *J. Arthroplast.* **2020**, *35*, S313–S318. [CrossRef]
39. Gómez-Barrena, E.; Warren, T.; Walker, I.; Jain, N.; Kort, N.; Loubignac, F.; Newman, S.; Perka, C.; Spinarelli, A.; Whitehouse, M.R.; et al. Prevention of Periprosthetic Joint Infection in Total Hip and Knee Replacement: One European Consensus. *J. Clin. Med.* **2022**, *11*, 381. [CrossRef]
40. Hinarejos, P.; Guirro, P.; Leal, J.; Monserrat, F.; Pelfort, X.; Sorli, M.L.; Horcajada, J.P.; Piug, L. The use of erythromycin and colistin-loaded cement in total knee arthroplasty does not reduce the incidence of infection: A prospective randomized study in 3000 knees. *J. Bone Jt. Surg. Am.* **2013**, *95*, 769–774. [CrossRef]
41. Chiu, F.-Y.; Chen, C.-M.; Lin, C.-F.J.; Lo, W.-H. Cefuroxime-impregnated cement in primary total knee arthroplasty: A prospective, randomized study of three hundred and forty knees. *J. Bone Jt. Surg. Am.* **2002**, *84*, 759–762. [CrossRef]
42. Chiu, F.-Y.; Lin, C.-F.J. Antibiotic-Impregnated Cement in Revision Total Knee Arthroplasty. *J. Bone Jt. Surg.* **2009**, *91*, 628–633. [CrossRef] [PubMed]
43. Chiu, F.-Y.; Lin, C.-F.J.; Chen, C.-M.; Lo, W.-H.; Chaung, T.-Y. Cefuroxime-impregnated cement at primary total knee arthroplasty in diabetes mellitus. *J. Bone Jt. Surgery. Br. Vol.* **2001**, *83*, 691–695. [CrossRef]
44. Calkins, T.E.; Culvern, C.; Nam, D.; Gerlinger, T.L.; Levine, B.R.; Sporer, S.M.; Della Valle, C.J. Dilute Betadine Lavage Reduces the Risk of Acute Postoperative Periprosthetic Joint Infection in Aseptic Revision Total Knee and Hip Arthroplasty: A Randomized Controlled Trial. *J. Arthroplast.* **2020**, *35*, 538–543.e1. [CrossRef] [PubMed]
45. Kunutsor, S.; Whitehouse, M.; Blom, A.W.; Beswick, A.; Team, I. Patient-Related Risk Factors for Periprosthetic Joint Infection after Total Joint Arthroplasty: A Systematic Review and Meta-Analysis. *PLoS ONE* **2016**, *11*, e0150866. [CrossRef]
46. Adams, A.L.; Paxton, E.W.; Wang, J.Q.; Johnson, E.S.; Bayliss, E.A.; Ferrara, A.; Nakasato, C.; Bini, S.A.; Namba, R.S. Surgical Outcomes of Total Knee Replacement According to Diabetes Status and Glycemic Control, 2001 to 2009. *J. Bone Jt. Surg.* **2013**, *95*, 481–487. [CrossRef]
47. Nelson, C.L.; Elkassabany, N.M.; Kamath, A.F.; Liu, J. Low Albumin Levels, More Than Morbid Obesity, Are Associated with Complications After TKA. *Clin. Orthop. Relat. Res.* **2015**, *473*, 3163–3172. [CrossRef]
48. Peersman, G.; Laskin, R.; Davis, J.; Peterson, M. Infection in total knee replacement: A retrospective review of 6489 total knee replacements. *Clin. Orthop. Relat. Res.* **2001**, *392*, 15–23. [CrossRef]
49. Bohl, D.D.; Shen, M.R.; Kayupov, E.; Cvetanovich, G.L.; Della Valle, C.J. Is Hypoalbuminemia Associated with Septic Failure and Acute Infection After Revision Total Joint Arthroplasty? A Study of 4517 Patients from the National Surgical Quality Improvement Program. *J. Arthroplast.* **2016**, *31*, 963–967. [CrossRef]
50. Walls, J.D.; Abraham, D.; Nelson, C.L.; Kamath, A.F.; Elkassabany, N.M.; Liu, J. Hypoalbuminemia More Than Morbid Obesity is an Independent Predictor of Complications After Total Hip Arthroplasty. *J. Arthroplast.* **2015**, *30*, 2290–2295. [CrossRef]
51. Rai, J.; Gill, S.S.; Kumar, B.R.J.S. The influence of preoperative nutritional status in wound healing after replacement arthroplasty. *Orthopedics* **2002**, *25*, 417–421. [CrossRef] [PubMed]
52. Buzby, G.P.; Mullen, J.L.; Matthews, D.C.; Hobbs, C.L.; Rosato, E.F. Prognostic nutritional index in gastrointestinal surgery. *Am. J. Surg.* **1980**, *139*, 160–167. [CrossRef]
53. Onodera, T.; Goseki, N.; Kosaki, G. Prognostic nutritional index in gastrointestinal surgery of malnourished cancer patients. *Nihon Geka Gakkai Zasshi* **1984**, *85*, 1001–1005. (In Japanese) [PubMed]
54. Tei, M.; Ikeda, M.; Haraguchi, N.; Takemasa, I.; Mizushima, T.; Ishii, H.; Yamamoto, H.; Sekimoto, M.; Doki, Y.; Mori, M. Risk factors for postoperative delirium in elderly patients with colorectal cancer. *Surg. Endosc.* **2010**, *24*, 2135–2139. [CrossRef] [PubMed]
55. Tokunaga, R.; Sakamoto, Y.; Nakagawa, S.; Miyamoto, Y.; Yoshida, N.; Oki, E.; Watanabe, M.; Baba, H. Prognostic Nutritional Index Predicts Severe Complications, Recurrence, and Poor Prognosis in Patients with Colorectal Cancer Undergoing Primary Tumor Resection. *Dis. Colon Rectum* **2015**, *58*, 1048–1057. [CrossRef]
56. Kirschbaum, S.; Erhart, S.; Perka, C.; Hube, R.; Thiele, K. Failure Analysis in Multiple TKA Revisions—Periprosthetic Infections Remain Surgeons' Nemesis. *J. Clin. Med.* **2022**, *11*, 376. [CrossRef]
57. Muwanis, M.; Barimani, B.; Luo, L.; Wang, C.K.; Dimentberg, R.; Albers, A. Povidone-iodine irrigation reduces infection after total hip and knee arthroplasty. *Arch. Orthop. Trauma. Surg.* **2022**, *online ahead of print*. [CrossRef]
58. Buchalter, D.B.; Nduaguba, A.; Teo, G.M.; Kugelman, D.; Aggarwal, V.K.; Long, W.J. Cefazolin remains the linchpin for preventing acute periprosthetic joint infection following primary total knee arthroplasty. *Bone Jt. Open* **2022**, *3*, 35–41. [CrossRef]
59. Parkulo, T.D.; Likine, E.; Ong, K.L.; Watson, H.; Smith, L.S.; Malkani, A.L. Manipulation Following Primary Total Knee Arthroplasty is Associated with Increased Rates of Infection and Revision. *J. Arthroplast.* **2022**, *online ahead of print*. [CrossRef]
60. Kurtz, S.M.; Mont, M.A.; Chen, A.F.; Della Valle, C.; Sodhi, N.; Lau, E.; Ong, K.L. Intra-Articular Corticosteroid or Hyaluronic Acid Injections Are Not Associated with Periprosthetic Joint Infection Risk following Total Knee Arthroplasty. *J. Knee Surg.* **2022**, *35*, 983–996. [CrossRef]
61. Avila, A.; Acuña, A.J.; Do, M.T.; Samuel, L.T.; Kamath, A.F. Intra-articular injection receipt within 3 months prior to primary total knee arthroplasty is associated with increased periprosthetic joint infection risk. *Knee Surg. Sport. Traumatol. Arthrosc.* **2022**, *online ahead of print*. [CrossRef] [PubMed]
62. Yang, X.; Li, L.; Ren, X.; Nie, L. Do preoperative intra-articular injections of corticosteroids or hyaluronic acid increase the risk of infection after total knee arthroplasty? A meta-analysis. *Bone Jt. Res.* **2022**, *11*, 171–179. [CrossRef] [PubMed]

63. Shin, K.-H.; Han, S.-B.; Song, J.-E. Risk of Periprosthetic Joint Infection in Patients with Total Knee Arthroplasty Undergoing Colonoscopy: A Nationwide Propensity Score Matched Study. *J. Arthroplast.* **2022**, *37*, 49–56. [CrossRef] [PubMed]
64. Rahardja, R.; Morris, A.J.; Hooper, G.J.; Grae, N.; Frampton, C.M.; Young, S.W. Surgical Helmet Systems Are Associated with a Lower Rate of Prosthetic Joint Infection After Total Knee Arthroplasty: Combined Results from the New Zealand Joint Registry and Surgical Site Infection Improvement Programme. *J. Arthroplast.* **2022**, *37*, 930–935.e1. [CrossRef] [PubMed]
65. Blanchard, N.P.; Browne, J.A.; Werner, B.C. The Timing of Preoperative Urinary Tract Infection Influences the Risk of Prosthetic Joint Infection Following Primary Total Hip and Knee Arthroplasty. *J. Arthroplast.* **2022**, *19*, S0883–S5403. [CrossRef]
66. Fisher, N.D.; Bi, A.S.; Singh, V.; Sicat, C.S.; Schwarzkopf, R.; Aggarwal, V.K.; Rozell, J.C. Are patient-reported drug allergies associated with prosthetic joint infections and functional outcomes following total hip and knee arthroplasty? *J. Arthroplast.* **2022**, *37*, 26–30. [CrossRef] [PubMed]

Complications and Implant Survival of Total Knee Arthroplasty in People with Hemophilia

Emerito Carlos Rodriguez-Merchan [1,2,*], Hortensia De la Corte-Rodriguez [3], Teresa Alvarez-Roman [4], Primitivo Gomez-Cardero [1], Carlos A. Encinas-Ullan [1] and Victor Jimenez-Yuste [4]

1. Department of Orthopedic Surgery, La Paz University Hospital-IdiPaz, 28046 Madrid, Spain
2. Osteoarticular Surgery Research, Hospital La Paz Institute for Health Research—IdiPAZ (La Paz University Hospital—Autonomous University of Madrid), 28046 Madrid, Spain
3. Department of Physical and Rehabilitation Medicine, La Paz University Hospital-IdiPaz, 28046 Madrid, Spain
4. Department of Hematology, La Paz University Hospital-IdiPaz, 28046 Madrid, Spain
* Correspondence: ecrmerchan@hotmail.com

Abstract: Total knee arthroplasty (TKA) is a commonly used option in advanced stages of knee arthropathy in people with hemophilia (PWH). The objective of this article is to determine what the complication rates and implant survival rates in PWH are in the literature. A literature search was carried out in PubMed (MEDLINE), Cochrane Library, Web of Science, Embase and Google Scholar utilizing the keywords "hemophilia TKA complications" on 20 October 2022. It was found that the rate of complications after TKA in PWH is high (range 7% to 30%), although it has improved during the last two decades, possibly due to better perioperative hematologic treatment. However, prosthetic survival at 10 years has not changed substantially, being in the last 30 years approximately 80% to 90% taking as endpoint the revision for any reason. Survival at 20 years taking as endpoint the revision for any reason is 60%. It is possible that with a precise perioperative control of hemostasis in PWH, the percentage of complications after TKA can be diminished.

Keywords: hemophilia; knee; total knee arthroplasty; complications; implant survival

1. Introduction

Total knee arthroplasty (TKA) is a surgical intervention that frequently has to be performed in people with hemophilia (PWH) when they suffer from very painful advanced arthropathy whose pain does not subside with conservative treatment (hematologic prophylaxis, analgesics, anti-inflammatory drugs, Physical Medicine and Rehabilitation (PMR), and intra-articular injections of hyaluronic acid or platelet-rich plasma (PRP). In addition, TKA usually works well in PWH in terms of pain and improved quality of life (QoL) [1,2].

It is essential that TKA is always performed with adequate control of hemostasis by the hematologists in charge of the patient, which is accomplished by intravenous administration of clotting factor deficiency factor (F) VIII or FIX at doses deemed necessary by the hematologists and for as long as they deem appropriate [3–6].

According to Escobar et al. planning and carrying out TKA in PWH is most effective with the implication of a specialist and expert multidisciplinary team (MDT) at a hemophilia hospital. Rehabilitation after surgery must start soon, with focus on management of hemostasis and pain. Surgery in PWH and inhibitors needs even more cautious planning [7]. However, despite carrying out this kind of surgery with the support of an MDT, complications after TKA in PWH are frequent. Logically, such complications are even more frequent if TKA is performed in a center not specialized in the treatment of hemophilia [1,2].

In osteoarthritis (OA), the survival rate of 10 years for revision published in 2022 by Ueyama et al. was 98% [8]. In OA, the reported survival of 20 years for revision was 96% [9]. The reported complication rate in OA was 7% [10].

The hypothesis of this article is that PWH have a higher rate of complications and lower implant survival than people without hemophilia. The research questions were the following: Do PWH have more complications when implanted with a TKA than people without hemophilia? Is implant survival different in PWH than in people without hemophilia? The aim of the study is to determine whether PWH have more complications than people without hemophilia when implanted with a TKA and whether prosthetic survival is lower in PWH than in people without hemophilia.

2. Methods

A PubMed (MEDLINE), Cochrane Library, Web of Science, Embase and Google Scholar search of reports on complications after TKA in PWH was conducted. The key words utilized were "hemophilia TKA complications". The main inclusion criteria were reports focused on the complications after TKA in PWH. Studies not focused on such risk factors were disregarded. The searches were dated from the creation of the search engines until 20 October 2022. From the 5138 articles (2870 in the Web of Science, 2030 in Google Scholar, 159 in Embase, 77 in PubMed (MEDLINE), 2 in The Cochrane Library), we chose those that seemed most directly related to the title of this article (53 articles).

Medical subject headings (MeSH) terms were "hemophilia", "TKA" and "complications" and the strig was the following: "hemophilia" OR TKA OR "complications"; "hemophilia" AND (TKA OR "complications"); ("hemophilia" AND TKA) OR "complications". Inclusion and exclusion criteria: The articles that were most directly related to the title of the article were subjectively included; the rest were excluded. Duplicate references were highlighted. To delete duplicate citations we right-clicked on any highlighted reference. Then, we selected "move references to trash". To achieve data extraction we used the three steps of the ETL process (extraction, transformation, and loading).

This article is not a systematic literature review, but a narrative review of the literature of the articles found in the various existing databases that, according to our criteria, were considered to be closely related to the title of the article.

3. Results

3.1. Published Series

In 1989, Figgie et al. analyzed 19 TKAs carried out in PWH. The average follow-up was of 9.5 years [11]. A total of 13 knees had good or excellent outcomes, and 6 knees had poor results. Those subjects with excellent outcomes had sustained good function and pain alleviation. Four of the six poor results were found in the first seven TKAs carried out, when only 80% FVIII coverage was utilized in the perioperative phase. Since the utilization of 100% FVIII coverage began, the rate of poor results diminished. A total of 10 of the 19 knees experienced adverse events: 1 periprosthetic joint infection (PJI), 6 superficial skin necroses, 3 nerve paralyses, 7 postoperative hemorrhages, and 1 transfusion reaction. Six of the seven knees that experienced TKA under 80% factor VIII coverage suffered adverse events. Once 100% FVIII coverage was initiated, the only adverse events were one skin necrosis and three postoperative hemorrhages. The percentage of radiographic failure was high, with progressive radiolucent lines in 13 of 19 tibial components, associated with tibial component displacement in 3 knees. The aforementioned radiographic findings did not correlate with clinical outcomes. However, pain alleviation and ameliorated function were preserved at longer follow-up periods. The best outcomes were attained under 100% FVIII coverage utilizing a posterior stabilized (PS) design and patellar resurfacing [11].

In 1990, Kjaersgaard-Andersen et al. analyzed 13 semiconstrained TKAs carried out in 9 males with hemophilia A with a mean age of 38 years [12]. The average FVIII amount during hospital stay was 84,222 units, and the average hospitalization period was 33 days. Four patients (44%) died during the study period, three from acquired immunodeficiency syndrome (AIDS) and one from sudden cardiac arrest. At the time of TKA, one of the subjects who died from AIDS had a positive test for human immunodeficiency virus (HIV). He died 3 months after surgery. The other two patients acquired AIDS 1 year and 4 years after surgery. The average follow-up period was 43 months. Utilizing the Hospital for Special Surgery (HSS) knee rating scale, the results were excellent in nine knees and good in three knees. All subjects were fully alleviated of pain. TKA in hemophiliacs seemed to be an efficacious treatment for hemophilic arthropathy [12].

In 2003, Legroux-Gérot et al. assessed the outcomes of 17 TKAs (12 patients) and its influence on both QoL and clotting factor utilization [13]. The TKAs were carried out between 1986 and 1996, and the mean follow-up was 54 months. Mean age at the time of TKS was 39 years. QoL was assessed utilizing the Short Form 36 (SF-36). In 94% of the subjects the outcomes were good or excellent. The amelioration was greatest for pain. Recurrent joint hemorrhages in six subjects and development of an inhibitor in two subjects were the only adverse events during the postoperative period. Clotting factor utilization did not diminish substantially after TKA. Legroux-Gérot et al. expressed that TKA for hemophilic arthropathy provided good outcomes that translated into QoL gains [13].

In 2004, Sheth et al. reported the outcomes of 14 TKAs in 9 PWH utilizing posterior cruciate ligament (PCL)-sacrificing designs [14]. The mean follow-up in surviving subjects (13 knees) was 77 months. Pain, functional score, flexion deformity, and flexion range improved significantly. Nine adverse events happened in 6 knees. One subject died from HIV-related adverse events. No subject seroconverted to HIV during the follow-up time [14].

The outcomes of 24 modular Genesis II (Smith & Nephew, Memphis, TN, USA) TKAs, carried out in 20 subjects (mean age, 36 years) with hemophilia, were prospectively reviewed in 2007 by Innocenti et al. [15]. The mean follow-up was 4.4 years. Knee score, the mean knee flexion contracture and the mean total flexion arc ameliorated. The outcomes of this report showed that the use of modular design improved the functional outcomes of TKA in hemophilic arthropathy, which led to a better range of motion (ROM) and lower flexion contracture [15].

In 2008, Chiang et al. assessed the clinical and functional results of TKA and reasons of prosthetic failure in 26 PWH (35 TKAs) [16]. The mean age was 34.2 years and the mean follow-up was 82.2 months. Three subjects required manipulation under anesthesia (MUA) because of an inadequate ROM. Three infections were managed with debridement and one of them experienced knee fusion after removal of prosthesis. Two subjects experienced revision TKA. One of them was due to loosening of the femoral component. The other one experienced revision TKA due to wear of the insert. Chiang et al. stated that TKA seemed to be an effective procedure to accomplish pain alleviation and to improve function in PWH [16].

In 2009, Massin et al. published the outcomes of 128 TKAs from 5 specialized centers. Only knees with preoperative flexion less than 90° were included [17]. Adverse events were 3 skin necroses, 2 infections, 2 femoral fractures, and 1 sciatic nerve paralysis. TKA rendered substantial flexion improvement. It frequently needed tibial tuberosity osteotomy to ameliorate exposure and preclude injury to the extensor mechanism [17].

In 2012, Feng et al. assessed the results of 25 TKAs (19 subjects) [18]. Average patella thickness was 16.3 mm and all patellas were managed by patelloplasty. The subjects were followed for an average postoperative period of 41 months. The preoperative HSS (Hospital for Special Surgery) score was 51 on average. The postoperative HSS score was 91. ROM was modified to 82°, compared with 55° preoperatively. A total of 13 subjects with flexion contracture were corrected from 19° to 2.7°. Four subjects complained of mild but sustainable pain in the anterior part of the knee joint [18].

In 2014, Westberg et al. studied clinical results and adverse events of 107 TKAs in 74 hemophilic subjects with special focus on prosthetic survival and PJI [19]. Mean follow-up was 11.2 years. Percentages of survival at 5 years and 10 years, with component removal for any cause as the end point, were 92% and 88%, respectively. A total of 28 TKAs were removed after 10 years on average. The most common reason of failure was aseptic loosening (14 knees) and PJI (seven knees). The infection rate was 6.5%. A painless knee was found in 93% of the TKAs at the final follow-up. The medium and long-run outcomes of primary TKA showed good prosthetic survival at 5 and 10 years with an excellent alleviation of pain. PJI was still a primary concern compared to patients without hemophilia [19].

In 2015, Strauss et al. assessed the clinical results of 23 TKAs carried out in 21 hemophilic subjects with preoperative ROM of 50° or less [20]. Mean follow-up was 8.3 years. There were one late PJI, and one aseptic implant loosening (8.7% complication rate). Nine subjects who required VY-quadricepsplasty for knee exposure suffered a mean postoperative extensor lag of 7°. Strauss et al. affirmed that although the clinical result was inferior compared to nonstiff knees previously published, TKA can be successfully carried out in PWH [20].

In 2015, Rodriguez-Merchan analyzed 74 PWH treated with TKA (N = 88) over a period of 13 years [21]. The same kind of design was utilized in all cases. A total of 14 subjects had 2-stage bilateral TKAs. The mean subject age was 38.2 years. A total of 14 subjects were positive for HIV and 32 for hepatitis C virus (HCV). The mean follow-up was 8 years. The percentage of prosthetic survival with implant removal for any cause regarded as final endpoint was 92%. Reasons of TKA failure were PJI (6.8%) and aseptic loosening (2.2%). Clinical outcomes of the primary TKAs in this report showed good prosthetic survival and excellent pain alleviation [21].

In 2017, Ernstbrunner et al. provided clinical and radiological long-run outcomes of 43 TKAs implanted in 30 PWH (study with level 4 of evidence) [22]. After a mean of 18 years, 15 subjects (21 knees) with a mean age of 58 years were accessible for follow-up. In 13 (30%) of the 43 knees, revision arthroplasty was required due to PJI or aseptic loosening among which 8 (19%) were due to aseptic loosening and 5 (12%) were due to hematogenous infection. The estimated survival percentages of 20 years, with revision for any cause or infection as the end points, were 59 and 82%, respectively. A total of 86% rated their outcome as either good or excellent. TKA in hemophilic subjects was associated with high revision, loosening and infection percentages after 18 years [22].

In 2017, Szmyd et al. analyzed 40 TKAs in 35 subjects. The mean follow-up was 19.4 months. The mean age of subjects was 36.7 years. The pain intensity was considerably diminished 12 months after the surgery. A significant improvement in patients' functioning was recorded. TKA seemed to be a very good therapy for subjects with advanced hemophilic arthropathy. TKA considerably diminished pain intensity. TKA markedly improved subjects' functioning in daily life. Subjects were very satisfied with the results of TKA [23].

In 2018, Song et al. assessed mid-run results and adverse events of TKA in hemophilic arthropathy [24]. They retrospectively reviewed 131 primary TKAs. The mean age was 41 years, and the mean follow-up was 6.8 years. Adverse events happened in 17 knees (13%): 7 articular hemorrhages, 4 periprosthetic fractures, 3 PJIs, 2 stiffness, and 1 medial collateral ligament injury. The mid-run outcomes of TKA in PWH were satisfactory in pain alleviation, ameliorated function and diminished flexion contracture [24].

A total of 18 TKAs carried out in 15 subjects with hemophilia during a period of 24 years were analyzed in 2019 by Santos Silva et al. Mean follow-up was 11.3 years. The survival percentage of 10 years with TKA removal as end point was 94.3%. Only two subjects needed perioperative transfusion. The rate of postoperative adverse events was 27.8% (two PJIs, two knee stiffness, and one case of recurrent articular hemorrhage) [25].

In 2022, Oyarzun et al. analyzed 41 TKAs (19 cases were bilateral) [26]. Six patients needed revision (6.66%) due to PJI. The percentage of TKA survival at 5 years was 92% (range 82–96%) [26].

In 2020, Bae et al. analyzed a series of 78 TKAs in 56 PWH [27]. The mean age was 38.7 years old and the mean follow up was 10.2 years. Postoperative adverse events happened in 12 knees (15.4%). The percentage of hospital readmission in the 30 days after discharge was 6.4%. Revision TKA was carried out in 3 knees for PJI and in 1 knee for loosening of the tibial component loosening. The prosthesis survival rates at 10 years and 13 years were 97.1% and 93.2%, respectively [27].

In 2022, Kleiboer et al. analyzed 98 TKAs in PWH of which 25% were complicated by major bleeding [28]. The risk of major bleeding was augmented by the presence of an inhibitor, increased body mass index (BMI), and non-use of an antifibrinolytic medication. Neither continuous clotting factor infusion (versus bolus infusion) nor pharmacologic thromboprophylaxis were associated with bleeding risk. Use of antifibrinolytic medications was associated with diminished risk [28].

In 2022, Wang et al. assessed the mid-run results of 32 TKAs (28 patients) for end-stage hemophilic arthropathy [29]. The follow-up was 69.1 months. Significant differences between the preoperative and final follow-up values of flexion contracture, ROM, clinical KSS (Knee Society Score), functional KSS, and VAS (Visual Analog score) were found. The incidence of adverse events was 15.6% and the rate of satisfaction was 100% [29].

In a population-based study published in 2022, Chen et al. analyzed 103 primary TKAs (75 subjects). Unilateral TKA was carried out on 47 subjects and bilateral TKAs on the remaining 28 subjects, including 12 simultaneous and 16 staged surgeries. The mean age of patients was 32.3 years, and the mean follow-up was 77.9 months. Failure occurred in eight subjects (8.5%) at mean 32.8 months after surgery. Four subjects suffered aseptic loosening and four experienced PJI. The prosthesis survivorship of 10 years was 88.6%. For subjects experiencing unilateral TKA, the mean length of stay (LOS) was 14 days. The prosthesis survivorship of 10 years was 88.6%. [30].

Table 1 summarizes the main series reported on TKA in PWH. Figure 1 shows the rate of complications reported between 1989 and 2022. Figure 2 depicts the rates of postoperative bleeding after TKA in PWH. Figure 3 shows the rates of PJI after TKA in PWH. Figure 4 depicts the survival rates of TKA in PWH.

Table 1. Series of total knee arthroplasty (TKA) in people with hemophilia (PWH) published in the literature.

Authors [Reference]	Year	Number of TKAs/Patients	Average Age (Years)	Average Follow-Up	Complications	TKA Survival Rate
Figgie et al. [11]	1989	19/NA	NA	9.5 years	RATE OF COMPLICATIONS: 52,6% (10/19: 1 PJI, 6 superficial skin necroses, 3 nerve palsies, 7 postoperative bleedings, 1 transfusion reaction).	NA
Kjaersgaard-Andersen et al. [12]	1990	13/19	38	3.6 years	NA	NA
Legroux-Gérot et al. [13]	2003	17/12	39	4.5 years	RATE OF COMPLICATIONS: 47% (recurrent hemarthrosis in 6 patients and development of an anticoagulant in 2 patients).	NA
Sheth et al. [14]	2004	14/9	NA	6.4 years	RATE OF COMPLICATIONS: 64.3% (9/14).	NA
Innocenti et al. [15]	2007	24/20	36	4.4 years	NA	NA
Chiang et al. [16]	2008	35/26	34.2	6.8 years	RATE OF COMPLICATIONS: 7% (3 patients underwent MUA because of an inadequate ROM; 3 PJIs).	NA

Table 1. Cont.

Authors [Reference]	Year	Number of TKAs/Patients	Average Age (Years)	Average Follow-Up	Complications	TKA Survival Rate
Massin et al. [17]	2009	128/NA	NA	NA	RATE OF COMPLICATIONS: 7% (3 skin necroses, 2 PJIs, 2 femoral fractures, 1 rupture of patellar tendon, 1 sciatic nerve palsy).	NA
Feng et al. [18]	2012	25/19	NA	3.4 years	RATE OF COMPLICATIONS: 16% (4 patients complained mild but endurable anterior knee pain).	NA
Westberg et al. [19]	2014	107/74	NA	11.2 years	RATE OF COMPLICATIONS: 6.5% (PJI in 7 knees).	FIVE-YEAR: 92%. TEN-YEAR: 88%. With component removal for any reason as the end point.
Strauss et al. [20]	2015	23/21	NA	8.3 years	RATE OF COMPLICATIONS: 8.7% (1 late PJI, and 1 aseptic implant loosening; 9 patients who required VY-quadricepsplasty for knee exposure developed a mean postoperative extensor lag of 7°).	NA
Rodriguez-Merchan [21]	2015	88/74	38.2	8 years	RATE OF COMPLICATIONS: 10% (PJI 6.8%; aseptic loosening 2.2%).	92% (with implant removal for any reason regarded as final endpoint).
Ernstbrunner et al. [22]	2017	43/30	58	18 years	RATE OF COMPLICATIONS: 12% (5 hematogenous PJIs).	20-YEAR: 59% (with revision for any reason as the endpoint). 20-YEAR: 82% (with infection as the endpoint).
Szmyd et al. [23]	2017	40/35	36.7	1.6 years	NA	NA
Song et al. [24]	2018	131/NA	41	6.8 years	RATE OF COMPLICATIONS: 13% (7 hemarthroses, 1 medial collateral ligament injury, 2 stiffness, 3 PJIs, 4 periprosthetic fractures).	NA
Santos Silva et al. [25]	2019	18/15	NA	11.3 years	RATE OF COMPLICATIONS: 27.8% (2 PJIs, 2 prosthesis stiffness, 1 recurrent hemarthrosis).	10-YEAR: 94.3% (with prosthesis removal as end point).
Oyarzun et al. [26]	2020	41/22	NA	NS	RATE OF COMPLICATIONS: 6.6% (6 PJIs).	5-YEAR: 92%
Bae et al. [27]	2020	78/56	38.7	10.2 years	RATE OF COMPLICATIONS: 15.4%.	10-YEAR: 97.1%. 13-YEAR: 93.2%.
Kleiboer et al. [28]	2022	98/NA	NA	NA	RATE OF COMPLICATIONS: 25% (major bleeding).	NA

Table 1. Cont.

Authors [Reference]	Year	Number of TKAs/Patients	Average Age (Years)	Average Follow-Up	Complications	TKA Survival Rate
Wang et al. [29]	2022	32/28	NA	5.1 years	RATE OF COMPLICATIONS: 15.6%.	NA
Chen et al. [30]	2022	103/75	32.3	6.5 years	RATE OF COMPLICATIONS: 3.9% (PJI).	10-YEAR: 88.6%.

NA = Not available; PJI = Periprosthetic joint infection; MUA = Mobilization under anesthesia; ROM = Range of motion.

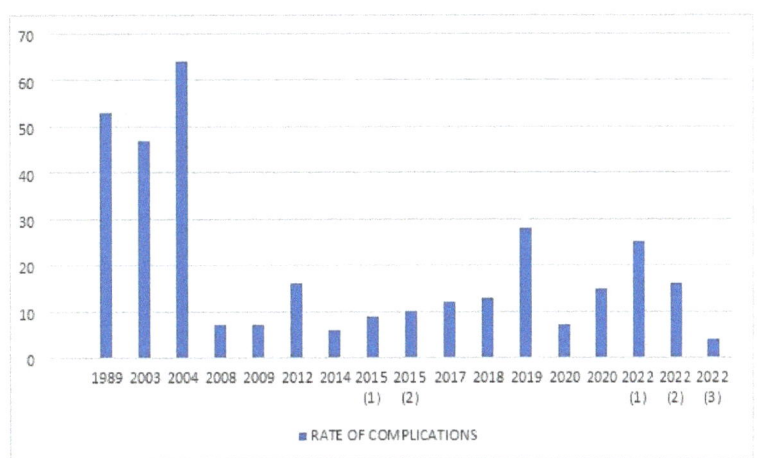

Figure 1. Rates of complications of total knee arthroplasty (TKA) in people with hemophilia (PWH) from 1989 to 2022. In 2015 there were two articles ((1) and (2)), while in 2022 there were three articles ((1)–(3)).

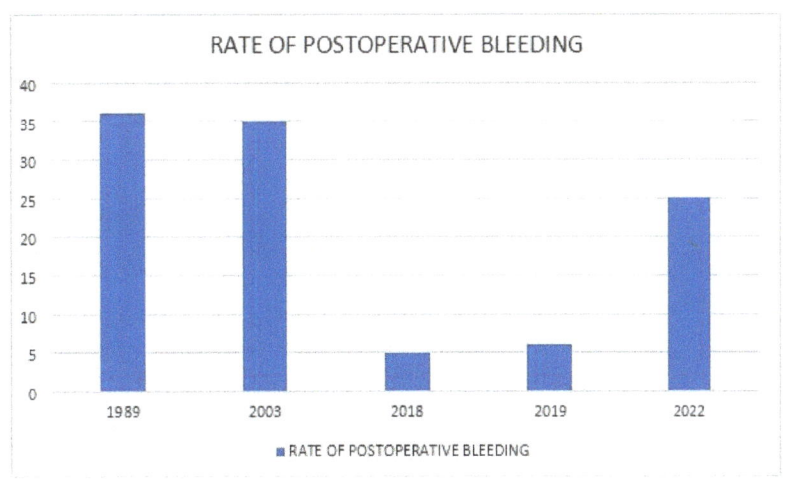

Figure 2. Rates of postoperative bleeding after total knee arthroplasty (TKA) in people with hemophilia (PWH) from 1989 to 2022.

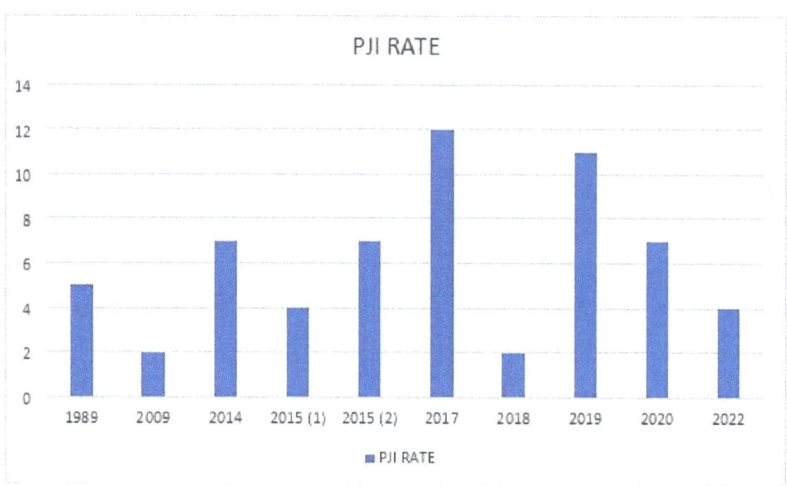

Figure 3. Rates of periprosthetic joint infection (PJI) after total knee arthroplasty (TKA) in people with hemophilia (PWH) from 1989 to 2022. In 2015 there were two articles [(1) and (2)].

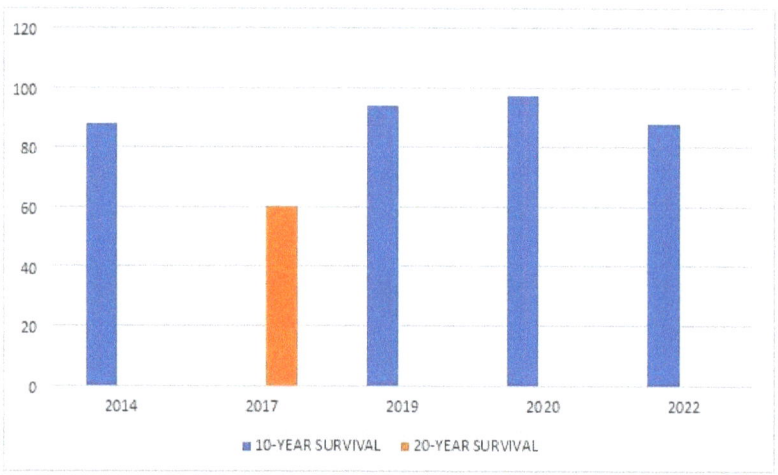

Figure 4. 10-year-, 13-year- and 20-year-rates of implant survival of total knee arthroplasty (TKA) in people with hemophilia (PWH) from 2014 to 2022.

3.2. Venous Thromboembolism (VTE)

In 2019, Peng et al. reported a 1.5% prevalence of clinically significant VTE in PWH experiencing TKA without chemoprophylaxis and a modified coagulation factor substitution [31]. They affirmed that given the low incidence of clinically significant VTE in their study, routine chemoprophylaxis in PWH experiencing TKA might not be required [31].

3.3. Arterial Pseudoaneurysms

An arterial pseudoaneurysm must be suspected when after the surgical procedure there is severe bleeding that does not cease with adequate management with intravenous injection of the deficient coagulation factor [32,33]. The diagnosis and treatment of a pseudoaneurysm have to be done quickly to prevent complications. The diagnosis must be confirmed by duplex ultrasonography (US), standard angiogram, computed tomography

(CT) angiogram or magnetic resonance angiography. There are several options for the treatment of pseudoaneurysms. Small pseudoaneurysms can be solved with conservative noninterventional treatment. It includes outside pressing, US probe pressing or US-guided thrombin injections. In bigger pseudoaneurysms, endovascular techniques, such as coil embolization, are now favored. If the aforementioned techniques are futile, standard surgical treatment with simple ligation or arterial reconstruction have to be performed [32,33].

3.4. Case Reports

3.4.1. Intraoperative Popliteal Artery Injury

In 2017, Feng et al. reported the case of a 48-year-old male subject with severe hemophilia A and stiff knees that experienced bilateral TKAs [34]. Left popliteal artery injury was detected at the end of the left TKA. Urgent angiography confirmed the diagnosis of the left popliteal artery transection. With clotting FVIII replacement treatment, open repair was carried out by end-to-end vascular bypass with the autograft of the large saphenous vein. Left lower limb was reperfused 4 h after the beginning of the ischemia. The subject recovered uneventfully. Postoperative Doppler examination demonstrated the left popliteal artery remained patent [34].

3.4.2. Brucella Infection

In 2017, Mortazavi et al. reported a 28-year-old man with *Brucella* infection of TKA, who at first experienced conservative management but then required a two-stage revision TKA [35].

3.4.3. Postoperative Flexion Contracture

In 2021, Liawrungrueang et al. reported the successful treatment of flexion contracture after primary TKA in a 20-year-old-man with hemophilia A by open soft tissue contracture releasing and serial casting [36]. Table 2 summarizes the complications of TKA in PWH.

Table 2. Complications of total knee arthroplasty (TKA) in people with hemophilia (PWH).

Complications
Postoperative bleeding
Early hematoma
Arterial pseudoaneurysm
Periprosthetic joint infection (PJI)
Superficial skin necrosis
Inadequate range of motion (ROM): postoperative extensor lag, stiffness, postoperative flexion contracture
Periprosthetic fracture
Nerve palsy
Popliteal artery injury
Rupture of the patellar tendon
Medial collateral ligament (MCL) injury
Heterotopic ossification
Deep vein thrombosis (DVT)
Pulmonary embolism
Transfusion reaction
Acquired immunodeficiency syndrome (AIDS)
Development of an inhibitor
Mild but endurable anterior knee pain
Aseptic loosening

3.5. Is Drain after TKA Necessary?

In a prospective study, Haghpanah et al. compared the outcomes of drain protocol (42 TKAs in 39 subjects, mean age 35.5 years) with no-drain-protocol (38 TKAs in 27 subjects, mean age 35.7 years) [37]. Patients were followed for at least 1 year. There was no statistical difference between the two groups in terms of knee scores, blood loss, postoperative pain, fever, time to regain the ROM and infection. Two subjects in the drain group and one subject in the no drain group were reoperated due to PJI. No subjects required blood transfusion in each group [37]. In a prospective randomized clinical trial, 176 subjects with hemophilia who experienced TKA were analyzed by Mortazavi et al. [38]. The study group consisted of 88 subjects (108 knees) in which we did not insert suction drain and the control group included 88 subjects (106 knees) in which drain was inserted at the end of the surgery. No differences in the mean VAS value between both groups were observed. Mortazavi et al. concluded that there was no basis for the utilization of drain after primary TKA in PWH [38].

3.6. Special Scenarios

3.6.1. Computer-Navigated TKA

In 2013, Cho et al. assessed the outcomes of 27 computer-navigated TKAs in 25 patients with hemophilic arthropathy [39]. The clinical results were substantially ameliorated after the surgery. There were no adverse events specific to the computer-navigated TKA [39].

3.6.2. Robot-Assisted TKA

In 2016, Kim et al. assessed 32 robot-assisted TKAs in 29 hemophilia subjects [40]. The mean follow-up period was 5 years. Adverse events included early hematoma in three knees, heterotopic ossification in three knees, and PJI in two knees [40].

3.6.3. TKA in Patients with Inhibitors

In 2021 Carulli et al. assessed the results of 18 hemophilic patients with inhibitors (26 TKAs) [41]. Subjects were divided in two groups: group A (primary total TKA): 13 subjects underwent 19 TKAs; and B (revision): 5 subjects underwent 3 revision TKAs. All subjects received the same hematological prophylaxis (recombinant factor VII activated-rFVIIa). The median follow-up was 12.2 years for group A, 8.6 years for group B. Few adverse events were found; the survival rate was 94.7% at 15 years. All patients reported satisfaction, pain alleviation and ameliorated functional ability. The use of continuous infusion of rFVIIa showed an appropriate hemostatic effect and low percentage of complications. Revision TKAs were more susceptible to complications compared to primary TKA [41].

3.6.4. Simultaneous Bilateral TKA

A study showed that bilateral TKA was a safe and cost-effective procedure for hemophilic arthropathy with similar medium-run outcomes compared to unilateral TKA [42].

3.6.5. Medicare Beneficiaries with a Diagnosis of Hemophilia

A study found that adverse medical events were more common among PWH: postoperative bleeding, deep vein thrombosis (DVT), pulmonary embolism and blood transfusions. PWH showed higher odds of PJI (1.78 versus 0.98%). Reimbursements of 90 days were higher for subjects with hemophilia (mean: $22,249 versus $13,017) [43].

3.6.6. TKA for a Stiff Knee of PWH

In a study, 67 primary TKAs for PWH (mean age, 48 years) were carried out, and incisional approaches to joint were standard (58 cases) and V-Y quadricepsplasty (V-Y) (9 cases). Preoperative ROM and flexion were significantly associated with V-Y. Ono et al. affirmed that primary TKA for PWH utilizing a standard approach might be carried out before the phase preoperative flexion < 45° and ROM < 35° [44].

3.7. Comparative Studies

3.7.1. Continuous Infusion versus Bolus Injection

In 2017 Park et al. assessed the efficacy of continuous infusion (CI) of coagulation factor concentrates during the perioperative period compared to bolus infusion (BI) [45]. A total of 42 TKAs were carried out in 31 subjects with severe hemophilia A. Although good control of hemostasis was accomplished utilizing either method during the perioperative period of TKA, CI appeared to be more tolerable and effective than BI to provide perioperative blood management in PWH experiencing TKA [45].

3.7.2. Hemophilia versus Non-Hemophilia

In 2011 Sikkema et al. compared the outcomes of TKA in subjects with and without hemophilia retrospectively [46]. The adverse events and long-run outcomes of 21 TKAs carried out in 22 hemophilia subjects were compared with those of 42 TKAs in subjects without hemophilia. Subjects were matched for gender, year of surgery and age. Hemarthrosis happened in 52% of the TKAs carried out in the hemophilia subjects, while hemarthrosis occurred in 7% of the TKAs of the control group. In the hemophilia group, the rate of PJI was 7%, while it was 13% in the control group. Subjective function was good in 76% of TKAs in hemophilia subjects versus 71% in TKAs in controls [46].

In 2019 Wang et al. assessed the risk of complications of PWH who experienced TKA utilizing information from the National Health Insurance Research Database [47]. PWH had longer LOS and greater total hospital expenses compared to people without hemophilia. There were no differences between the rates of adverse events of 30 days and 90 days, a PJI of 1 year, reoperation and mortality between PWH and people without hemophilia [47].

3.7.3. Hemophilia versus Osteoarthritis and Rheumatoid Arthritis

In 2020 Li et al. analyzed the adverse events of 2083 TKA in 1515 PWH compared with osteoarthritis (OA) and rheumatoid arthritis (RA) [10]. The overall rate of adverse events in the hemophilic arthropathy group was 21.79%, which was much greater than the OA or RA group (7.08% and 8.70%, respectively). The main adverse events were loosening of the implant and wound dehiscence. For PWH, more adverse events happened in the period more than 1 year after TKA, when compared with OA (33.33% vs. 11.43%). Among the potential risk factors, subjects with hemophilia B and severe hemophilia had substantially greater percentages of adverse events [10].

3.8. Meta-Analysis

In 2016 Moore et al. published a meta-analysis of 20 studies (336 TKAs in 254 PWH). The mean follow-up was 6.3 years. Statistically significant ROM improvements were encountered. Knee scores showed statistically significant improvements. A 31.5% rate of adverse events was found [48].

4. Discussion

TKA is contemplated as the management of choice for end stage arthropathy in PWH. Compared to other subjects experiencing TKA, PWH have specific characteristics, such as a bleeding trend, younger age, preoperative limited ROM, altered anatomy, and increased adverse events [1]. The use of a multimodal blood loss prevention approach that includes intra-articular tranexamic acid (TXA) (MBLPM-TXA) in PWH who experience TKA is effective in reducing the percentages of transfusion [49].

Perioperative treatment with expert orthopedic and hematological counsel is advised to optimize results in PWH [50]. TKA (both primary and revision) should be carried out in hospitals specialized in orthopedic surgery, physical and rehabilitation medicine, and hematology [2].

A coagulation factor level <93.5% or hematocrit level of <38.2% might be a substantial risk factor for increasing perioperative blood loss [51]. Adequate intra- and postoperative care to avert postoperative residual contracture is needed in PWH [52]. In the last 30 years, there has been a decrease in the rate of TKA, probably indicating the impact of extensive utilization of tertiary hematological prophylaxis [53].

It seems logical to think that inadequate hemostasis at the time of surgery will not only cause the patient to bleed more in the postoperative period but will also increase the risk of prosthetic infection (since blood is an excellent breeding ground for bacteria). Such infection can appear more or less early, often leading to septic loosening of the implant. In fact, it is well known that the average infection rate after TKA in PWH is 7% (compared to 1–2% in people without hemophilia). This would suggest that the percentage of prostheses still in situ in the long term is probably lower in PWH than in persons without hemophilia, since an average of 7 out of 100 prostheses in PWH can loosen due to infection versus 1–2 out of 100 in persons without hemophilia. In other words, although there is no irrefutable evidence that inadequate hemostasis during surgery is the cause of late loosening of the implant, in our opinion it seems a logical assumption that will undoubtedly have to be confirmed in the future with clinical evidence.

The main limitations of this article are that although the major databases (PubMed, Cochrane Library, Embase, Web of Science, and Google Scholar) have been used, it is not a systematic review of the literature but a narrative review of the literature. Furthermore, the selection of articles was carried out subjectively, considering only those closely related to the title of the article. Therefore, it is possible that some important articles on the topic were not included.

5. Conclusions

The rate of adverse events after TKA in PWH remains high (range 7% to 30%), although it has improved during the last two decades, possibly due to better perioperative hematologic treatment. However, prosthetic survival at 10 years has not changed substantially, being in the last 30 years approximately 80% to 90% taking as an endpoint the revision for any reason. Survival at 20 years taking as an endpoint the revision for any reason is 60%. It is possible that with an exquisite perioperative control of hemostasis in PWH, the percentage of complications after TKA can be reduced.

Author Contributions: All authors participated equally in all tasks: Conceptualization; methodology; writing—original draft preparation; writing—review and editing. All authors have read and agreed to the published version of the manuscript.

Funding: This research received no external funding.

Conflicts of Interest: The authors declare no conflict of interest.

References

1. Mortazavi, S.J.; Bagheri, N.; Farhoud, A.; Hadi Kalantar, S.; Ghadimi, E. Total knee arthroplasty in patients with hemophilia: What do we know? *Arch. Bone Jt. Surg.* **2020**, *8*, 470–478. [CrossRef]
2. Rodriguez-Merchan, E.C.; De la Corte-Rodriguez, H.; Alvarez-Roman, T.; Gomez-Cardero, P.; Encinas-Ullan, C.A.; Jimenez-Yuste, V. Total knee arthroplasty in hemophilia: Lessons learned and projections of what's next for hemophilic knee joint health. *Expert Rev. Hematol.* **2022**, *15*, 65–82. [CrossRef]
3. Jimenez-Yuste, V.; Rodriguez-Merchan, E.C.; Matsushita, T.; Holme, P.A. Concomitant use of bypassing agents with emicizumab for people with haemophilia A and inhibitors undergoing surgery. *Haemophilia* **2021**, *27*, 519–530. [CrossRef] [PubMed]
4. Hermans, C.; Apte, S.; Santagostino, E. Invasive procedures in patients with haemophilia: Review of low-dose protocols and experience with extended half-life FVIII and FIX concentrates and non-replacement therapies. *Haemophilia* **2021**, *27* (Suppl. 3), 46–52. [CrossRef] [PubMed]
5. Valentino, L.A.; Cooper, D.L.; Goldstein, B. Surgical Experience with rFVIIa (NovoSeven) in congenital haemophilia A and B patients with inhibitors to factors VIII or IX. *Haemophilia* **2011**, *17*, 579–589. [CrossRef] [PubMed]
6. Escobar, M.; Maahs, J.; Hellman, E.; Donkin, J.; Forsyth, A.; Hroma, N.; Young, G.; Valentino, L.A.; Tachdjian, R.; Cooper, D.L.; et al. Multidisciplinary management of patients with haemophilia with inhibitors undergoing surgery in the United States: Perspectives and best practices derived from experienced treatment centres. *Haemophilia* **2012**, *18*, 971–981. [CrossRef]
7. Escobar, M.A.; Brewer, A.; Caviglia, H.; Forsyth, A.; Jimenez-Yuste, V.; Laudenbach, L.; Lobet, S.; McLaughlin, P.; Oyesiku, J.O.O.; Rodriguez-Merchan, E.C.; et al. Recommendations on multidisciplinary management of elective surgery in people with haemophilia. *Haemophilia* **2018**, *24*, 693–702. [CrossRef] [PubMed]

8. Ueyama, H.; Kanemoto, N.; Minoda, Y.; Yamamoto, N.; Taniguchi, Y.; Nakamura, H. No difference in postoperative knee flexion and patient joint awareness between cruciate-substituting and cruciate-retaining medial pivot total knee prostheses: A 10-year follow-pp study. *J. Arthroplast.* **2022**, *37*, 279–285. [CrossRef] [PubMed]
9. Kim, Y.H.; Park, J.W.; Jang, Y.S. 20-year minimum outcomes and survival rate of high-flexion versus standard total knee arthroplasty. *J. Arthroplast.* **2021**, *36*, 560–565. [CrossRef] [PubMed]
10. Li, Z.; Feng, B.; Du, Y.; Wang, Y.; Bian, Y.; Weng, X. Complications of total knee arthroplasty in patients with haemophilia compared with osteoarthritis and rheumatoid arthritis: A 20-year single-surgeon cohort. *Haemophilia* **2020**, *26*, 861–866. [CrossRef] [PubMed]
11. Figgie, M.P.; Goldberg, V.M.; Figgie, H.E., 3rd; Heiple, K.G.; Sobel, M. Total knee arthroplasty for the treatment of chronic hemophilic arthropathy. *Clin. Orthop. Relat. Res.* **1989**, *248*, 98–107.
12. Kjærsgaard-Andersen, P.; Christiansen, S.E.; Ingerslev, J.; Sneppen, O. Total knee arthroplasty in classic hemophilia. *Clin. Orthop. Relat. Res.* **1990**, *256*, 137–146. [CrossRef]
13. Legroux-Gérot, I.; Strouk, G.; Parquet, A.; Goodemand, J.; Gougeon, F.; Duquesnoy, B. Total knee arthroplasty in hemophilic arthropathy. *Jt. Bone Spine* **2003**, *70*, 22–32. [CrossRef]
14. Sheth, D.S.; Oldfield, D.; Ambrose, C.; Clyburn, T. Total knee arthroplasty in hemophilic arthropathy. *J. Arthroplast.* **2004**, *19*, 56–60. [CrossRef]
15. Innocenti, M.; Civinini, R.; Carulli, C.; Villano, M.; Linari, S.; Morfini, M. A modular total knee arthroplasty in haemophilic arthropathy. *Knee* **2007**, *14*, 264–268. [CrossRef]
16. Chiang, C.C.; Chen, P.Q.; Shen, M.C.; Tsai, W. Total knee arthroplasty for severe haemophilic arthropathy: Long-term experience in Taiwan. *Haemophilia* **2008**, *14*, 828–834. [CrossRef]
17. Massin, P.; Lautridou, C.; Cappelli, M.; Petit, A.; Odri, G.; Ducellier, F.; Sabatier, C.; Hulet, C.; Canciani, J.; Letenneur, J.; et al. Total knee arthroplasty with limitations of flexion. *Orthop. Traumatol. Surg. Res.* **2009**, *95* (Suppl. 1), S1–S6. [CrossRef]
18. Feng, B.; Weng, X.S.; Lin, J.; Qian, W.W.; Wei, W.; Sheng, L.; Zhai, J.-L.; Bian, Y.-Y.; Qiu, G.-X. Outcome of total knee arthroplasty combined patelloplasty for end-stage type A hemophilic arthropathy. *Knee* **2012**, *19*, 107–111. [CrossRef]
19. Westberg, M.; Paus, A.C.; Holme, P.A.; Tjønnfjord, G.E. Haemophilic arthropathy: Long-term outcomes in 107 primary total knee arthroplasties. *Knee* **2014**, *21*, 147–150. [CrossRef]
20. Strauss, A.C.; Schmolders, J.; Friedrich, M.J.; Pflugmacher, R.; Müller, M.; Goldmann, G.; Oldenburg, J.; Pennekamp, P.H. Outcome after total knee arthroplasty in haemophilic patients with stiff knees. *Haemophilia* **2015**, *21*, e300–e305. [CrossRef]
21. Rodriguez-Merchan, E.C. Total knee arthroplasty in hemophilic arthropathy. *Am. J. Orthop.* **2015**, *44*, E503–E507. [PubMed]
22. Ernstbrunner, L.; Hingsammer, A.; Catanzaro, S.; Sutter, R.; Brand, B.; Wieser, K.; Fucentese, S.F. Long-term results of total knee arthroplasty in haemophilic patients: An 18-year follow-up. *Knee Surg. Sports Traumatol. Arthrosc.* **2017**, *25*, 3431–3438. [CrossRef] [PubMed]
23. Szmyd, J.; Jaworski, J.M.; Kaminski, P. Outcomes of total knee arthroplasty in patients with bleeding disorders. *Ortop. Traumatol. Rehabil.* **2017**, *19*, 361–371. [CrossRef] [PubMed]
24. Song, S.J.; Bae, J.K.; Park, C.H.; Yoo, M.C.; Bae, D.K.; Kim, K.I. Mid-term outcomes and complications of total knee arthroplasty in haemophilic arthropathy: A review of consecutive 131 knees between 2006 and 2015 in a single institute. *Haemophilia* **2018**, *24*, 299–306. [CrossRef]
25. Santos Silva, M.; Rodrigues-Pinto, R.; Rodrigues, C.; Morais, S.; Costa e Castro, J. Long-term results of total knee arthroplasty in hemophilic arthropathy. *J. Orthop. Surg.* **2019**, *27*, 2309499019834337. [CrossRef]
26. Oyarzun, A.; Barrientos, C.; Barahona, M.; Martinez, A.; Soto-Arellano, V.; Courtin, C.; Cruz-Montecinos, C. Knee haemophilic arthropathy care in Chile: Midterm outcomes and complications after total knee arthroplasty. *Haemophilia* **2020**, *26*, e179–e186. [CrossRef]
27. Bae, J.K.; Kim, K.I.; Lee, S.H.; Yoo, M.C. Mid-to long-term survival of total knee arthroplasty in hemophilic arthropathy. *J. Clin. Med.* **2020**, *9*, 3247. [CrossRef]
28. Kleiboer, B.; Layer, M.A.; Cafuir, L.A.; Cuker, A.; Escobar, M.; Eyster, M.E.; Kraut, E.; Leavitt, A.D.; Lentz, S.R.; Quon, D.; et al. Postoperative bleeding complications in patients with hemophilia undergoing major orthopedic surgery: A prospective multicenter observational study. *J. Thromb. Haemost.* **2022**, *20*, 857–865. [CrossRef]
29. Wang, R.; Wang, Z.; Gu, Y.; Zhang, J.; Wang, P.; Tong, P.; Lv, S. Total knee arthroplasty in patients with haemophilic arthropathy is effective and safe according to the outcomes at a mid-term follow-up. *J. Orthop. Traumatol.* **2022**, *23*, 31. [CrossRef]
30. Chen, C.F.; Yu, Y.B.; Tsai, S.W.; Chiu, J.W.; Hsiao, L.T.; Gau, J.P.; Hsu, H.C. Total knee replacement for patients with severe hemophilic arthropathy in Taiwan: A nationwide population-based retrospective study. *J. Chin. Med. Assoc.* **2022**, *85*, 228–232. [CrossRef]
31. Peng, H.-M.; Wang, L.-C.; Zhai, J.-L.; Jiang, C.; Weng, X.-S.; Feng, B.; Gao, N. Incidence of symptomatic venous thromboembolism in patients with hemophilia undergoing hip and knee joint replacement without chemoprophylaxis: A retrospective study. *Orthop. Surg.* **2019**, *11*, 236–240. [CrossRef] [PubMed]
32. Rodriguez-Merchan, E.C.; Jimenez-Yuste, V.; Gomez-Cardero, P.; Rodriguez, T. Severe postoperative haemarthrosis following a total knee replacement in a haemophiliac patient caused by a pseudoaneurysm: Early treatment with arterial embolization. *Haemophilia* **2014**, *20*, e86–e89. [CrossRef] [PubMed]

33. Rodriguez-Merchan, E.C. Enormous articular hemorrhage following arthroscopy, total joint replacement and other surgical operations in hemophilic patients due to arterial pseudoaneurysms: Diagnosis and treatment. *Arch. Bone Jt. Surg.* 2021, *9*, 475–479. [CrossRef] [PubMed]
34. Feng, B.; Xiao, K.; Shao, J.; Fan, Y.; Weng, X. Open repair of intraoperative popliteal artery injury during total knee arthroplasty in a patient with severe hemophilia A: A case report and literature review. *Medicine* 2017, *96*, e8791. [CrossRef] [PubMed]
35. Mortazavi, S.M.J.; Sobhan, M.R.; Mazoochy, H. Brucella arthritis following total knee arthroplasty in a patient with hemophilia: A case report. *Arch. Bone Jt. Surg.* 2017, *5*, 342–346. [CrossRef] [PubMed]
36. Liawrungrueang, W.; Tangtrakulwanich, B.; Yuenyongviwat, V. Soft tissue releasing and serial casting for management of flexion contracture after primary total knee arthroplasty in a patient with hemophilia. *Int. J. Surg. Case Rep.* 2021, *83*, 105995. [CrossRef]
37. Haghpanah, B.; Mortazavi, S.M.J.; Kaseb, M.H.; Ebrahiminasab, S.M. Drain after total knee arthroplasty in patients with hemophilia: A necessary practice? *Haemophilia* 2016, *22*, 88.
38. Mortazavi, S.M.J.; Firoozabadi, M.A.; Najafi, A.; Mansouri, P. Evaluation of outcomes of suction drainage in patients with haemophilic arthropathy undergoing total knee arthroplasty. *Haemophilia* 2017, *23*, e310–e315. [CrossRef]
39. Cho, K.Y.; Kim, K.I.; Khurana, S.; Cho, S.W.; Kang, D.G. Computer-navigated total knee arthroplasty in haemophilic arthropathy. *Haemophilia* 2013, *19*, 259–266. [CrossRef]
40. Kim, K.I.; Kim, D.K.; Juh, H.S.; Khurana, S.; Rhyu, K.H. Robot-assisted total knee arthroplasty in haemophilic arthropathy. *Haemophilia* 2016, *22*, 446–452. [CrossRef]
41. Carulli, C.; Innocenti, M.; Linari, S.; Morfini, M.; Castaman, G.; Innocenti, M. Joint replacement for the management of haemophilic arthropathy in patients with inhibitors: A long-term experience at a single Haemophilia centre. *Haemophilia* 2021, *27*, e93–e101. [CrossRef] [PubMed]
42. Jiang, C.; Zhao, Y.; Feng, B.; Zhai, J.; Bian, Y.; Qiu, G.; Weng, X. Simultaneous bilateral total knee arthroplasty in patients with end-stage hemophilic arthropathy: A mean follow-up of 6 years. *Sci. Rep.* 2018, *8*, 1608. [CrossRef] [PubMed]
43. Rosas, S.; Buller, L.T.; Plate, J.; Higuera, C.; Barsoum, W.K.; Emory, C. Total knee arthroplasty among Medicare beneficiaries with hemophilia A and B is associated with increased complications and higher costs. *J. Knee Surg.* 2021, *34*, 372–377. [CrossRef] [PubMed]
44. Ono, K.; Hirose, J.; Noguchi, M.; Asano, K.; Yasuda, M.; Takedani, H. Extension contracture stiff knee in hemophilia: Surgical timing and procedure for total knee arthroplasty. *Mod. Rheumatol.* 2022, roac067. [CrossRef] [PubMed]
45. Park, Y.S.; Shin, W.J.; Kim, K.I. Comparison of continuous infusion versus bolus injection of factor concentrates for blood management after total knee arthroplasty in patients with hemophilia. *BMC Musculoskelet. Disord.* 2017, *18*, 356. [CrossRef] [PubMed]
46. Sikkema, T.; Boerboom, A.L.; Meijer, K. A comparison between the complications and long-term outcome of hip and knee replacement therapy in patients with and without haemophilia; a controlled retrospective cohort study. *Haemophilia* 2011, *17*, 300–303. [CrossRef] [PubMed]
47. Wang, S.H.; Chung, C.H.; Chen, Y.C.; Cooper, A.M.; Chien, W.C.; Pan, R.Y. Does hemophilia increase risk of adverse outcomes following total hip and knee arthroplasty? A propensity score–matched analysis of a nationwide, population-based study. *J. Arthroplast.* 2019, *34*, 2329–2336.e1. [CrossRef]
48. Moore, M.F.; Tobase, P.; Allen, D.D. Meta-analysis: Outcomes of total knee arthroplasty in the haemophilia population. *Haemophilia* 2016, *22*, e275–e285. [CrossRef]
49. Rodriguez-Merchan, E.C.; Encinas-Ullan, C.A.; Gomez-Cardero, P. Intra-articular tranexamic acid in primary total knee arthroplasty decreases the rate of post-operative blood transfusions in people with hemophilia: A retrospective case-control study. *HSS J. Musculoskelet. J. Hosp. Spéc. Surg.* 2020, *16*, 218–221. [CrossRef]
50. Mohan, K.; Broderick, J.M.; Raftery, N.; McAuley, N.F.; McCarthy, T.; Hogan, N. Perioperative haematological outcomes following total knee arthroplasty in haemophiliacs. *J. Orthop. Surg.* 2021, *29*, 23094990211033999. [CrossRef]
51. Kim, M.S.; Kim, J.H.; Kim, K.I. Risk factors for increased perioperative blood loss during total knee arthroplasty in patients with haemophilia. *Haemophilia* 2022, *28*, 491–496. [CrossRef] [PubMed]
52. Lee, H.W.; Park, C.H.; Bae, D.K.; Song, S.J. How much preoperative flexion contracture is a predictor for residual flexion contracture after total knee arthroplasty in hemophilic arthropathy and rheumatoid arthritis? *Knee Surg. Relat. Res.* 2022, *34*, 20. [CrossRef] [PubMed]
53. Lin, C.Y.; Hosseini, F.; Squire, S.; Jackson, S.; Sun, H.L. Trends of outcomes and healthcare utilization following orthopaedic procedures in adults with haemophilia: A 3-decade retrospective review. *Haemophilia* 2022, *28*, 151–157. [CrossRef] [PubMed]

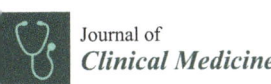

Review

New Horizons of Cementless Total Knee Arthroplasty

Giuseppe Polizzotti [1,*], Alfredo Lamberti [2], Fabio Mancino [3,4] and Andrea Baldini [2,*]

1. Istituto Chirurgico Ortopedico Traumatologico (ICOT), Sapienza University of Rome, 00185 Rome, Italy
2. Istituto Fiorentino di Cura e Assistenza, 50139 Florence, Italy
3. University College London Hospital, London NW1 2BU, UK
4. The Princess Grace Hospital, London W1U 5NY, UK
* Correspondence: giuseppepolizzotti2@gmail.com (G.P.); drbaldiniandrea@yahoo.it (A.B.)

Abstract: Background: Considering the increasing number of young and active patients needing TKA, orthopedic surgeons are looking for a long-lasting and physiological bond for the prosthetic implant. Multiple advantages have been associated with cementless fixation including higher preservation of the native bone stock, avoidance of cement debris with subsequent potential third-body wear, and the achievement of a natural bond and osseointegration between the implant and the bone that will provide a durable and stable fixation. Discussion: Innovations in technology and design have helped modern cementless TKA implants to improve dramatically. Better coefficient of friction and reduced Young's modulus mismatch between the implant and host bone have been related to the use of porous metal surfaces. Moreover, biologically active coatings have been used on modern implants such as periapatite and hydroxyapatite. These factors have increased the potential for ingrowth by reducing micromotion and increasing osteoconductive properties. New materials with better biocompatibility, porosity, and roughness have been introduced to increase implant stability. Conclusions: Innovations in technology and design have helped modern cementless TKA implants improve primary stability in both the femur and tibia. This means that short-term follow-up are comparable to cemented. These positive prognostic factors may lead to a future in which cementless fixation may be considered the gold-standard technique in young and active patients.

Keywords: cementless; total knee arthroplasty; survivorship; biomaterials

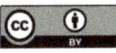

1. Introduction

Total Knee Arthroplasty (TKA) has been widely recognized as the gold standard treatment for end-stage knee osteoarthritis [1]. This procedure is performed in more than 600,000 patients per year in the United States (US) and the number is projected to remarkably grow by 2030 [2].

The current literature is debatable regarding the efficacy and results of cementless TKA when compared to conventional cemented TKA. It has been often stated that press-fit fixation performs similarly or worse than cemented fixation depending on the selection criteria of patients [3,4]. Moreover, despite several cohort studies detecting comparable outcomes between the two types of fixations, higher costs have limited the widespread diffusion of cementless implants, leaving the conventional technique as the widely recognized gold standard [5,6].

One of the greatest concerns regarding cementless fixation was the increased risk of tibial component early aseptic loosening [7–10]. However, the development of new implant designs and materials has turned cementless fixation into an interesting and reliable option, especially in younger patients with good bone quality [11]. In addition, radiostereometric analysis (RSA) showed promising results that will be thoroughly analyzed in the following sections [12,13].

Despite the excellent reported outcomes of conventional cemented fixation, young and active patients have been frequently associated with a higher risk for implant revision, refs. [14–16] leading to a growing interest in a more durable fixation method.

1.1. Mechanical Characteristics of Cementless TKA

Considering the increasing number of young and active patients needing TKA [17], orthopedic surgeons are looking for a long-lasting and physiological bond for the prosthetic implant.

Multiple advantages have been associated with cementless fixation including higher preservation of the native bone stock, avoidance of cement debris with subsequent potential third-body wear, and the achievement of a natural bond and osseointegration between the implant and the bone that will provide a durable and stable fixation. This fixation is based on the migration of osteoblasts and mesenchymal cells towards the implant and the osseointegration through the roughened surface of the implant [18,19]. It has been reported that the minimum requirement for pore size is considered to be approximately 100 µm due to cell size, migration requirements, and transport. However, pore sizes >300 µm are recommended, due to enhanced new bone formation and the formation of capillaries. Moreover, considering that it has been shown that adequate primary stability is a prerequisite for a successful long-term fixation of uncemented implants [20], a rough surface has a double effect: firstly, on primary stability by increasing the shear-load bearing capacity at the bone-implant interface in the direct post-operative period [21,22], and secondly, on secondary fixation providing a mechanical interlock between bone and implant [22]. However, careful attention must be taken when using a highly rough surface because of potential complications related to the surgical procedure such as required higher insertion forces that may lead to periprosthetic fracture [23] and malseating of the implant [24,25]. Indeed, primary fixation remains crucial in both influencing long-term fixation [26] and in achieving osseointegration by limiting the amount of micromotions [27,28].

1.2. First Generation of Cementless TKA

First, the generation of cementless TKA has been associated with numerous design flaws that led to early failure. When evaluating the prosthetic components, the femoral component reached better outcomes than the tibial and patellar counterparts. Femoral component failures were mainly associated with fatigue fractures of the thin areas [29]. Moreover, other pitfalls included the use of sintered beads or mesh coating, non-continuous fixation surfaces, short pegs, poor polyethylene locking mechanisms, and sterilization methods, and the use of metal-backed patellar components that showed poor survivorship [9].

1.3. New Materials

Innovations in technology and design have helped modern cementless TKA implants improve dramatically. The better coefficient of friction and reduced Young's modulus mismatch between the implant and host bone have been related to the use of porous metal surfaces. Moreover, biologically active coatings have been used on modern implants such as periapatite and hydroxyapatite. These factors have increased the potential for ingrowth by reducing micromotion and increasing osteoconductive properties. New materials with better biocompatibility, porosity, and roughness have been introduced to increase implant stability.

1.3.1. Hydroxyapatite

Hydroxyapatite (HA) represented a promising material with the potential to achieve biological fixation of implants. HA coating, in comparison to press fit fixation or porous coating, is an osteoconductive calcium phosphate molecule that can encourage the biological growth of the bone even in the presence of gaps or partially unstable conditions [30]. Moreover, similar micromotions at one to two years have been reported between HA-augmented and cemented implants [31]. In addition, several clinical studies have shown reliable fixation of HA-coated implants in TKA [32,33]. Nelissen et al. [33] compared HA-coated cementless implants with non-coated and cemented TKA reporting better performance in terms of micromotion in the HA and cemented groups in the longitudinal, transverse, and sagittal axes. Similarly, Cross et al. [32], reported on 1000 HA-coated cementless TKA with a cumulative survivorship at ten years of 99% (95% confidence interval [CI] 92.5 to 99.8), supporting the reliability of HA in cementless TKA. Finally, Voigt et al. [34], after evaluating 14 randomized controlled trials (RCT), stated that in patients < 70 years of age, an HA-coated tibial implant may provide better durability than other forms of tibial fixation.

1.3.2. Trabecular Metal

More recently, Trabecular Metal™ (Zimmer Inc., Warsaw, IN, USA) (Figure 1), a newer biomaterial made of tantalum, has been introduced as being similar in porosity to cancellous bone. It has been extensively associated with excellent mechanical and biological properties, including predictable ingrowth and osseointegration, primary stability, and maintenance of bone mineral density (BMD). However, clinical results at the mid-to-long-term follow-up with tibial monoblock components have been controversial [35–38]. In a recent meta-analysis by Hu et al. [11] on six studies involving 977 patients, the authors stated that the use of cementless porous tantalum monoblock tibial component achieved no substantial superiority over conventional cemented modular tibia at the 5-year follow-up. However, excellent mid-term outcomes have been reported by Niemeläinen et al. [39] on 1143 primary cementless TKAs based on the Finnish Arthroplasty Registry at a mean of 7 years follow-up. The authors reported a survivorship of 100% (95% CI 99–100) at 1, 5, and 7 years postoperatively using revision for aseptic loosening of the tibial component as an endpoint in a population-based setting.

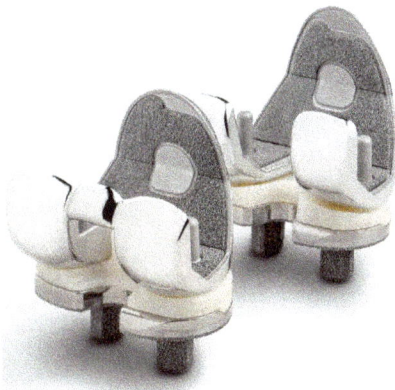

Figure 1. Persona Posterior Stabilized and Medially Congruent cementless with tantalum coating (Zimmer Biomet Inc., Warsaw, IN, USA).

To the best of the author's knowledge, only a few RCTs have been performed at different follow-ups. Dunbar et al. [40] compared the outcomes of porous monoblock and cemented tibial components in 70 randomized patients at a 24-month follow-up. A subset of the TM components migrated extensively in the postoperative period, but all stabilized by one year with 0.0 implants (95% confidence interval, 0.0 to 0.12) considered to be at risk for early aseptic loosening, whilst four cemented components were considered to be at risk (proportion at risk, 0.19; 95% confidence interval, 0.08 to 0.4). The same cohort of patients was then re-evaluated at a 5-year follow-up [12], reporting similar tibial motions between the 2 groups ($p = 0.9$) and a similar proportion of implants "at risk" (2 of 18 in the cemented group and 0 of 27 in the TM group; $p = 0.2$), suggesting that the TM implants provide solid fixation at mid-term follow-up despite high levels of initial migration. Moreover, Fernandez-Fairen et al. [41], randomized 145 patients into two groups receiving either a TM cementless tibial component or a cemented conventional one reporting similar outcomes at a 5-year follow-up in terms of clinical scores, complication rate, and survivorship from aseptic loosening. Similarly, Pulido et al. [42] randomized 397 patients and evaluated the outcomes at a 5-year follow-up reporting that no highly porous metal tibial components were revised for aseptic loosening and that they provided similar durable fixation and reliable pain relief and restoration of function when compared with a traditional cemented modular tibia in TKA. Finally, Hampton et al. [43] randomized 90 patients into receiving either cementless TKA with TM monoblock tibial component or hybrid fixation TKA at an up-to-15-year follow-up and reported better clinical outcomes ($p = 0.001$) and better radiological analysis compared with the cemented group ($p < 0.001$) despite both groups having excellent survivorship at the final follow-up.

Recently, modular trabecular metal tibial components have become available for clinical use. Fricka et al. [44] randomized 100 patients to receive either the cementless or cemented version (50 patients each) and evaluated survivorship and clinical outcomes at a 2-year follow-up. Despite comparable results, one implant in the cementless group was revised due to implant-related failure; moreover, four other implants experienced a mean 3° varus subsidence and further stabilized with clear signs of osseointegration, while 15% of the cementless implants (7 out of 47) reported some radiolucencies (RLL). The authors assumed that the higher rate of RLL with respect to the non-modular design was probably related to the stiffer titanium baseplate and inflexibility as compared to the flexibility of the metaphyseal bone, suggesting further evaluation to determine their long-term stability.

1.3.3. BIOFOAM

BIOFOAM (Microport Orthopedics, Inc., Arlington, TN, USA) is a cancellous titanium foam that can be manufactured to reach a porosity of up to 80% to increase mechanical properties. Cancellous titanium is a porous reticulated titanium material developed for load-bearing orthopedic implants with a compressive modulus similar to bone and it shows improved material properties with increased porosity and friction coefficient which enhances early stability and osseointegration [45]. Promising short-term outcomes have been reported by Waddell et al. [46] in a retrospective cohort of patients with no cases of implant-related failures and no progressive radiolucencies at 24-month follow-up. Further analysis has been described by Karachalios et al. [45], who retrospectively evaluated two groups of 54 patients treated with cemented and titanium cancellous-foam cementless implants and reported comparable results at a 9-year follow-up, with no cases of implant-related failures in the cementless group and satisfactory radiological outcomes.

1.3.4. Tritanium

A novel modular cementless tibial component (Triathlon® Tritanium®, Stryker Orthopedics, Mahwah, NJ, USA) has been introduced. It is made up of a highly porous titanium coating applied by 3-dimensional printing to create a biological fixation surface with a triangular keel and 4 cruciform 9-mm-long pegs coated solely at the base of each peg. This device has been compared in a cadaveric study with a two-peg TM monoblock baseplate reporting reduced rocking motions and liftoff, supporting higher potentials for biological fixation [47]. Clinical results on the same prosthetic implant have been retrospectively reported by Miller et al. [6] on 400 patients with a revision rate due to aseptic loosening of 0.5% at a minimum 2-year follow-up (comparable to the cemented control group) with areas of increased bone density at the pegs of the tibial baseplate. In addition, the same Tritanium implant has been tested in a consecutive series of 406 primary cementless TKA in obese patients and matched 1:1 with a group of the same cemented implant, reporting a high 7-year survivorship free from aseptic revision (99.0% vs. 99.5%, $p = 0.665$) [48]. Nam et al. [29], prospectively randomized 147 patients (67 cemented and 80 cementless) and evaluated the outcomes at a mean 2-year follow-up. The authors reported comparable early outcomes in terms of clinical scores and survivorship with no signs of progressive radiolucencies or component subsidence in either group.

1.4. Implant Migration and RSA Analysis

Radiostereometric analysis (RSA) represents a valid method to evaluate implant fixation to bone and early migration, especially within the first two postoperative years, providing a prediction to long-term outcomes. Cementless fixation has shown a pattern of high initial migration called "settling", followed by stabilization after approximately one year, compared with lower initial migration for cemented components [49]. However, cemented fixation can be affected by late degenerative processes to the cement mantle such as delamination that can compromise implant fixation [5]. Moreover, Pijls et al. [49] reported a clinically relevant association between early migration, as measured with RSA, and long-term clinical failure resulting in revision for aseptic loosening, stating that each mm of migration was associated with an increase in the 5-year revision rate of 8%.

Laende et al. [50] compared the long-term migration of 79 patients with cemented (58 TKA) and cementless (21 TKA) tibial components at a mean of 12 years postoperatively. The authors reported a significant correlation between one-year and long-term migration, especially for cementless components. In addition, the long-term migration was comparable but the inducible displacement (single-leg stance weight bearing) at 10 years was significantly higher for the cemented components (0.2 [range, 0.2–0.4] vs. 0.1 [range, 0.1–0.2]; $p < 0.001$), suggesting at least equivalent, if not superior, long-term fixation of the press-fit technique. Similar findings were detected by Henricson et al. [51] in their RSA analysis at 10 years postoperatively between 26 TM tibial monoblock implants and 21 cemented counterparts. The authors reported that TM implants continued to be firmly fixed to bone at the final follow-up, with stabilization from 3 months onwards after the early initial migration, suggesting that the pattern of migration represents a more reliable factor for analysis of the implant fixation than the magnitude of fixation itself. Therefore, stabilization after the initial settling should be considered as a positive sign for long-lasting fixation, conversely to continuous migration which represents an unfavorable sign. The magnitude of migration at 1 year postoperatively should not be considered as an indicator of potential future loosening of cementless implants. Similarly, Hasan et al. [52] evaluated the RSA analysis of the novel 3D-printed highly porous Tritanium implants, randomizing 72 patients to receive either a cementless (35 patients) or cemented (34 patients) TKA. One 71-year-old female had to be revised for migration of the tibial component 20 months postoperatively in the cementless group, however, despite a higher migration in the first three months, all the press-fit implants resulted well stabilized at a two-year evaluation. Conversely, three cemented implants were initially stable but showed continuous migration between one and two years of follow-up. In addition, the authors reported that the novel 3D-printed cementless TKA showed promising results as the initial migration seemed to be lower than other cementless designs, probably due to the additional four pegs of the baseplate design.

1.5. Implant Loosening in Obese and Young Patients

The increasing interest in cementless TKA is additionally related to the higher failure rate of cemented implants in particular subcategories of patients such as young, obese, and active. The mechanisms of failure in obese patients are believed to be related with increased sheer forces and stress at the bone–cement interface, leading to micromotion and aseptic loosening or osteolysis [53]. Whiteside and Viganò [54], reported on a first cementless generation implant comparing the outcomes at a mean of 7 years follow-up of 122 young and heavy patients (<55 years, >90 kg) with 122 older and lighter ones (>65 years, <80 kg), showing no cases of implant loosening and no difference of implant survivorship, suggesting that press-fit fixation is safe in young, overweight patients. In addition, Bagsby et al. [53] retrospectively compared the outcomes in 292 morbidly obese patients (BMI > 40), 154 cemented TKA and 245 cementless. When evaluating aseptic revisions, the authors reported a statistically significant higher incidence of aseptic loosening in the cemented cohort (5.8%) compared with the cementless cohort (9 vs. 0 TKAs, p 1/4 0.005) at a mean follow-up of 6.1 years in the former and 3.6 in the latter. Therefore, the authors suggested that cementless fixation may provide biologic bony ingrowth and a subsequent more durable implant–bone interface, which may better tolerate the added mechanical stress generated in this population. Similarly, Sinicrope et al. [55] retrospectively compared 108 cementless TKA with 85 cemented, all in morbidly obese patients (BMI > 40). The authors noted survivorship with aseptic loosening as the endpoint of 99.1% (1 failure) in the former and 88.2% (16 failures) in the latter at a 8-year follow-up ($p = 0.02$), suggesting that cementless fixation may represent a promising alternative to mechanical cement fixation in this category of patients.

Regarding the outcomes in young patients (<55 years), Kim et al. [56] compared, in a prospective high-quality RCT, cemented and cementless implants in bilateral, sequential, and simultaneous TKAs in 80 patients at a mean follow-up of 16.6 years using a first generation cementless device. The authors noted comparable results in terms of clinical outcomes and implant survivorship with one (1.3%) reported case of early mechanical failure (within the first year) in the cementless group. However, the difference was not significant, suggesting a reliable survivorship in young patients in the long-term for both investigated implants. Furthermore, the same group of authors [57] reported a mean follow-up of 23.8 years of 261 patients (522 knees) which randomly underwent simultaneous bilateral TKA with cementless and cemented implants and reported comparable outcomes with 97% and 98% survivorship, respectively. The prevalence of aseptic loosening and osteolysis were similar in both groups, suggesting no substantial differences between the two fixation techniques.

1.6. Best Biology for Secondary Fixation

It has been reported that thermal injury to bone is time and temperature dependent, with temperatures below 44° not being associated with osseous injury but with temperatures between 47° and 50° that are maintained for more than 60 s being associated with bone reabsorption and osteonecrosis, increasing the risk of early migration and subsequent failure [49]. A cadaveric study by Vertullo et al. [58] showed that the modern tibial cementing technique has been associated with temperatures below the safety cutoff, despite the narrow thermal safety margin for osseous injury of 4.95° (95% CI ± 4.31) and that cement penetration depth did not correlate with the maximum cement temperature. Moreover, besides the thermal damage potentially generated by cement polymerization, thermal osteonecrosis could be induced by the heat generated by cutting tools such as a saw or burr. Tawy et al. [59] reported in a cadaveric study that mean bone temperatures above 47° were maintained for more than 60 s in non-irrigated bone as well as in bone burred with room temperature irrigation, while uncooled irrigation was effective in reducing the mean temperature of sawed bone to <47° ($p < 0.05$) and the usage of cooled irrigation would prevent the bone from reaching temperatures beyond 47°, either in burred or sawed. Therefore, the authors suggested that irrigation with saline solution at room temperature is effective in reducing the likelihood of thermal osteonecrosis in sawed bone.

1.7. Our Surgical Technique Tips

We start with tibia resection, using a 1.27 mm saw blade and we irrigate it with saline water at room temperature, while also trying not to spend so much time on the resection in order to not warm up the bone. In our opinion, reducing the time for cutting, blade thickness, irrigation with saline water, and bone pre-cooling are very good tips to not overheat the bone. Minimizing heat shock is important because thermal necrosis at 60° can cause an immediate cellular depletion and a slow cell recovery [60]. After the resection, the tibia plane should be symmetric and flat. Distal femur resection is performed with the same irrigation and sawing technique. Once again, the flatness of the surface is primary to avoid no contact areas with the implant. After appropriate femoral sizing, different from the original technique, we start from chamfer resections and AP are made later on. We believe the "chamfer first" technique is crucial to avoid imperfect femur resection, which can be the reason why the implant does not seat very well into the bone.

AP resections are parallel cuts and they are less sensitive to small micro-movements of the jig. After that, we complete the posterior condylar resection, changing the saw with a thinner one for the posterolateral bone resection in order to save the popliteus ligament.

The next step is the research of the optimal fit of the baseplate in tibial sizing, close to the cortical ream. After tibial sizing, we complete the tibia by reverse drilling where the bone is softer and normal drilling where the bone is harder. At the end, the impaction of the tibia baseplate should be symmetric: medial and lateral, anterior, and posterior. During the femur implantation, the surgeon must raise the hand while pushing the femoral component. The aim is to achieve no space area around the corner of the femoral component prosthesis, even if less than 2 mm of gap is accepted. Knee stability is tested throughout a complete ROM. At last, we use the intraoperative "pull-out lift-off" (POLO) test to check the appropriate tension of PCL.

1.8. Short Term Follow Up of a Novel 3D Printed Cementless TKA

Among the 370 primary total knee replacements performed in the period 2021 to 2022 at our institution, 127 received GKS prosthesis and they were included in a perspective study, 60 patients received a 3D-printed cementless TKA (Figure 2). All the patients were evaluated at 3, 6, and 12 months by recording the VAS score, the Oxford Knee Score, the Knee Society Score, and the Forgotten Knee Score. No significant differences between the two groups were reported. The mean time to reach a VAS score < 3 was 6 months in 70% of the patients. The mean FJS was 67 at 3 months, 76 at 6 months, and 79 at 12 months post-operatively.

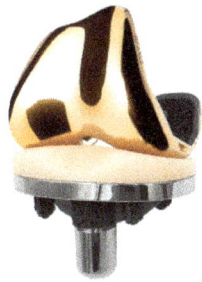

Figure 2. GKS Prime Flex Traser (Permedica, Merate, Italy).

1.9. Cost Analysis

Cementless implants are surely more expensive than their cemented counterparts, potentially creating an obstacle to their diffusion in a cost-sensitive health system. Moreover, considering that prosthetic implants account for the single largest expense in the 90-day episode of care for TKA, making up about 25% of the total cost, the use of higher-cost implants may be limited or restricted [61]. However, Laurie et al. [62] compared 80 cementless and 67 cemented single-design TKA and showed that although the general cost of cemented TKA implants is lower than the cementless, the actual cost of the procedure is less for the press-fit technique when considering the costs of operating theatre time, cement, and cementing accessories. Indeed, despite the increased charge of USD 366 between the two implants, the authors reported longer operative time for cemented TKA (11.6 min at USD 35 per minute; $p = 0.001$) with cement and accessories costs ranging from USD 170 to USD 625 reaching an additional cost related to the cementation of USD 588 to USD 1043. Similar findings were reported by Yayac et al. [63] among 2426 TKA, with higher cementless implant costs (USD 3047.80 vs. USD 2808.73, $p < 0.0001$) but lower supply costs (USD 639.49 vs. USD 815.57, $p < 0.0001$) and lower operating room personnel costs (USD 982.01 vs. USD 1238.26, $p < 0.0001$) outlined that, at their institution, cementless TKA did not significantly increase total procedural costs when compared to traditional cemented TKA. Conversely, Gwam et al. [64] reported on a National Inpatient Sample (NIS) analysis of 167,930 TKAs that cementless TKA (4870) was associated with higher inpatient hospital costs (USD 17,357 vs. USD 16,888) and charges (USD 67,366 vs. USD 64,190; $p < 0.001$), despite its association with a lower mean length of stay (2.63 vs. 2.71 days; $p < 0.001$), and higher odds of being discharged to home (OR = 1.99; $p = 0.002$).

2. Conclusions

There are large amounts of proof that innovations in technology and design have helped modern cementless TKA implants improve primary stability in both the femur and tibia. This means that short-term and mid-term revision rates are comparable to cemented implants [65]. All of these positive prognostic factors may lead orthopedic surgeons into a future where cementless fixation may be considered the gold-standard technique in TKA in young and active patients.

Author Contributions: G.P. wrote and structured the paper; A.L. analyzed literature data and helped to write the paper; F.M. reviewed the literature; A.B. conceived the study, coordinated and helped to draft the manuscript. All authors have read and agreed to the published version of the manuscript.

Funding: The authors received no financial support for the authorship and publication of this article.

Institutional Review Board Statement: Not applicable.

Data Availability Statement: Data supporting this study are openly available on PubMed.

Conflicts of Interest: G.P. and F.M. declare that they have no conflict of interest. A.L. is consultant for Zimmer Biomet. A.B. is consultant for Zimmer Biomet and Permedica.

References

1. Bourne, M.H.; Miller, T.L.; Mariani, E.M. Cumulative Incidence of Revision for a Balanced Knee System at a Mean 8-Year Follow-Up: A Retrospective Review of 500 Consecutive Total Knee Arthroplasties. *Adv. Orthop.* **2019**, *2019*, 9580586. [CrossRef]
2. Kurtz, S.; Ong, K.; Lau, E.; Mowat, F.; Halpern, M. Projections of primary and revision hip and knee arthroplasty in the United States from 2005 to 2030. *J. Bone Jt. Surg Am.* **2007**, *89*, 780–785. [CrossRef]
3. Franceschetti, E.; Torre, G.; Palumbo, A.; Papalia, R.; Karlsson, J.; Ayeni, O.R.; Samuelsson, K.; Franceschi, F. No difference between cemented and cementless total knee arthroplasty in young patients: A review of the evidence. *Knee Surg. Sports Traumatol. Arthrosc.* **2017**, *25*, 1749–1756. [CrossRef]
4. Gandhi, R.; Tsvetkov, D.; Davey, J.R.; Mahomed, N.N. Survival and clinical function of cemented and uncemented prostheses in total knee replacement: A meta-analysis. *J. Bone Jt. Surg. Br.* **2009**, *91*, 889–895. [CrossRef]
5. Dalury, D.F. Cementless total knee arthroplasty: Current concepts review. *Bone Jt. J.* **2016**, *98*, 867–873. [CrossRef]
6. Miller, A.J.; Stimac, J.D.; Smith, L.S.; Feher, A.W.; Yakkanti, M.R.; Malkani, A.L. Results of Cemented vs Cementless Primary Total Knee Arthroplasty Using the Same Implant Design. *J. Arthroplast.* **2018**, *33*, 1089–1093. [CrossRef]
7. Bassett, R.W. Results of 1000 Performance knees: Cementless versus cemented fixation. *J. Arthroplast.* **1998**, *13*, 409–413. [CrossRef]
8. Duffy, G.P.; Berry, D.J.; Rand, J.A. Cement versus cementless fixation in total knee arthroplasty. *Clin. Orthop. Relat. Res.* **1998**, *356*, 66–72. [CrossRef]
9. Berger, R.A.; Lyon, J.H.; Jacobs, J.J.; Barden, R.M.; Berkson, E.M.; Sheinkop, M.B.; Rosenberg, A.G.; Galante, J.O. Problems with cementless total knee arthroplasty at 11 years followup. *Clin. Orthop. Relat. Res.* **2001**, *392*, 196–207. [CrossRef]
10. Carlson, B.J.; Gerry, A.S.; Hassebrock, J.D.; Christopher, Z.K.; Spangehl, M.J.; Bingham, J.S. Clinical outcomes and survivorship of cementless triathlon total knee arthroplasties: A systematic review. *Arthroplasty* **2022**, *4*, 25. [CrossRef]
11. Hu, B.; Chen, Y.; Zhu, H.; Wu, H.; Yan, S. Cementless Porous Tantalum Monoblock Tibia vs Cemented Modular Tibia in Primary Total Knee Arthroplasty: A Meta-Analysis. *J. Arthroplast.* **2017**, *32*, 666–674. [CrossRef] [PubMed]
12. Wilson, D.A.; Richardson, G.; Hennigar, A.W.; Dunbar, M.J. Continued stabilization of trabecular metal tibial monoblock total knee arthroplasty components at 5 years-measured with radiostereometric analysis. *Acta Orthop.* **2012**, *83*, 36–40. [CrossRef] [PubMed]

13. Henricson, A.; Wojtowicz, R.; Nilsson, K.G.; Crnalic, S. Uncemented or cemented femoral components work equally well in total knee arthroplasty. *Knee Surg. Sports Traumatol. Arthrosc.* **2019**, *27*, 1251–1258. [CrossRef] [PubMed]
14. Niemeläinen, M.J.; Mäkelä, K.T.; Robertsson, O.; W-Dahl, A.; Furnes, O.; Fenstad, A.M.; Pedersen, A.B.; Schrøder, H.M.; Reito, A.; Eskelinen, A. The effect of fixation type on the survivorship of contemporary total knee arthroplasty in patients younger than 65 years of age: A register-based study of 115,177 knees in the Nordic Arthroplasty Register Association (NARA) 2000–2016. *Acta Orthop.* **2020**, *91*, 184–190. [CrossRef] [PubMed]
15. Julin, J.; Jämsen, E.; Puolakka, T.; Konttinen, Y.T.; Moilanen, T. Younger age increases the risk of early prosthesis failure following primary total knee replacement for osteoarthritis. A follow-up study of 32,019 total knee replacements in the Finnish Arthroplasty Register. *Acta Orthop.* **2010**, *81*, 413–419. [CrossRef]
16. Meehan, J.P.; Danielsen, B.; Kim, S.H.; Jamali, A.A.; White, R.H. Younger age is associated with a higher risk of early periprosthetic joint infection and aseptic mechanical failure after total knee arthroplasty. *J. Bone Jt. Surg. Am.* **2014**, *96*, 529–535. [CrossRef]
17. Kurtz, S.M.; Ong, K.L.; Schmier, J.; Zhao, K.; Mowat, F.; Lau, E. Primary and revision arthroplasty surgery caseloads in the United States from 1990 to 2004. *J. Arthroplast.* **2009**, *24*, 195–203. [CrossRef]
18. Bobyn, J.D.; Pilliar, R.M.; Cameron, H.U.; Weatherly, G.C. The optimum pore size for the fixation of porous-surfaced metal implants by the ingrowth of bone. *Clin. Orthop. Relat. Res.* **1980**, *150*, 263–270. [CrossRef]
19. Karageorgiou, V.; Kaplan, D. Porosity of 3D biomaterial scaffolds and osteogenesis. *Biomaterials* **2005**, *26*, 5474–5491. [CrossRef]
20. Huddleston, J.I.; Wiley, J.W.; Scott, R.D. Zone 4 femoral radiolucent lines in hybrid versus cemented total knee arthroplasties: Are they clinically significant? *Clin. Orthop. Relat. Res.* **2005**, *441*, 334–339. [CrossRef] [PubMed]
21. Harrison, A.K.; Gioe, T.J.; Simonelli, C.; Tatman, P.J.; Schoeller, M.C. Do porous tantalum implants help preserve bone?: Evaluation of tibial bone density surrounding tantalum tibial implants in TKA. *Clin. Orthop. Relat. Res.* **2010**, *468*, 2739–2745. [CrossRef] [PubMed]
22. Overgaard, S.; Lind, M.; Glerup, H.; Grundvig, S.; Bünger, C.; Søballe, K. Hydroxyapatite and fluorapatite coatings for fixation of weight loaded implants. *Clin. Orthop. Relat. Res.* **1997**, *336*, 286–296. [CrossRef]
23. Nowak, M.; Kusz, D.; Wojciechowski, P.; Wilk, R. Risk factors for intraoperative periprosthetic femoral fractures during the total hip arthroplasty. *Pol. Orthop. Traumatol.* **2012**, *77*, 59–64. [PubMed]
24. Sikorski, J.M. Alignment in total knee replacement. *J. Bone Jt. Surg. Br.* **2008**, *90*, 1121–1127. [CrossRef] [PubMed]
25. Jeffery, R.S.; Morris, R.W.; Denham, R.A. Coronal alignment after total knee replacement. *J. Bone Jt. Surg. Br.* **1991**, *73*, 709–714. [CrossRef] [PubMed]
26. Berahmani, S.; Janssen, D.; Wolfson, D.; Rivard, K.; de Waal Malefijt, M.; Verdonschot, N. The effect of surface morphology on the primary fixation strength of uncemented femoral knee prosthesis: A cadaveric study. *J. Arthroplast.* **2015**, *30*, 300–307. [CrossRef]
27. Søballe, K.; Hansen, E.S.; Brockstedt-Rasmussen, H.; Bünger, C. Hydroxyapatite coating converts fibrous tissue to bone around loaded implants. *J. Bone Jt. Surg. Br.* **1993**, *75*, 270–278. [CrossRef]
28. Cameron, H.U.; Pilliar, R.M.; MacNab, I. The effect of movement on the bonding of porous metal to bone. *J. Biomed. Mater. Res.* **1973**, *7*, 301–311. [CrossRef]
29. Nam, D.; Lawrie, C.M.; Salih, R.; Nahhas, C.R.; Barrack, R.L.; Nunley, R.M. Cemented Versus Cementless Total Knee Arthroplasty of the Same Modern Design: A Prospective, Randomized Trial. *J. Bone Jt. Surg. Am. Vol.* **2019**, *101*, 1185–1192. [CrossRef]
30. Søballe, K.; Hansen, E.S.; Brockstedt-Rasmussen, H.; Pedersen, C.M.; Bünger, C. Hydroxyapatite coating enhances fixation of porous coated implants: A comparison in dogs between press fit and noninterference fit. *Acta Orthop. Scand.* **1990**, *61*, 299–306. [CrossRef]
31. Onsten, I.; Nordqvist, A.; Carlsson, A.S.; Besjakov, J.; Shott, S. Hydroxyapatite augmentation of the porous coating improves fixation of tibial components. A randomised RSA study in 116 patients. *J. Bone Jt. Surg. Br. Vol.* **1998**, *80*, 417–425. [CrossRef]
32. Cross, M.J.; Parish, E.N. A hydroxyapatite-coated total knee replacement—Prospective analysis of 1000 patients. *J. Bone Jt. Surg. Br. Vol.* **2005**, *87*, 1073–1076. [CrossRef] [PubMed]
33. van der Voort, P.; Nulent ML, K.; Valstar, E.R.; Kaptein, B.L.; Fiocco, M.; Nelissen, R.G. Long-term migration of a cementless stem with different bioactive coatings. Data from a "prime" RSA study: Lessons learned. *Acta Orthop.* **2020**, *91*, 660–668. [CrossRef]
34. Voigt, J.D.; Mosier, M. Hydroxyapatite (HA) coating appears to be of benefit for implant durability of tibial components in primary total knee arthroplasty. *Acta Orthop.* **2011**, *82*, 448–459. [CrossRef] [PubMed]
35. Meneghini, R.M.; de Beaubien, B.C. Early failure of cementless porous tantalum monoblock tibial components. *J. Arthroplast.* **2013**, *28*, 1505–1508. [CrossRef]
36. DeFrancesco, C.J.; Canseco, J.A.; Nelson, C.L.; Israelite, C.L.; Kamath, A.F. Uncemented Tantalum Monoblock Tibial Fixation for Total Knee Arthroplasty in Patients Less Than 60 Years of Age: Mean 10-Year Follow-up. *J. Bone Jt. Surg. Am. Vol.* **2018**, *100*, 865–870. [CrossRef]
37. De Martino, I.; D'Apolito, R.; Sculco, P.K.; Poultsides, L.A.; Gasparini, G. Total Knee Arthroplasty Using Cementless Porous Tantalum Monoblock Tibial Component: A Minimum 10-Year Follow-Up. *J. Arthroplast.* **2016**, *31*, 2193–2198. [CrossRef]

38. Gerscovich, D.; Schwing, C.; Unger, A. Long-term results of a porous tantalum monoblock tibia component: Clinical and radiographic results at follow-up of 10 years. *Arthroplast. Today* **2017**, *3*, 192–196. [CrossRef]
39. Niemeläinen, M.; Skyttä, E.T.; Remes, V.; Mäkelä, K.; Eskelinen, A. Total Knee Arthroplasty with an Uncemented Trabecular Metal Tibial Component A Registry-Based Analysis. *J. Arthroplast.* **2013**, *29*, 57–60. [CrossRef]
40. Dunbar, M.J.; Wilson, D.A.; Hennigar, A.W.; Amirault, J.D.; Gross, M.; Reardon, G.P. Fixation of a trabecular metal knee arthroplasty component. A prospective randomized study. *J. Bone Jt. Surg. Am. Vol.* **2009**, *91*, 1578–1586. [CrossRef] [PubMed]
41. Fernandez-Fairen, M.; Hernández-Vaquero, D.; Murcia, A.; Torres, A.; Llopis, R. Trabecular metal in total knee arthroplasty associated with higher knee scores: A randomized controlled trial. *Clin. Orthop. Relat. Res.* **2013**, *471*, 3543–3553. [CrossRef]
42. Pulido, L.; Abdel, M.P.; Lewallen, D.G.; Stuart, M.J.; Sanchez-Sotelo, J.; Hanssen, A.D.; Pagnano, M.W. The Mark Coventry Award: Trabecular metal tibial components were durable and reliable in primary total knee arthroplasty: A randomized clinical trial. *Clin. Orthop. Relat. Res.* **2015**, *473*, 34–42. [CrossRef] [PubMed]
43. Hampton, M.; Mansoor, J.; Getty, J.; Sutton, P.M. Uncemented tantalum metal components versus cemented tibial components in total knee arthroplasty: 11- to 15-year outcomes of a single-blinded randomized controlled trial. *Bone Jt. J.* **2020**, *102*, 1025–1032. [CrossRef] [PubMed]
44. Fricka, K.B.; Sritulanondha, S.; McAsey, C.J. To cement or not? Two-year results of a prospective, randomized study comparing cemented vs. cementless total knee arthroplasty (TKA). *J. Arthroplast.* **2015**, *30*, 55–58. [CrossRef] [PubMed]
45. Karachalios, T.; Komnos, G.; Amprazis, V.; Antoniou, I.; Athanaselis, S. A 9-Year Outcome Study Comparing Cancellous Titanium-Coated Cementless to Cemented Tibial Components of a Single Knee Arthroplasty Design. *J. Arthroplast.* **2018**, *33*, 3672–3677. [CrossRef] [PubMed]
46. Waddell, D.D.; Sedacki, K.; Yang, Y.; Fitch, D.A. Early radiographic and functional outcomes of a cancellous titanium-coated tibial component for total knee arthroplasty. *Musculoskelet. Surg.* **2016**, *100*, 71–74. [CrossRef] [PubMed]
47. Bhimji, S.; Meneghini, R. Micromotion of Cementless Tibial Baseplates: Keels with Adjuvant Pegs Offer More Stability Than Pegs Alone. *J. Arthroplast.* **2014**, *29*, 1503–1506. [CrossRef]
48. Goh, G.S.; Fillingham, Y.A.; Sutton, R.M.; Small, I.; Courtney, P.M.; Hozack, W.J. Cemented Versus Cementless Total Knee Arthroplasty in Obese Patients with Body Mass Index $\geq$35 kg/m^2: A Contemporary Analysis of 812 Patients. *J. Arthroplast.* **2022**, *37*, 688–693.e1. [CrossRef]
49. Pijls, B.G.; Valstar, E.R.; Kaptein, B.L.; Fiocco, M.; Nelissen, R.G. The beneficial effect of hydroxyapatite lasts: A randomized radiostereometric trial comparing hydroxyapatite-coated, uncoated, and cemented tibial components for up to 16 years. *Acta Orthop.* **2012**, *83*, 135–141. [CrossRef]
50. Laende, E.K.; Richardson, C.G.; Dunbar, M.J. Predictive value of short-term migration in determining long-term stable fixation in cemented and cementless total knee arthroplasties. *Bone Jt. J.* **2019**, *101*, 55–60. [CrossRef] [PubMed]
51. Henricson, A.; Nilsson, K. Trabecular metal tibial knee component still stable at 10 years. *Acta Orthop.* **2016**, *87*, 1–7. [CrossRef] [PubMed]
52. Hasan, S.; van Hamersveld, K.T.; Marang-van de Mheen, P.J.; Kaptein, B.L.; Nelissen RG, H.H.; Toksvig-Larsen, S. Migration of a novel 3D-printed cementless versus a cemented total knee arthroplasty: Two-year results of a randomized controlled trial using radiostereometric analysis. *Bone Jt. J.* **2020**, *102*, 1016–1024. [CrossRef] [PubMed]
53. Bagsby, D.T.; Issa, K.; Smith, L.S.; Elmallah, R.K.; Mast, L.E.; Harwin, S.F.; Mont, M.A.; Bhimani, S.J.; Malkani, A.L. Cemented versus cementless total knee arthroplasty in morbidly obese patients. *J. Arthroplast.* **2016**, *31*, 1727–1731. [CrossRef] [PubMed]
54. Whiteside, L.A.; Viganò, R. Young and heavy patients with a cementless TKA do as well as older and lightweight patients. *Clin. Orthop. Relat. Res.* **2007**, *464*, 93–98. [CrossRef]
55. Sinicrope, B.J.; Feher, A.W.; Bhimani, S.J.; Smith, L.S.; Harwin, S.F.; Yakkanti, M.R.; Malkani, A.L. Increased Survivorship of Cementless versus Cemented TKA in the Morbidly Obese. A Minimum 5-Year Follow-Up. *J. Arthroplast.* **2019**, *34*, 309–314. [CrossRef] [PubMed]
56. Kim, Y.H.; Park, J.W.; Lim, H.M.; Park, E.S. Cementless and cemented total knee arthroplasty in patients younger than fifty five years. Which is better? *Int. Orthop.* **2014**, *38*, 297–303. [CrossRef]
57. Kim, Y.H.; Park, J.W.; Jang, Y.S. The 22 to 25-Year Survival of Cemented and Cementless Total Knee Arthroplasty in Young Patients. *J. Arthroplast.* **2021**, *36*, 566–572. [CrossRef]
58. Vertullo, C.J.; Zbrojkiewicz, D.; Vizesi, F.; Walsh, W.R. Thermal Analysis of the Tibial Cement Interface with Modern Cementing Technique. *Open Orthop. J.* **2016**, *10*, 19–25. [CrossRef]
59. Tawy, G.F.; Rowe, P.J.; Riches, P.E. Thermal Damage Done to Bone by Burring and Sawing with and without Irrigation in Knee Arthroplasty. *J. Arthroplast.* **2016**, *31*, 1102–1108. [CrossRef]
60. Dolan, E.B.; Haugh, M.G.; Tallon, D.; Casey, C.; McNamara, L.M. Heat-shock-induced cellular responses to temperature elevations occurring during orthopaedic cutting. *J. R. Soc. Interface* **2012**, *9*, 3503–3513. [CrossRef]
61. Navathe, A.S.; Troxel, A.B.; Liao, J.M.; Nan, N.; Zhu, J.; Zhong, W.; Emanuel, E.J. Cost of Joint Replacement Using Bundled Payment Models. *JAMA Intern. Med.* **2017**, *177*, 214–222. [CrossRef] [PubMed]
62. Lawrie, C.M.; Schwabe, M.; Pierce, A.; Nunley, R.M.; Barrack, R.L. The cost of implanting a cemented versus cementless total knee arthroplasty. *Bone Jt. J.* **2019**, *101*, 61–63. [CrossRef] [PubMed]
63. Yayac, M.; Harrer, S.; Hozack, W.J.; Parvizi, J.; Courtney, P.M. The Use of Cementless Components Does Not Significantly Increase Procedural Costs in Total Knee Arthroplasty. *J. Arthroplast.* **2020**, *35*, 407–412. [CrossRef] [PubMed]

4. Gwam, C.U.; George, N.E.; Etcheson, J.I.; Rosas, S.; Plate, J.F.; Delanois, R.E. Cementless versus Cemented Fixation in Total Knee Arthroplasty: Usage, Costs, and Complications during the Inpatient Period. *J. Knee Surg.* **2019**, *32*, 1081–1087. [CrossRef]
5. Quispel, C.R.; Duivenvoorden, T.; Beekhuizen, S.R.; Verburg, H.; Spekenbrink-Spooren, A.; Van Steenbergen, L.N.; Pasma, J.H.; De Ridder, R. Comparable mid-term revision rates of primary cemented and cementless total knee arthroplasties in 201,211 cases in the Dutch Arthroplasty Register (2007–2017). *Knee Surg. Sports Traumatol. Arthrosc. Off. J. ESSKA* **2021**, *29*, 3400–3408. [CrossRef]

Disclaimer/Publisher's Note: The statements, opinions and data contained in all publications are solely those of the individual author(s) and contributor(s) and not of MDPI and/or the editor(s). MDPI and/or the editor(s) disclaim responsibility for any injury to people or property resulting from any ideas, methods, instructions or products referred to in the content.

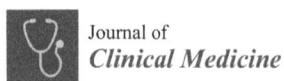

Article

Pain Course after Total Knee Arthroplasty within a Standardized Pain Management Concept: A Prospective Observational Study

Melanie Schindler [1,*], Stephanie Schmitz [1], Jan Reinhard [1], Petra Jansen [2], Joachim Grifka [1] and Achim Benditz [1,3]

[1] Department of Orthopedics, University Medical Center Regensburg, Asklepios Klinikum Bad Abbach, 93077 Bad Abbach, Bavaria, Germany
[2] Department of Sport Science, University of Regensburg, 93053 Regensburg, Bavaria, Germany
[3] Department of Orthopedics, Klinikum Fichtelgebirge, 95615 Marktredwitz, Bavaria, Germany
* Correspondence: melanie.schindler@klinik.uni-regensburg.de

Abstract: Background: Joint replacement surgeries have been known to be some of the most painful surgical procedures. Therefore, the options for postoperative pain management are of great importance for patients undergoing total knee arthroplasty (TKA). Despite successful surgery, up to 30% of the patients are not satisfied after the operation. The aim of this study is to assess pain development within the first 4 weeks after TKA in order to gain a better understanding and detect possible influencing factors. Methods: A total of 103 patients were included in this prospective cohort study. Postoperative pain was indicated using a numeric rating scale (NRS). Furthermore, demographic data and perioperative parameters were correlated with the reported postoperative pain. Results: The evaluation of postoperative pain scores showed a constant decrease in the first postoperative week (mean NRS score of 5.8 on day 1 to a mean NRS score of 4.6 on day 8). On day 9, the pain increased again. Thereafter, a continuous decrease in pain intensity from day 10 on was noted (continuous to a mean NRS score of 3.0 on day 29). A significant association was found between postoperative pain intensity and gender, body mass index (BMI), and preoperative leg axis. Conclusions: The increasing pain score after the first postoperative week is most likely due to more intensive mobilization and physiotherapy in the rehabilitation department. Patients that were female, had a low BMI, and a preoperative valgus leg axis showed a significantly higher postoperative pain scores. Pain management should consider these results in the future to improve patient satisfaction in the postoperative course after TKA.

Keywords: total knee arthroplasty; postoperative pain; numeric rating scale; influencing factors

Citation: Schindler, M.; Schmitz, S.; Reinhard, J.; Jansen, P.; Grifka, J.; Benditz, A. Pain Course after Total Knee Arthroplasty within a Standardized Pain Management Concept: A Prospective Observational Study. *J. Clin. Med.* 2022, 11, 7204. https://doi.org/10.3390/jcm11237204

Academic Editor: Stephen Vogt

Received: 6 November 2022
Accepted: 2 December 2022
Published: 4 December 2022

Publisher's Note: MDPI stays neutral with regard to jurisdictional claims in published maps and institutional affiliations.

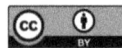

Copyright: © 2022 by the authors. Licensee MDPI, Basel, Switzerland. This article is an open access article distributed under the terms and conditions of the Creative Commons Attribution (CC BY) license (https://creativecommons.org/licenses/by/4.0/).

1. Introduction

Knee osteoarthritis causes pain and limited mobility. Hence, it is the main indication for total knee arthroplasty (TKA). TKA relieves pain, improves mobility, and thus increases quality of life. In Germany, primary TKA is one of the most frequently performed surgical procedures [1]. The total number of TKA procedures in Germany is expected to increase by 45%, from 168,772 procedures in 2016 to 244,714 procedures in 2040 [2]. As a result, it is all the more important that this stressful surgical procedure is successful for the patients. Surgical procedures are influenced by many factors, including patient and surgeon preferences. Pain is the most important factor in patient satisfaction [3]. Most patients achieve postoperative pain reduction with a good clinical outcome [1]. 10–20% of patients are dissatisfied with the surgical outcome and report persistent chronic pain postoperatively (CPSP) [4]. This can lead to delayed mobilization, a longer duration of hospitalization, and thus higher costs for the health care system. Therefore, multidisciplinary pain management is of high significance. It is crucial to have a better understanding of this dissatisfaction and the factors that influence it. Patients with early postoperative persistent pain had a lower chance of being pain-free after one year than patients who reported no or only little pain. [5]. A detailed assessment of the postoperative pain course with a pain curve has not been performed up to now. The early postoperative phase and the rehabilitation phase both represent a particular challenge for patients and their reintegration.

Prolonged postoperative pain leads to increased consumption of analgesics and a longer rehabilitation stay. Therefore, the aim of this study is to evaluate postoperative pain development and detect possible factors influencing postoperative pain after TKA.

2. Material and Methods

This work is a prospective study of a single center of orthopedic surgery at a university hospital, including patients undergoing primary TKA between October 2020 and July 2021. The patients were enrolled on the day of preoperative preparation, which in our department usually takes place a few days before the surgical performance.

Patients received cemented PFC Sigma (Depuy Synthes, Warsaw, IN, USA) or cemented nickel-free NexGen® knee prostheses (Zimmer Biomet Inc., Warsaw, IN, USA). Patellar resection arthroplasty with circumpatellar electrocautery and osteophyte removal was performed on all of the patients. Patellar resurfacing was not performed. Patients who received primary TKA, anesthesia via peripheral nerve block, sedation with propofol, and inpatient rehabilitation in our department were included in the study. The follow-up for patients became easier as the rehabilitation treatment was standardized. Patients with chronic pain syndromes preoperatively and/or an intraoperative change to general anesthesia were excluded.

A standardized pain management regimen was given to all patients: Preoperatively, patients were given 7.5 mg of midazolam orally one hour before surgery. The psoas compartment block was performed with 20 mL of ropivacaine 0.75% and the ischiatic nerve proximal dorsal block (transgluteal) with 20 mL of prilocaine 1%. The peripheral nerve block was placed using neurostimulation, and the feedback was expected to be a twitch of the leg. During surgery, patients were sedated with propofol. In the intermediate care unit, 10 mL of ropivacaine 0.75% were administered to the patients via the psoas block at regular intervals during the first 12 h after surgery. Furthermore, patients use the pain catheter at 45 min intervals with 10 mL of ropivacaine 0.75% if needed. In cases of severe pain, the ischiatic nerve block was maintained with ropivacaine 0.2 6 mL/hr.

The standard oral analgesic medication, which was also given during the analgesic therapy via catheter, was metamizole 500 mg four times daily and ibuprofen 600 mg three times daily. In case of pain exacerbation, tramadol 100 mg (40 gtt) was provided, which could be repeated after 30 min when the NRS was 3–6. Also, oxycodone 20 mg could be given and repeated after 1 h in the case of an NRS of 7–10. If the patient used all therapy options, the standard analgesic medication was adjusted. Cold packs were also provided for the knee. Full weight bearing with crutches was allowed directly after surgery.

The preoperative clinical status and the results one week and four weeks postoperatively were evaluated according to the Knee Society Score and Function Score (KSS and FS) [6].

A whole-leg radiograph was performed preoperatively and a few days after surgery. The measured radiographic parameters included the anatomical axis of the leg. It connects the anatomical femoral axis with the anatomical tibial axis and forms a physiological angle of 5° to 10° valgus. A positive degree value corresponds to a valgus position, a negative one to a varus position.

All patients documented their postoperative pain four times a day (morning, lunchtime, evening, and nighttime) and the maximum pain of the day using the numerous rating scale (NRS 0 = no pain; 10 = worst imaginable pain). In our department, the patients received physiotherapy once a day, including continuous passive motion (CPM) therapy. They got an intense rehabilitation program during the following stationary rehabilitation.

The study was approved by the local ethics committee (16-101-0204). Information was supplied to all potential patients, and participation was voluntary. A written informed consent was received from every subject.

IBM SPSS Statistics 25 (IBM Corp., Armonk, NY, USA) was used for analysis. Demographics and clinical characteristics were presented as means and standard deviations. Predictors of postoperative pain were analyzed using linear regression models. Leg axis and function scores were evaluated using paired t-tests. A p-value < 0.05 was considered as statistically significant.

3. Results

Initially, 139 patients were included in the study. 15% of the initial data could not be used because of incomplete/missing pain sheets (n = 7), discontinuation of rehabilitation treatment due to SARS-CoV-2 infection/contact (n = 8), or a second surgical procedure on account of a complication (n = 3). The complications that led to a revision surgery included wound healing disorder (n = 1), early infection (n = 1), and arthrofibrosis (n = 1). Finally, a participation rate of 85% (n = 103) was achieved.

The mean age of patients was 66.5 ± 8.7 years. Most of the patients were female (n = 56, 54.4%). According to the classification of the World Health Organization (WHO), 8.7% of the patients were of normal weight, 34% were pre-obese, and 57.3% were obese. Indications for performing TKA were osteoarthritis (88.3%) and post-traumatic osteoarthritis (11.7%). In general, 29.1% underwent a knee arthroscopy preoperatively and 32% had already a total hip or contralateral knee arthroplasty before. One third of the patients (35%) took painkillers daily, 35.9% casually, and 29.1% of the patients did not take any painkillers preoperatively. Most patients (68%) had an ASA score (American Society of Anesthesiologists) of 2, 22.4% had an ASA score of 3, and 9.7% had an ASA score of 1.

The mean duration of surgery was 82.7 ± 18.6 min (minimum 47, maximum 150). 84.5% received a cemented PFC Sigma total knee arthroplasty, and 15.5% received a cemented nickel-free NexGen implant. 61.2% of the operations were computer-assisted, and 38.8% were conventional TKAs.

The pain catheter was removed at day 2.7 + 0.71 (min 1, max 5 days) on average.

The mean anatomical axis of the leg showed a significant difference from 4.3 ± 7.2° (min −1°, max 25°) preoperatively to 7.2 ± 3.4° (min −2°, max 16°) postoperatively ($p = 0.001$).

The clinical outcome showed a preoperative KSS of 46 ± 15 points and FS of 56 ± 16 points, 1 week postoperatively 61 ± 16 ($p = 0.001$) and 41 ± 17 ($p = 0.001$), and after 4 weeks 69 ± 17 ($p = 0.001$) and 55 ± 11 ($p = 0.735$). Accordingly, the improvement was significant even without the last FS.

In the following postoperative period, the mean pain score was measured on days 1 to 29 (Table 1; Figure 1). The maximum and minimum pain of the day, documented by the patients, were then evaluated (Figure 2). In general, influencing factors were sex, BMI, and anatomical axis. Female gender (Figure 3), low BMI, and valgus leg axis showed a significant correlation with more severe postoperative pain scores. In contrast, age, ASA score, surgical duration, KS score, and FS score did not influence the pain score (Table 1).

Table 1. Linear regression of pain after TKA, based on mean pain levels of the first postoperative week in the acute hospital (T1), the second week until the fourth postoperative week in the rehabilitation unit (T2), and the total analyzed postoperative time (T3); KSS1: knee society score preoperative; FS1: functional score preoperative; KSS2 and FS2 after one week in the acute hospital; and KSS3 and FS2 after four weeks in a rehabilitation unit.

Predictor	B (95% CI)	p-Value	R^2 Value
Sex			
T1	−0.999 (−1.84, −0.16)	0.020	−0.257
T2	−1.548 (−2.41, −0.69)	0.001	−0.375
T3	−1.417 (−2.23, −0.61)	0.001	−0.362

Table 1. Cont.

Predictor	B (95% CI)	p-Value	R^2 Value
Age			
T1	−0.026 (−0.08, 0.02)	0.280	−0.118
T2	−0.026 (−0.08, 0.02)	0.290	−0.112
T3	−0.027 (−0.07, 0.02)	0.250	−0.121
BMI			
T1	−0.105 (−0.19, −0.03)	0.010	−0.309
T2	−0.124 (−0.21, −0.04)	0.003	−0.343
T3	−0.120 (−0.20, −0.04)	0.003	−0.349
ASA Score			
T1	0.311 (−0.44, 1.06)	0.409	0.089
T2	0.669 (−0.09, 1.43)	0.085	0.180
T3	0.589 (−0.13, 1.31)	0.110	0.166
Surgical duration			
T1	0.004 (−0.02, 0.03)	0.768	0.035
T2	0.017 (−0.01, 0.04)	0.166	0.158
T3	0.014 (−0.01, 0.04)	0.236	0.134
Paincatheter duration			
T1	0.026 (−0.50, 0.56)	0.922	0.010
T2	0.251 (−0.29, 0.79)	0.359	0.087
T3	0.203 (−0.31, 0.71)	0.432	0.075
Previous surgery			
T1	0.037 (−0.85, 0.92)	0.935	0.009
T2	−0.413 (−1.31, 0.49)	0.366	−0.091
T3	−0.303 (−1.16, 0.55)	0.483	−0.071
Operation type			
T1	0.387 (−0.39, 1.17)	0.328	0.097
T2	0.377 (−0.45, 1.21)	0.369	0.089
T3	0.380 (−0.41, 1.17)	0.340	0.095
Anatomical axis 1			
T1	0.065 (0.01, 0.12)	0.020	0.240
T2	0.062 (0.01, 0.12)	0.030	0.215
T3	0.061 (0.01, 0.11)	0.022	0.226
Anatomical axis 2			
T1	0.026 (−0.09, 0.14)	0.648	0.044
T2	0.008 (−0.11, 0.12)	0.888	0.013
T3	0.014 (−0.09, 0.12)	0.794	0.024
KSS 1			
T1	0.011 (−0.01, 0.04)	0.378	0.086
T2	−0.004 (−0.03, 0.02)	0.733	−0.032
T3	−0.001 (−0.03, 0.02)	0.961	−0.005

Table 1. Cont.

Predictor	B (95% CI)	p-Value	R² Value
FS 1			
T1	−0.002 (−0.03, 0.02)	0.897	−0.014
T2	−0.006 (−0.03, 0.02)	0.666	−0.046
T3	−0.005 (−0.03, 0.02)	0.694	−0.042
KSS 2			
T1	−0.027 (−0.06, 0.00)	0.055	−0.231
T2	−0.027 (−0.06, 0.00)	0.064	−0.214
T3	−0.027 (−0.05, 0.00)	0.051	−0.225
FS 2			
T1	−0.012 (−0.05, 0.02)	0.476	−0.073
T2	−0.018 (−0.05, 0.02)	0.292	−0.104
T3	−0.016 (−0.05, 0.02)	0.319	−0.098
KSS 3			
T1	−0.007 (−0.03, 0.02)	0.612	−0.060
T2	−0.008 (−0.04, 0.02)	0.577	−0.064
T3	−0.008 (−0.03, 0.02)	0.549	−0.068
FS 3			
T1	0.009 (−0.03, 0.05)	0.655	0.052
T2	0.022 (−0.02, 0.06)	0.276	0.122
T3	0.019 (−0.02, 0.06)	0.326	0.109

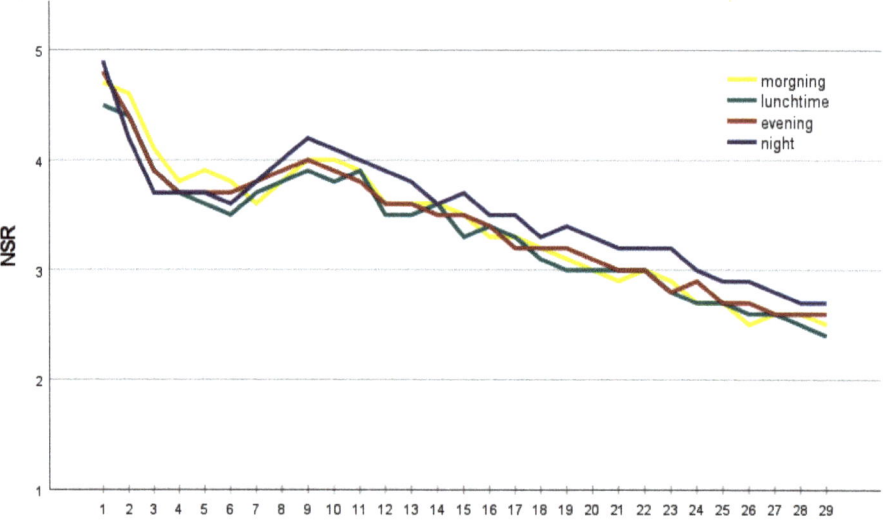

Figure 1. Graph represents the mean pain and maximum pain on days 1–29 on an NRS scale. The mean pain calculation is based on morning, lunchtime, evening, and nighttime pain values.

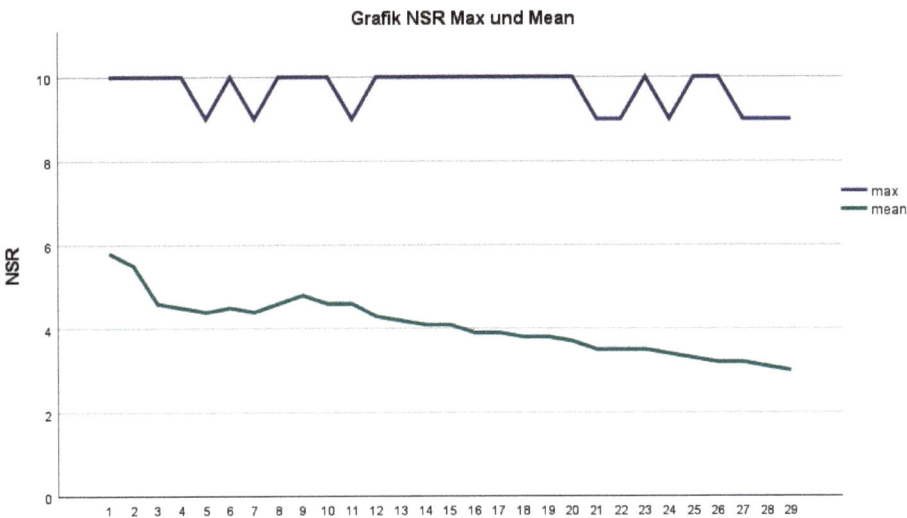

Figure 2. Graph represents the morning, lunchtime, evening, and nighttime pain on days 1–29 on an NRS scale.

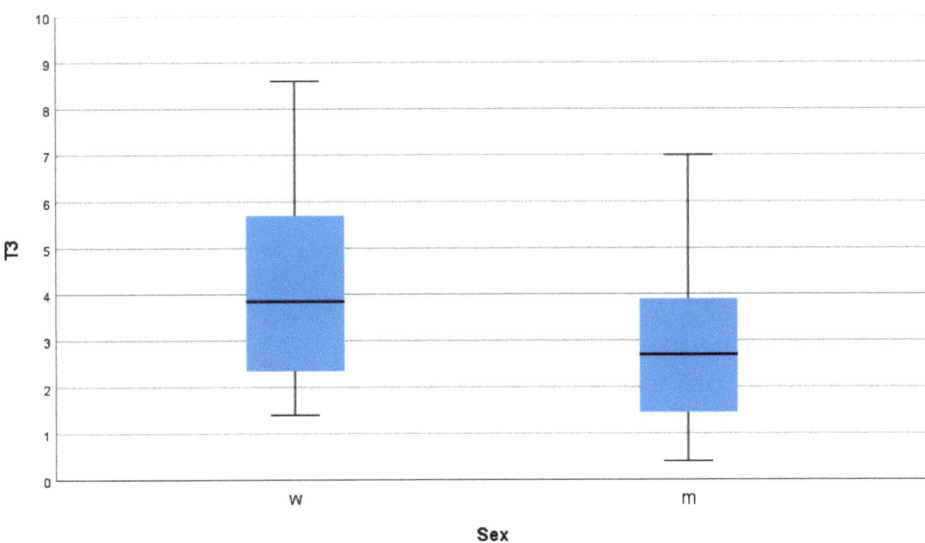

Figure 3. Boxplot over the total analyzed postoperative time and gender (w = women; m = men).

4. Discussion
4.1. Postoperative Pain Course

Overall, postoperative pain decreases significantly after TKA. In the first postoperative week, the lowest pain scores were on day 8 with an NRS of 4.6. This increased to 4.8 on day 9. The reason for the increase in pain progression may be related to the start of the intensive rehabilitation program. Subsequently, there was a constant decrease in the pain level from day 10 to day 29. Another study showed a comparable mean maximum pain of 5.44 ± 1.83 on the first postoperative day [7]. Here, the NSR was 5.8 ± 2.8. An increase from the middle of the first postoperative week to the end of the week had already been observed in another study [8].

An identical study design has already been published for primary total hip arthroplasty. They described the postoperative pain over a course of four weeks as well as possible factors influencing pain intensity after primary total hip arthroplasty [9]. Comparable to our study, the pain intensity was lowest on day 8, with an NSR of 2.3, and increased to 2.6 on day 9, when they were transferred from the acute hospital to the rehabilitation unit.

There are numerous studies that have compared preoperative pain with postoperative pain outcomes. High preoperative knee pain, anxiety, and anticipated pain were the most important predictive factors and had the most influence on satisfaction one year postoperatively [10]. None of the studies found a correlation between preoperative KSS/FS and postoperative pain intensity.

In the future, special attention should be paid to the timing of increasing pain, as the high rate of chronic postoperative pain (CPSP) is alarming. High postoperative pain scores are associated with a higher likelihood of developing CSPS 3 months to a year after the operation [3]. If the pain curve increases by more than 2.8 points, the probability is 33.3% 1 year postoperatively [11]. This study shows the greatest increase in pain on the first day of rehabilitation. However, it confirms that the first few weeks after surgery are the most critical.

4.2. Gender of the Patient

When analyzing gender as a possible predictor of postoperative pain intensity, women reported significantly higher pain scores at each surveyed level. This difference is in line with other studies [12,13]. Furthermore, women demonstrated poorer clinical outcomes and lower satisfaction after surgery [14,15]. The gender difference has also been analyzed in other reviews, concluding that women are at increased risk for developing more severe postoperative pain conditions and subsequent CSPS [16]. One reason for this could be because women have more sensory pain fibers [17]. Women report having higher levels of general anxiety as well as factors that capture pain-related stress [16]. Another aspect is that women generally undergo surgery later compared to men and often have greater movement limitations preoperatively [18]. This suggests that earlier treatment in women would improve postoperative outcomes. All in all, several psychosocial, biological, and sociocultural mechanisms may play an important role in the emergence of gender differences in pain.

4.3. BMI at Surgery

Another known risk factor for the development of knee osteoarthritis is a high BMI [19,20]. This study population has a total of 91.3% overweight patients (BMI > 30 kg/m^2). In Germany, 67.1% of men and 53.0% of women are overweight [21]. Therefore, our patients are well above the German average. In the present study, BMI was investigated as a possible influencing factor on the postoperative pain course after TKA. Normal-weight patients reported significantly more severe pain in the postoperative period up to four weeks compared to overweight patients. Here, there was no correlation between gender and BMI. One explanation could be the increased motivation to move and the associated more severe postoperative pain in normal-weight patients. This theory cannot be substantiated in this work. The literature on the effects of BMI on pain and functional outcomes after TKA is somewhat inconsistent. Several studies have shown that the risk of revision after TKA is higher in obese patients than in nonobese patients [22,23]. Chen et al. [23] reported similar clinical outcomes after TKA. Compared with normal-weight patients, obese patients showed significantly higher improvement in the Oxford Knee Score (OKS) and KSS two years after surgery. Another study that evaluated preoperative and 12-month postoperative clinical scores demonstrated greater improvement in overweight patients [24]. High BMI, as well as female gender, Indian/Malay race, and use of general anesthesia compared with regional anesthesia, are identified as influencing factors of "severe pain" [25]. It is important to note that this study did not consider the increased complication rate in obese patients. All in all, a clear benefit of surgery can be obtained regardless of weight.

4.4. Age at Surgery

The predictor age was analyzed, and no association was found in this study. Previous work, however, showed partly different results. For example, a patient aged over 70 years showed statistically significantly worse EQ-5D and WOMAC scores [15].

4.5. Operation Type

In our evaluation, the type of operation was not a risk factor for more severe pain progression. Preexisting studies also found no clinically important differences between computer-assisted and conventionally performed TKR [26–28]. Kim et al. [28] prospectively compared patients who received a computer-navigated knee arthroplasty in one knee and a knee arthroplasty without computer navigation in the other knee. Both groups had similar clinical function, position, and component survival. In contrast, a randomized, double-blind responder analysis showed that more patients with computer-assisted TKR were pain free and had better function after two years than in the conventional group [29].

4.6. Perioperative Factors

Surgical time as a possible cause for increased pain intensity was also analyzed, as the duration of the operation may reflect the complexity of the implantation. The repeated resection of bone or the more frequent placement of trial implants during the procedure may influence postoperative pain development. Nevertheless, this hypothesis found no support in the present study report. The same conclusion was also reached in another prospective study [30].

Perioperative blood loss and postoperative pain after TKA could also be issues preventing early mobilization of patients [31]. The effect of tranexamic acid in reducing perioperative blood loss has been described extensively in the past. Several studies have shown a significant reduction in blood loss when using tranexamic acid [32,33].

In the evaluation of the possible influence of the ASA score on the postoperative pain level, no correlation was found.

The duration of the pain catheter was not found to be a possible cause of increased pain intensity. Another study [34] showed that continuous femoral nerve block for at least 72 h resulted in good control of acute postoperative pain as well as early joint mobilization. In the first 24 h after surgery, the 243 patients included reported a VAS of 0-1. All patients achieved 90 degrees of flexion by postoperative day 7. The proximal peripheral nerve block is a commonly used method in pain control after TKA because of its excellent analgesic effect and is considered the gold standard for postoperative analgesia after TKA. However, it may decrease quadriceps strength, which is essential for early mobilization. The adductor canal block might be a reasonable alternative, providing a predominantly sensory block with greater quadriceps strength. [35,36]

The influence of mental health on physical well-being and pain was not investigated in this study, but it also has a major role in postoperative outcome. Anxiety symptoms and depression are likely risk factors for poor outcomes [37]. Similarly, preoperative sleep quality correlates with clinical outcomes (i.e., pain, ROM, function, and length of hospital stay) after total joint arthroplasty [38]. Patients living alone also have a longer hospital stay [39].

4.7. Radiological Parameters

About 10% of all TKA patients had a valgus deformity [40]. Valgus of the knee is one of the main reasons for knee joint disease and bears many complications. With this type of deformity, the surgeon must achieve proper alignment, stability, and balance to achieve successful clinical outcomes. The study showed a significant correlation between a valgus leg axis and higher postoperative pain scores. Similar trends could be found in the literature. A study that looked at the factors influencing the prolonged postoperative hospital length of stay noted that preoperative valgus deformity of the knee was a risk factor [41]. Another study compared the postoperative outcomes of valgus and varus leg axes. This showed that patients with a valgus deformity had a WOMAC stiffness score that was significantly worse than the valgus one year postoperatively [42]. Thus, patients with increasing valgus deformity should not wait too long to receive surgical care.

4.8. Limitations

The main limitation of the study is the single center setting. Possible important predictors such as psychosocial factors or the radiological severity of knee osteoarthritis were not recorded. The standardized rehabilitation treatment in our rehabilitation facility could be considered a possible selection bias. Also, further information on pain progression, such as pain severity, was not collected at the 3-month follow-up visits. Another limitation is the inclusion of patients during the COVID-19 pandemic. Patients with SARS-CoV-2 infection or contact had to be excluded because they had to stop stationary therapy earlier, both in the acute hospital and in the rehabilitation clinic.

5. Conclusions

In this study, the course of pain after total knee arthroplasty showed another peak after nine days. Female gender, low BMI, and preoperative valgus deformity as risk factors resulted in significantly higher postoperative pain scores. This knowledge should be taken into account by surgeons in the future to reduce patient dissatisfaction and prevent chronic pain after primary total knee arthroplasty informing the patient and by counteracting the risk factors at an early stage.

Hereafter, studies should also consider psychological factors, as the perception of pain is individual.

Author Contributions: M.S.: conceptualization, methodology, data curation, software, and writing—original draft preparation; S.S.: conceptualization, methodology, and data curation; J.R.: supervision and writing—reviewing; P.J.: software and validation; J.G.: supervision; A.B.: writing—reviewing and editing. All authors have read and agreed to the published version of the manuscript.

Funding: This research did not receive any specific grant from funding agencies in the public, commercial, or not-for-profit sectors.

Institutional Review Board Statement: The study was approved by the local ethics committee (16-101-0204). Information was supplied to all potential patients and participation was voluntary.

Informed Consent Statement: Informed consent was obtained from all subjects involved in the study. Written informed consent has been obtained from the patients to publish this paper.

Data Availability Statement: The datasets generated for this study are available on request to the corresponding author.

Conflicts of Interest: The authors declare no conflict of interest.

References

1. Carr, A.J.; Robertsson, O.; Graves, S.; Price, A.J.; Arden, N.K.; Judge, A.; Beard, D.J. Knee replacement. *Lancet* **2018**, *392*, 1672–1682. [CrossRef] [PubMed]
2. Rupp, M.; Lau, E.; Kurtz, S.M.; Alt, V. Projections of Primary TKA and THA in Germany from 2016 through 2040. *Clin. Orthop. Relat. Res.* **2020**, *478*, 1622–1633. [CrossRef] [PubMed]
3. Lavand'homme, P.M.; Grosu, I.; France, M.N.; Thienpont, E. Pain trajectories identify patients at risk of persistent pain after knee arthroplasty: An observational study. *Clin. Orthop. Relat. Res.* **2014**, *472*, 1409–1415. [CrossRef] [PubMed]
4. Wylde, V.; Beswick, A.; Bruce, J.; Blom, A.; Howells, N.; Gooberman-Hill, R. Chronic pain after total knee arthroplasty. *EFORT Open Rev.* **2018**, *3*, 461–470. [CrossRef] [PubMed]
5. Harmelink, K.E.M.; Dandis, R.; der Van der Wees Pj, P.J.; Zeegers, A.V.C.M.; der Sanden, M.W.; Staal, J.B. Recovery trajectories over six weeks in patients selected for a high-intensity physiotherapy program after Total knee Arthroplasty: A latent class analysis. *BMC Musculoskelet Disord.* **2021**, *22*, 179. [CrossRef]

6. Insall, J.N.; Dorr, L.D.; Scott, R.D.; Scott, W.N. Rationale of the Knee Society Clinical Rating System. Available online: http://www.orthopaedicscore.com/scorepages/knee_society_score.html (accessed on 16 June 2022).
7. Benditz, A.; Drescher, J.; Greimel, F.; Zeman, F.; Grifka, J.; Meißner, W.; Völlner, F. Implementing a benchmarking and feedback concept decreases postoperative pain after total knee arthroplasty: A prospective study including 256 patients. *Sci. Rep.* **2016**, *6*, 38218. [CrossRef]
8. Benditz, A.; Völlner, F.; Baier, C.; Götz, J.; Grifka, J.; Keshmiri, A. Schmerzverlauf nach operativer orthopädischer Intervention: Charakterisierung am Beispiel der Knieendoprothetik. *Schmerz* **2016**, *30*, 181–186. [CrossRef]
9. Greimel, F.; Dittrich, G.; Schwarz, T.; Kaiser, M.; Krieg, B.; Zeman, F.; Grifka, J.; Benditz, A. Course of pain after total hip arthroplasty within a standardized pain management concept: A prospective study examining influence, correlation, and outcome of postoperative pain on 103 consecutive patients. *Arch. Orthop. Trauma. Surg.* **2018**, *138*, 1639–1645. [CrossRef]
10. Rice, D.A.; Kluger, M.T.; McNair, P.J.; Lewis, G.N.; Somogyi, A.A.; Borotkanics, R.; Barratt, D.T.; Walker, M. Persistent postoperative pain after total knee arthroplasty: A prospective cohort study of potential risk factors. *Br. J. Anaesth.* **2018**, *121*, 804–812. [CrossRef]
11. Imai, R.; Nishigami, T.; Kubo, T.; Ishigaki, T.; Yonemoto, Y.; Mibu, A.; Morioka, S.; Fujii, T. Using a postoperative pain trajectory to predict pain at 1 year after total knee arthroplasty. *Knee* **2021**, *32*, 194–200. [CrossRef] [PubMed]
12. Nandi, M.; Schreiber, K.L.; Martel, M.O.; Cornelius, M.; Campbell, C.M.; Haythornthwaite, J.A.; Smith, M.T.; Wright, J.; Aglio, L.S.; Edwards, R.R. Sex differences in negative affect and postoperative pain in patients undergoing total knee arthroplasty. *Biol. Sex Differ.* **2019**, *10*, 23. [CrossRef]
13. Huang, Y.; Lee, M.; Chong, H.C.; Ning, Y.; Lo, N.N.; Yeo, S.J. Reasons and Factors Behind Post-Total Knee Arthroplasty Dissatisfaction in an Asian Population. *Ann. Acad. Med. Singap.* **2017**, *46*, 303–309. [CrossRef]
14. Rissolio, L.; Sabatini, L.; Risitano, S.; Bistolfi, A.; Galluzzo, U.; Massè, A.; Indelli, P.F. Is It the Surgeon, the Patient, or the Device? A Comprehensive Clinical and Radiological Evaluation of Factors Influencing Patient Satisfaction in 648 Total Knee Arthroplasties. *J. Clin. Med.* **2021**, *10*, 2599. [CrossRef] [PubMed]
15. Götz, J.S.; Benditz, A.; Reinhard, J.; Schindler, M.; Zeman, F.; Grifka, J.; Greimel, F.; Leiss, F. Influence of Anxiety/Depression, Age, Gender and ASA on 1-Year Follow-Up Outcomes Following Total Hip and Knee Arthroplasty in 5447 Patients. *J. Clin. Med.* **2021**, *10*, 3095. [CrossRef] [PubMed]
16. Bartley, E.J.; Fillingim, R.B. Sex differences in pain: A brief review of clinical and experimental findings. *Br. J. Anaesth.* **2013**, *111*, 52–58. [CrossRef] [PubMed]
17. Peteler, R.; Schmitz, P.; Loher, M.; Jansen, P.; Grifka, J.; Benditz, A. Sex-Dependent Differences in Symptom-Related Disability Due to Lumbar Spinal Stenosis. *J. Pain Res.* **2021**, *14*, 747–755. [CrossRef]
18. Parsley, B.S.; Bertolusso, R.; Harrington, M.; Brekke, A.; Noble, P.C. Influence of gender on age of treatment with TKA and functional outcome. *Clin. Orthop. Relat. Res.* **2010**, *468*, 1759–1764. [CrossRef] [PubMed]
19. Zheng, H.; Chen, C. Body mass index and risk of knee osteoarthritis: Systematic review and meta-analysis of prospective studies. *BMJ Open* **2015**, *5*, e007568. [CrossRef]
20. Ackerman, I.N.; Kemp, J.L.; Crossley, K.M.; Culvenor, A.G.; Hinman, R.S. Hip and Knee Osteoarthritis Affects Younger People, too. *J. Orthop. Sports. Phys. Ther.* **2017**, *47*, 67–79. [CrossRef]
21. Mensink, G.B.M.; Schienkiewitz, A.; Haftenberger, M.; Lampert, T.; Ziese, T.; Scheidt-Nave, C. Übergewicht und Adipositas in Deutschland: Ergebnisse der Studie zur Gesundheit Erwachsener in Deutschland (DEGS1). *Bundesgesundheitsblatt Gesundh. Gesundh.* **2013**, *56*, 786–794. [CrossRef]
22. Vasso, M.; Corona, K.; Gomberg, B.; Marullo, M. Obesity increases the risk of conversion to total knee arthroplasty after unicompartimental knee arthroplasty: A meta-analysis. *Knee Surg. Sports Traumatol. Arthrosc.* **2021**, *30*, 3945–3957. [CrossRef] [PubMed]
23. Chen, J.Y.; Lo, N.N.; Chong, H.C.; Pang, H.N.; Tay, D.K.J.; Chia, S.L.; Yeo, S.J. The influence of body mass index on functional outcome and quality of life after total knee arthroplasty. *Bone Jt. J.* **2016**, *98*, 780–785. [CrossRef] [PubMed]
24. Giesinger, K.; Giesinger, J.M.; Hamilton, D.F.; Rechsteiner, J.; Ladurner, A. Higher body mass index is associated with larger postoperative improvement in patient-reported outcomes following total knee arthroplasty. *BMC Musculoskelet Disord.* **2021**, *22*, 635. [CrossRef]
25. Lo, L.W.T.; Suh, J.; Chen, J.Y.; Liow, M.H.L.; Allen, J.C.; Lo, N.N.; Koh, J.S.B. Early Postoperative Pain After Total Knee Arthroplasty Is Associated with Subsequent Poorer Functional Outcomes and Lower Satisfaction. *J. Arthroplast.* **2021**, *36*, 2466–2472. [CrossRef]
26. Cip, J.; Obwegeser, F.; Benesch, T.; Bach, C.; Ruckenstuhl, P.; Martin, A. Twelve-Year Follow-Up of Navigated Computer-Assisted Versus Conventional Total Knee Arthroplasty: A Prospective Randomized Comparative Trial. *J. Arthroplast.* **2018**, *33*, 1404–1411. [CrossRef]
27. Kim, A.G.; Bernhard, Z.; Acuña, A.J.; Wu, V.S.; Kamath, A.F. Use of intraoperative technology in total knee arthroplasty is not associated with reductions in postoperative pain. *Knee Surg. Sports Traumatol. Arthrosc.* **2022**. [CrossRef]
28. Kim, Y.-H.; Park, J.-W.; Kim, J.-S. The Clinical Outcome of Computer-Navigated Compared with Conventional Knee Arthroplasty in the Same Patients: A Prospective, Randomized, Double-Blind, Long-Term Study. *J. Bone Jt. Surg. Am.* **2017**, *99*, 989–996. [CrossRef]

29. Petursson, G.; Fenstad, A.M.; Gøthesen, Ø.; Dyrhovden, G.S.; Hallan, G.; Röhrl, S.M.; Aamodt, A.; Furnes, O. Computer-Assisted Compared with Conventional Total Knee Replacement: A Multicenter Parallel-Group Randomized Controlled Trial. *J. Bone Jt. Surg. Am.* **2018**, *100*, 1265–1274. [CrossRef]
30. Benditz, A.; Maderbacher, G.; Zeman, F.; Grifka, J.; Weber, M.; von Kunow, F.; Greimel, F.; Keshmiri, A. Postoperative pain and patient satisfaction are not influenced by daytime and duration of knee and hip arthroplasty: A prospective cohort study. *Arch. Orthop. Trauma. Surg.* **2017**, *137*, 1343–1348. [CrossRef] [PubMed]
31. Su, E.P.; Su, S. Strategies for reducing peri-operative blood loss in total knee arthroplasty. *Bone Jt. J.* **2016**, *98*, 98–100. [CrossRef]
32. Wang, D.; Luo, Z.-Y.; Yu, Z.-P.; Liu, L.X.; Chen, C.; Meng, W.K.; Zeng, W.N. The antifibrinolytic and anti-inflammatory effects of multiple doses of oral tranexamic acid in total knee arthroplasty patients: A randomized controlled trial. *J. Thromb. Haemost.* **2018**, *16*, 2442–2453. [CrossRef] [PubMed]
33. Luo, Z.Y.; Wang, H.Y.; Wang, D.; Zhou, K.; Pei, F.X.; Zhou, Z.K. Oral vs Intravenous vs Topical Tranexamic Acid in Primary Hip Arthroplasty: A Prospective, Randomized, Double-Blind, Controlled Study. *J. Arthroplast.* **2018**, *33*, 786–793. [CrossRef]
34. Cappiello, G.; Camarda, L.; Pulito, G.; Tarantino, A.; Martino, D.D.; Russi, V.; Stramazzo, L.; Ragusa, C.; Guarino, G.; Ripani, U. Continuous Femoral Catheter for Postoperative Analgesia After Total Knee Arthroplasty. *Med. Arch.* **2020**, *74*, 54–57. [CrossRef]
35. Pascarella, G.; Costa, F.; Del Buono, R.; Strumia, A.; Cataldo, R.; Agrò, F.; Carassiti, M. The para-sartorial compartments (PASC) block: A new approach to the femoral triangle block for complete analgesia of the anterior knee. *Anaesth. Rep.* **2022**, *10*, e12165. [CrossRef]
36. Koh, I.J.; Choi, Y.J.; Kim, M.S.; Koh, H.J.; Kang, M.S.; In, Y. Femoral Nerve Block versus Adductor Canal Block for Analgesia after Total Knee Arthroplasty. *Knee Surg. Relat. Res.* **2017**, *29*, 87–95. [CrossRef]
37. Kazarian, G.S.; Anthony, C.A.; Lawrie, C.M.; Barrack, R.L. The Impact of Psychological Factors and Their Treatment on the Results of Total Knee Arthroplasty. *J. Bone Jt. Surg. Am.* **2021**, *103*, 1744–1756. [CrossRef] [PubMed]
38. Luo, Z.-Y.; Li, L.-L.; Wang, D. Preoperative sleep quality affects postoperative pain and function after total joint arthroplasty: A prospective cohort study. *J. Orthop. Surg. Res.* **2019**, *14*, 378. [CrossRef] [PubMed]
39. Ding, Z.-C.; Xu, B.; Liang, Z.-M.; Wang, H.Y.; Luo, Z.Y.; Zhou, Z.K. Limited Influence of Comorbidities on Length of Stay after Total Hip Arthroplasty: Experience of Enhanced Recovery after Surgery. *Orthop. Surg.* **2020**, *12*, 153–161. [CrossRef]
40. Ranawat, A.S.; Ranawat, C.S.; Elkus, M.; Rasquinha, V.J.; Rossi, R.; Babhulkar, S. Total knee arthroplasty for severe valgus deformity. *J. Bone Jt. Surg. Am.* **2005**, *87* (Suppl. 1), 271–284.
41. Zhang, S.; Huang, Q.; Xie, J.; Xu, B.; Cao, G.; Pei, F. Factors influencing postoperative length of stay in an enhanced recovery after surgery program for primary total knee arthroplasty. *J. Orthop. Surg. Res.* **2018**, *13*, 29. [CrossRef]
42. Kahlenberg, C.A.; Trivellas, M.; Lee, Y.Y.; Padgett, D.E. Preoperative Valgus Alignment Does Not Predict Inferior Outcome of Total Knee Arthroplasty. *HSS J.* **2018**, *14*, 50–54. [CrossRef] [PubMed]

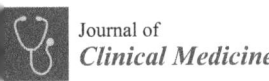

Article

Prognostic Factors in Staged Bilateral Total Knee Arthroplasty—A Retrospective Case Series Analysis

Krystian Kazubski [1], Łukasz Tomczyk [2], Andrzej Bobiński [1] and Piotr Morasiewicz [1,*]

[1] Department of Orthopaedic and Trauma Surgery, University Hospital in Opole, Institute of Medical Sciences, University of Opole, Witosa 26, 45-401 Opole, Poland
[2] Department of Food Safety and Quality Management, Poznan University of Life Sciences, Wojska Polskiego 28, 60-637 Poznan, Poland
* Correspondence: morasp@poczta.onet.pl; Tel.: +48-77-45-20-624

Abstract: Background: Bilateral osteoarthritis of the knee is an indication for a bilateral total knee replacement (TKR) procedure. The goal of our study was to assess the sizes of the implants used during the first and second stages of TKR procedures in order to compare their size and identify the prognostic factors for the second procedure. Methods: We evaluated 44 patients who underwent staged bilateral TKR procedures. We assess the following prognostic factors from the first and second surgery: duration of anesthesia, femoral component size, tibial component size, duration of hospital stay, tibial polyethylene insert size, and the number of complications. Results: All assessed prognostic factors did not differ statistically between the first and second TKR. A strong correlation was found between the size of femoral components and the size of tibial components used during the first and second total knee arthroplasty. The mean duration of the hospital stay associated with the first TKR surgery was 6.43 days, whereas the mean duration of the second hospital stay was 5.5 days ($p = 0.211$). The mean sizes of the femoral components used during the first and second procedures were 5.43 and 5.2, respectively ($p = 0.54$). The mean sizes of the tibial components used during the first and second TKR procedures were 5.36 and 5.25, respectively ($p = 0.382$). The mean sizes of the tibial polyethylene inserts used during the first and second procedures were 9.45 and 9.34 ($p = 0.422$), respectively. The mean duration of anesthesia during the first and second knee arthroplasty was 117.04 min and 118.06 min, respectively ($p = 0.457$). The mean rates of recorded complications associated with the first and second TKR procedures were 0.13 and 0.06 per patient ($p = 0.371$). Conclusions: We observed no differences between the two stages of treatment in terms of all analyzed parameters. We observed a strong correlation between the size of femoral components used during the first and second total knee arthroplasty. We noted a strong correlation between the size of tibial components used during the first and second procedure. Slightly weaker prognostic factors include the number of complications, duration of anesthesia and tibial polyethylene insert size.

Keywords: total knee replacement; two-stage; prognostic factors; bilateral; predictive factors

1. Introduction

Total knee replacement (TKR) procedures are an important proportion of all orthopedic surgeries worldwide [1,2], with approximately 1.5–2 million total hip replacement (THR) and TKR procedures in the United States being performed annually [1–3]. An estimated 2.34% to 4.55% of individuals aged 50 or more have undergone a total hip or knee replacement surgery [2].

Bilateral osteoarthritis of the knee is an indication for a bilateral TKR procedure [4–21]. Approximately 19–30% of patients with degenerative joint disease of the knee require bilateral total knee arthroplasty [8,11,17].

There are two management strategies available for patients diagnosed with bilateral knee osteoarthritis: simultaneous bilateral TKR or a staged treatment involving two

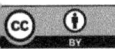

consecutive TKR procedures performed one at a time [7–21]. Many orthopedic surgeons consider either treatment strategy to be beneficial [8–10,19]. However, most authors choose the staged approach, which reduces loss of blood, the rate of complications, the extent of the procedure, and the required rehabilitation period and enables the patient to more rapidly resume physical activity [8–11,16,17,20]. Another potential advantage of the staged approach over simultaneous TKR is the opportunity to determine the prognostic factors for the second procedure [7,11,17,22].

Neither the postoperative symmetry of endoprosthetic parameter assessment following bilateral TKR procedures, nor the assessment of associated prognostic factors, has been extensively investigated, and literature data on these subjects are sparse [7,9,11,17]. To date, authors have compared the staged and simultaneous TKR procedures only in terms of the main complications and treatment outcomes [8–11,14,15,20,21]. Approximately 20% of patients following a unilateral TKR procedure are dissatisfied with the treatment and decide to forego the procedure in the other knee [17]. Therefore, it is imperative to identify the prognostic factors and assess the risk of complications for the second procedure. There have been no studies in which the data from the first TKR procedure were used to analyze the prognostic factors that could affect the subsequent procedure in the contralateral knee. A thorough understanding of the various factors involved in and resulting from single knee arthroplasty may considerably facilitate the course of the subsequent procedure in the other knee [7,11,22]. Knowing the parameters of the components already implanted during the first procedure (femoral component size, tibial component size, and tibial polyethylene insert size) may considerably facilitate the planning of the surgery for the other knee joint. This would also prepare the orthopedists for potential difficulties and complications, which would greatly improve the course of the procedure and the planning of rehabilitation [7,11,22].

In our study, we set two objectives: first, assess the sizes of the implants used during the first and second stages of TKR procedures; second, identify the prognostic factors for the second procedure in two-staged bilateral TKR procedures.

We hypothesized that the size of the implants used during the first and second stages of TKR procedures will be the same and that there will be a correlation between the parameters we evaluate during the first and second operations.

2. Materials and Methods

2.1. Study Design

This study was a retrospective case series analysis of TKR surgeries performed at a teaching healthcare facility that deals with comprehensive diagnostics, surgical treatment, postoperative follow-up, and rehabilitation.

2.2. Patients

In the period between 2017 and 2021, 50 patients underwent staged bilateral TKR procedures. All 50 patients were operated on due to advanced bilateral osteoarthritis of the knee and the associated severe pain, in the absence of improvement after the use of rehabilitation, analgesics, symptomatic slow-acting drugs for osteoarthritis (SySADOA) and lifestyle modification. Study inclusion criteria were a staged bilateral TKR procedure due to knee osteoarthritis, complete medical records, and complete radiographic data. The exclusion criteria were a unilateral TKR procedure, unicompartmental knee arthroplasty, distal femoral osteotomy or proximal tibial osteotomy, incomplete radiographic records, or incomplete medical records. The study was conducted in accordance with the Declaration of Helsinki, and the study protocol had been approved by the local ethics committee.

Six patients were excluded from the study due to the lack of complete radiological documentation. Once the inclusion and exclusion criteria were applied, a total of 44 patients (24 women, 20 men) were found to be eligible for our retrospective analysis. The mean age of those patients was 67 years (range 53–77 years). The TKR procedures in all patients were performed by one out of three experienced orthopedic surgeons. The staged procedure was performed by the same surgeon in the 1st and second surgery. The surgical technique (implant insertion and placement) was identical in all cases, and all patients had identical rehabilitation regimens.

2.3. Methods

We reviewed all medical and radiographic records in order to assess duration of anesthesia and hospital stay, femoral component size, tibial component size, tibial polyethylene insert size, and the number of complications (infection, prosthetic dislocation, delayed surgical wound healing, periprosthetic fracture, deep vein thrombosis, pulmonary embolism, hematoma, cardiac complications, respiratory complications).

We compared the first and second stage of TKR procedures in terms of all the evaluated prognostic factors. To identify the prognostic factors for the second surgery, we analyzed the correlation between the following parameters from the first- and second-stage procedure: femur implant size, tibia implant size, tibial polyethylene insert size, the duration of anesthesia, the duration of hospital stay, and the number of complications.

2.4. Statistical Analysis

Data were statistically analyzed using Statistica 13.1. The Shapiro–Wilk test was used to check for normality of distribution. The Wilcoxon signed-rank test was used to compare quantitative variables. A Spearman's rank correlation coefficient was used to test the correlation between the variables. The level of statistical significance was set at $p < 0.05$.

3. Results

We analyzed the outcomes of staged bilateral TKR surgeries in 44 patients. In 29 cases, the knee endoprosthesis was implanted first on the right side. In 15 patients, the left knee was operated on first. The outcomes have been presented in Tables 1–3.

Table 1. Characteristics of data from the first and second surgery.

Variable Mean ± Standard Deviation	First Operation	Second Operation	p-Value
Duration of hospital stay [days]	6.43 ± 1.98	5.5 ± 1.69	0.211 *
Time of anesthesia during surgery [minutes]	117.04 ± 9.23	118.06 ± 8.29	0.457 *
Femur implant size	5.43 ± 1.46	5.2 ± 1.28	0.54 *
Tibia implant size	5.36 ± 1.55	5.25 ± 1.52	0.382 *
Tibial polyethylene insert size	9.45 ± 0.66	9.34 ± 0.61	0.422 *
Number of complications per patient	0.13 ± 0.34	0.06 ± 0.25	0.371 *

* Wilcoxon signed-rank test; Data are medians and 5th–95th percentiles.

Table 2. Correlation between data from the first and second surgery.

Variable	Correlation Coefficient	p-Value *
Duration of hospital stay [days]	0.281	0.0640
Time of anesthesia during surgery [minutes]	0.464	0.0014
Femur implant size	0.790	$p < 0.0001$
Tibia implant size	0.820	$p < 0.0001$
Tibial polyethylene insert size	0.379	0.0109
Number of complications per patient	0.418	0.0047

* Spearman's rank correlation.

All assessed prognostic factors did not differ statistically between the first and second TKR. A strong correlation was found between the size of femoral components and the size of tibial components used during the first and second total knee arthroplasty. The mean duration of the hospital stay associated with the first TKR surgery was 6.43 days, whereas the mean duration of the second hospital stay was 5.5 days. This difference was not statistically significant ($p = 0.211$)—Table 1.

Table 3. Details data of all patients.

Patient Number	Duration of Hospital Stay [Days]		Femur Implant Size		Tibia Implant Size		Tibial Polyethylene Insert Size		Time of Anesthesia during Surgery [Minutes]		Complications		Order of Surgery	
	First Surgery	Second Surgery	First Surgery	Second Surgery	First Surgery	Second Surgery	First Surgery	Second Surgery	First Surgery	Second Surgery	First Surgery	Second Surgery	First	Second
1	10	7	7	6	7	6	11	9	135	140	1	0	R	L
2	10	10	10	6	7	7	10	9	155	130	1	1	R	L
3	7	4	6	6	7	7	9	9	120	115	0	0	R	L
4	6	5	6	6	7	7	9	9	115	110	0	0	R	L
5	5	4	6	7	6	7	9	9	115	120	0	0	R	L
6	7	4	3	4	2	4	10	9	105	130	0	0	R	L
7	12	10	6	7	4	6	10	10	130	130	1	1	R	L
8	5	6	5	4	5	4	9	9	110	110	0	0	R	L
9	6	7	8	7	8	7	9	10	110	110	0	0	R	L
10	4	4	3	4	4	4	9	9	100	110	0	0	R	L
11	4	5	6	6	6	6	9	9	120	120	0	0	R	L
12	7	4	6	6	6	5	9	9	110	110	0	0	R	L
13	10	7	6	4	3	3	10	9	120	125	1	0	R	L
14	9	7	5	4	5	5	9	9	110	115	1	0	R	L
15	5	6	4	3	4	4	10	9	115	110	0	0	R	L
16	6	7	6	5	6	5	10	11	110	120	0	0	R	L
17	5	6	7	7	6	6	9	9	115	120	0	0	R	L
18	8	4	4	4	4	4	10	10	110	115	0	0	R	L
19	6	4	6	6	7	7	9	9	115	120	0	0	R	L
20	4	5	6	6	6	5	9	9	110	110	0	0	R	L
21	5	6	4	4	4	3	9	9	110	120	0	0	R	L
22	8	6	3	4	4	3	9	9	115	110	0	0	R	L
23	7	5	7	7	8	8	10	9	110	120	0	0	R	L
24	6	7	6	5	6	5	11	10	115	120	0	0	R	L
25	5	6	7	7	6	6	9	9	120	120	0	0	R	L
26	8	4	4	4	6	6	9	9	115	115	0	0	R	L
27	6	4	6	6	7	7	10	10	120	120	0	0	R	L
28	4	5	6	6	7	7	9	9	115	115	0	0	R	L
29	7	6	3	4	3	4	9	9	110	110	0	0	R	L
30	8	4	4	4	3	4	9	11	120	120	0	0	L	R
31	7	8	7	8	8	8	11	9	120	140	0	0	L	R
32	5	5	4	4	4	4	11	11	120	140	0	0	L	R
33	7	9	5	6	5	5	9	9	110	115	0	1	L	R
34	4	6	3	3	4	2	9	9	130	110	0	0	L	R
35	3	5	7	5	7	7	9	10	110	110	0	0	L	R
36	9	4	6	6	6	6	9	9	130	120	1	0	L	R
37	6	4	6	4	7	4	10	9	120	110	0	0	L	R
38	7	4	6	6	5	5	9	9	130	120	0	0	L	R
39	5	4	4	4	3	4	10	10	110	110	0	0	L	R
40	8	6	5	4	4	6	9	10	120	115	0	0	L	R
41	8	7	5	6	6	6	10	10	115	120	0	0	L	R
42	4	5	5	6	5	6	9	9	115	110	0	0	L	R
43	5	3	5	4	4	3	9	9	120	115	0	0	L	R
44	5	3	5	4	4	3	9	9	120	120	0	0	L	R

The mean sizes of the femoral components used during the first and second procedures were 5.43 and 5.2, respectively. This difference was not significant ($p = 0.54$)—Table 1.

We observed a strong correlation between the femoral component size used during the first and second TKR procedure (correlation coefficient = 0.790)—Figure 1, Table 2.

The mean sizes of the tibial components used during the first and second TKR procedures were 5.36 and 5.25, respectively. There were no significant differences between the two procedures in terms of the tibial component size ($p = 0.382$)—Table 1. We observed a strong correlation between the tibial component size used during the first and second procedures (correlation coefficient = 0.820)—Figure 2, Table 2.

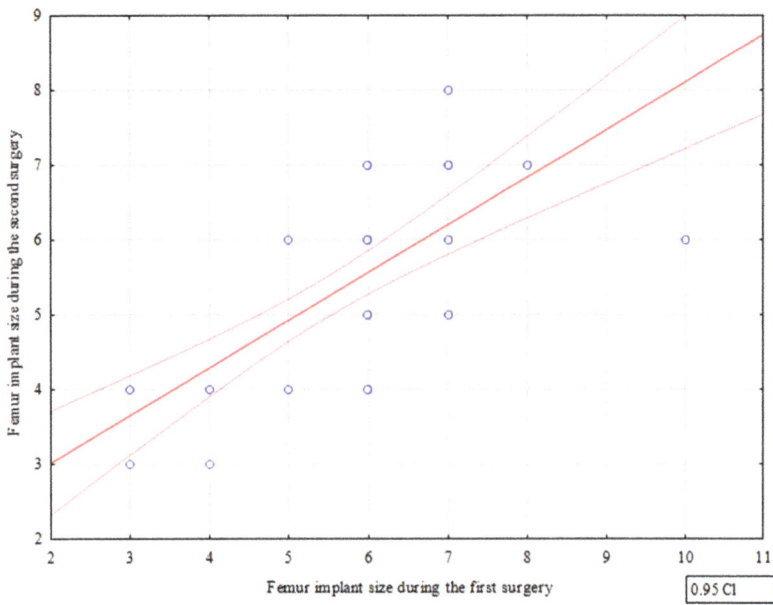

Figure 1. Correlation between femur implant sizes used during the first and second surgery.

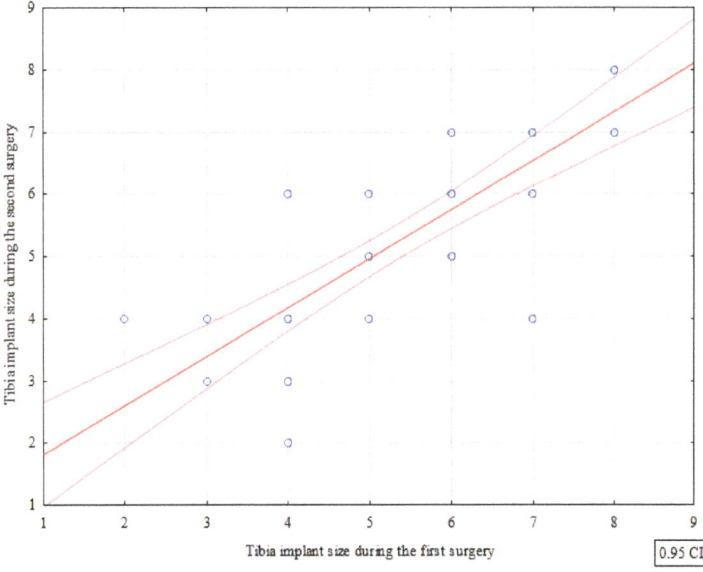

Figure 2. Correlation between tibia implant sizes used during the first and second surgery.

The mean sizes of the tibial polyethylene inserts used during the first and second procedures were 9.45 and 9.34, respectively. These differences were not statistically significant ($p = 0.422$)—Table 1.

The mean duration of anesthesia during the first and second knee arthroplasty was 117.04 min and 118.06 min, respectively. The two procedures showed no significant differences in terms of anesthesia duration ($p = 0.457$)—Table 1.

The mean rates of recorded complications associated with the first and second TKR procedures were 0.13 and 0.06 per patient. This difference was not statistically significant ($p = 0.371$)—Table 1. The first and second procedures combined were associated with nine cases of delayed surgical wound healing (due to hematoma reabsorption). In each of these cases the wound swab cultures done during the hospitalization were negative, and C-reactive protein (CRP) and procalcitonin levels were within normal limits. There were no cases of surgical wound infection, prosthetic dislocation, deep vein thrombosis, periprosthetic fracture, pulmonary embolism, hematoma, cardiac complications, or respiratory complications, either during the first or during the second hospital stay.

4. Discussion

In our study, we found no statistically significant differences between the two stages of TKR in terms of the duration of anesthesia, duration of hospital stay, femur implant size, tibia implant size, tibial polyethylene insert size, or the number of complications. We observed a strong correlation between the size of femoral components and the size of tibial components used during the first and second total knee arthroplasty.

The main purpose of TKR procedures is to improve the range of motion and pain in the knee joint, and consequently improve the motor function of the lower limb [1,4–6,12,18]. TKR procedures often help the patients become more physically active and improve their quality of life. According to the available data, 19%–30% of patients require bilateral total knee arthroplasty due to bilateral knee osteoarthritis [8,11,17]. The opinions on the surgical approach to patients with bilateral knee osteoarthritis are divided [7–13,15,17,20]. Some authors prefer simultaneous bilateral TKR procedures [12,13,15], whereas others choose the staged treatment for bilateral knee osteoarthritis [8–11,17,20].

The staged approach to knee osteoarthritis treatment may be better than simultaneous bilateral knee arthroplasty due to the possibility of identifying prognostic factors for the second procedure [7,11,17,22]. It may be important to identify and predict the risk factors for the second surgery in patients undergoing bilateral TKR procedures. Bilateral TKR procedures have not been extensively evaluated, particularly in terms of assessing the symmetry of implant size in both limbs and identifying the prognostic factors for the second surgery [7,11]. Most authors have focused on comparing simultaneous and staged TKR procedures in terms of complication rates and treatment outcomes [8–11,14,15,20,21]. Assessing the patients who undergo staged bilateral TKR procedures will help better prepare for the second stage, identify risk factors, and plan further stages of patient treatment and rehabilitation. Moreover, it will help the surgeon prepare for possible intraoperative difficulties and complications, which will considerably improve the course of treatment.

Scott observed no correlation in the level of patient satisfaction associated with the first and second TKR procedure [17]. Wang et al. compared 12 patients who underwent unicompartmental knee arthroplasty during the first stage and total knee arthroplasty during the second stage and 12 patients who underwent staged total knee arthroplasty [7]. Those authors observed no clinical, radiographic, or functional differences between the evaluated groups [7]. Warren et al. analyzed the complications of simultaneous bilateral TKR procedures and staged treatment [9]. The authors observed a lower risk of complications in the staged surgery group [9]. Another study analyzed 39 patients following unilateral total knee arthroplasty and 36 patients following simultaneous bilateral total knee arthroplasty [10]. Those authors reported higher rates of complications and blood transfusions in the simultaneous bilateral total knee arthroplasty group [10]. In their systematic review and meta-analysis, Liu et al. evaluated 73,617 patients following simultaneous bilateral total knee arthroplasty and 61,838 patients following staged total knee arthroplasty [8]. Their analysis of various complications showed neither of the two strategies to be superior in terms of safety [8]. Grace et al. analyzed 36,278 patients who had undergone staged bilateral total knee arthroplasty [11]. These authors reported that all types of complications observed during the first procedure significantly increased the risk of complications during the second procedure [11]. Our study showed a moderate correlation between the rates of complications associated with the first and the second procedure. Ahd observed complications in 13.5% of total knee arthroplasty patients [18], which was a higher proportion than that observed in our study (10.2%).

It seems important to assess the possibility of predicting the length of stay during the second TKR operation, knowing the length of stay during the first TKR operation. The period of hospital stay after surgery is important for patients, doctors and hospital administration. When planning surgery and admission to the hospital, patients want to know how long the hospitalization will last, how long they will be away from home, how much stuff (e.g., clothes, food) they should bring to the hospital, etc. The doctor, knowing the estimated duration of stay, is able to better manage the movement of patients and the occupancy of beds in the ward, and can better calculate the costs of treatment. The hospital administration, knowing the estimated duration of stay, can more accurately predict the cost of treatment and the staffing of doctors and nurses in the ward. The period of hospital stay in the population evaluated by Wang was 7.9 days [7] and in that evaluated by Ahd—12.7 days [18]. In a group of patients after TKR from Italy, the average period of hospitalization was 8.1 ± 2.4 days [23]. The average length of hospital stay in the group of patients after TKR from Pakistan was 7 days [24]. Halawi reported an average hospitalization period of 3 days among a group of patients from the United States after TKR [25]. In a group of Chinese patients after TKR, the average hospital stay was 8.3 days [26]. The period of hospitalization after TKR reported by other researchers [7,18,23–26] from different countries was similar to our results. Our study showed no significant differences between the first and second surgery of staged bilateral TKR procedures in terms of the duration of hospital stay. The correlation between the duration of the first and second hospitalization was weak.

In our study we observed no significant differences between the duration of anesthesia during the first and second procedure. There was a moderate correlation between the duration of anesthesia during the first and second TKR procedure.

We observed a strong correlation between the femoral component size during the first and second TKR surgery. Moreover, we noted a strong correlation between the tibial component size during the first and second procedure.

In our study, 29 patients had their right knee operated on first, and 15 patients had their left knee operated on first. The fact that 65% of patients first underwent right knee arthroplasty suggests a higher rate of degenerative changes in the right knee. Most of the evaluated patients had a dominant right lower limb, did physical labor, and were retired. It is possible that right lower limb dominance may have accelerated the development of degenerative chances in the right knee joint, in a similar way as that observed in the right hip joint [22]. However, the small sample size prevents us from drawing such conclusions and necessitates caution in data interpretation.

The limitations of our study were the relatively small sample size (44 patients), exclusive analysis of medical and radiographic records, and the retrospective nature of the study. Nonetheless, some other studies were also retrospective in nature [10,11,18,20,22] and involved populations of similar size [7,10,12,19,22].

The strengths of our study were the fact that the procedures were performed by one out of only three orthopedic surgeons with the use of the same surgical technique and had the same rehabilitation regimen. In the future, we are planning to conduct studies to assess the insertion and placement of the implant in detail and studies involving a larger patient population, for more accurate determination of prognostic factors following two-staged bilateral TKR procedures.

In this study we evaluated the inter-procedure similarity of sizes of the implants used during staged surgical treatment for bilateral knee osteoarthritis and identified the prognostic factors involved. This may help better plan surgeries and reduce the risk of complications during the second procedure, which would help achieve improve treatment outcomes and patient satisfaction after the second stage of bilateral knee arthroplasty.

This work will be useful for future researchers as it allows for the identification of prognostic factors when planning and executing a two-staged bilateral TKR. Orthopedists, analyzing the available medical and radiological documentation after the first TKR operation, will be able to predict the number of complications, duration of anesthesia, femoral component size, tibial component size and tibial polyethylene insert size.

5. Conclusions

We observed no differences between the two stages of treatment in terms of the duration of anesthesia, duration of hospital stay, femur implant size, tibia implant size, tibial polyethylene insert size, nor the number of complications.

We observed a strong correlation between the size of femoral components used during the first and second total knee arthroplasty. Moreover, we noted a strong correlation between the size of tibial components used during the first and second procedure.

Slightly weaker prognostic factors include the number of complications, duration of anesthesia and tibial polyethylene insert size.

Author Contributions: Conceptualization, K.K. and P.M.; methodology, K.K. and P.M.; software, K.K.; validation, K.K.; formal analysis, K.K.; investigation, K.K., Ł.T. and A.B.; resources, K.K.; data curation, K.K. and Ł.T.; writing—original draft preparation, K.K., A.B. and P.M.; writing—review and editing, K.K. and P.M; visualization, K.K.; supervision, K.K.; project administration, K.K. All authors have read and agreed to the published version of the manuscript.

Funding: This research received no external funding.

Institutional Review Board Statement: The study was conducted in accordance with the Declaration of Helsinki, and the study protocol had been and approved by the Institutional Review Board of Opole University (protocol code U)/0004/KB/2021, date of approval 17 June 2021.

Informed Consent Statement: Informed consent was obtained from all subjects involved in the study.

Data Availability Statement: The datasets used and/or analyzed during the current study are available from the corresponding author on reasonable request. The data are not publicly available due to privacy.

Conflicts of Interest: The authors declare no conflict of interest.

References

1. Sloan, M.; Premkumar, A.; Sheth, N.P. Projected Volume of Primary Total Joint Arthroplasty in the U.S., 2014 to 2030. *J. Bone Jt. Surg. Am.* **2018**, *100*, 1455–1460. [CrossRef] [PubMed]
2. Maradit Kremers, H.; Larson, D.R.; Crowson, C.S.; Kremers, W.K.; Washington, R.E.; Steiner, C.A.; Jiranek, W.A.; Berry, D.J. Prevalence of Total Hip and Knee Replacement in the United States. *J. Bone Jt. Surg. Am.* **2015**, *97*, 1386–1397. [CrossRef] [PubMed]
3. Bedard, N.A.; Elkins, J.M.; Brown, T.S. Effect of COVID-19 on Hip and Knee Arthroplasty Surgical Volume in the United States. *J. Arthroplast.* **2020**, *35*, S45–S48. [CrossRef]
4. Gademan, M.G.; Hofstede, S.N.; Vliet Vlieland, T.P.; Nelissen, R.G.; de Mheen, P.J.M.-v. Indication criteria for total hip or knee arthroplasty in osteoarthritis: A state-of-the-science overview. *BMC Musculoskelet. Disord.* **2016**, *17*, 463. [CrossRef] [PubMed]
5. Price, A.J.; Alvand, A.; Troelsen, A.; Katz, J.N.; Hooper, G.; Gray, A.; Carr, A.; Beard, D. Knee replacement. *Lancet* **2018**, *392*, 1672–1682. [CrossRef]
6. Chen, F.; Li, R.; Lall, A.; Schwechter, E.M. Primary Total Knee Arthroplasty for Distal Femur Fractures: A Systematic Review of Indications, Implants, Techniques, and Results. *Am. J. Orthop.* **2017**, *46*, E163–E171.
7. Wang, S.; Zhang, Y.; Li, J. Clinical application of unicompartmental knee arthroplasty and total knee arthroplasty in patient with bilateral knee osteoarthritis. *Zhongguo Xiu Fu Chong Jian Wai Ke Za Zhi* **2020**, *34*, 1568–1573. [CrossRef]
8. Liu, L.; Liu, H.; Zhang, H.; Song, J.; Zhang, L. Bilateral total knee arthroplasty: Simultaneous or staged? A systematic review and meta-analysis. *Medicine* **2019**, *98*, e15931. [CrossRef]
9. Warren, J.A.; Siddiqi, A.; Krebs, V.E.; Molloy, R.; Higuera, C.A.; Piuzzi, N.S. Bilateral Simultaneous Total Knee Arthroplasty May Not Be Safe Even in the Healthiest Patients. *J. Bone Jt. Surg. Am.* **2021**, *103*, 303–311. [CrossRef]
10. Obaid-ur-Rahman; Hafeez, S.; Amin, M.S.; Ameen, J.; Adnan, R. Unilateral versus simultaneous bilateral total knee arthro-plasty: A comparative study. *J. Pak. Med. Assoc.* **2021**, *71* (Suppl. S5), S21–S25.
11. Grace, T.R.; Tsay, E.L.; Roberts, H.J.; Vail, T.P.; Ward, D.T. Staged Bilateral Total Knee Arthroplasty: Increased Risk of Recurring Complications. *J. Bone Jt. Surg. Am.* **2020**, *102*, 292–297. [CrossRef] [PubMed]

12. Alghadir, A.H.; Iqbal, Z.A.; Anwer, S.; Anwar, D. Comparison of simultaneous bilateral versus unilateral total knee re-placement on pain levels and functional recovery. *BMC Musculoskelet. Disord.* **2020**, *21*, 246. [CrossRef] [PubMed]
13. Chen, J.Y.; Lo, N.N.; Jiang, L.; Chong, H.C.; Tay, D.K.; Chin, P.L.; Chia, S.L.; Yeo, S.J. Simultaneous versus staged bilateral unicom-partmental knee replacement. *Bone Jt. J.* **2013**, *95-B*, 788–792. [CrossRef] [PubMed]
14. Pfeil, J.; Hohle, P.; Rehbein, P. Bilateral endoprosthetic total hip or knee arthroplasty. *Dtsch. Arztebl. Int.* **2011**, *108*, 463–468. [CrossRef]
15. Kim, Y.H.; Choi, Y.W.; Kim, J.S. Simultaneous bilateral sequential total knee replacement is as safe as unilateral total knee replacement. *J. Bone Jt. Surg. Br.* **2009**, *91*, 64–68. [CrossRef]
16. Memtsoudis, S.G.; Ma, Y.; Chiu, Y.L.; Poultsides, L.; Gonzalez Della Valle, A.; Mazumdar, M. Bilateral total knee arthroplasty: Risk factors for major morbidity and mortality. *Anesth. Analg.* **2011**, *113*, 784–790. [CrossRef]
17. Scott, C.E.; Murray, R.C.; MacDonald, D.J.; Biant, L.C. Staged bilateral total knee replacement: Changes in expectations and outcomes between the first and second operations. *Bone Jt. J.* **2014**, *96-B*, 752–758. [CrossRef]
18. Ahd, J.H.; Kang, D.M.; Choi, K.J. Bilateral simultaneous unicompartmental knee arthroplasty versus unilateral total knee arthroplasty: A comparison of the amount of blood loss and transfusion, perioperative complications, hospital stay, and functional recovery. *Orthop. Traumatol. Surg. Res.* **2017**, *103*, 1041–1045. [CrossRef]
19. Rovňák, M.; Hrubina, M.; Šiarnik, P.; Sýkora, J.; Melišík, M.; Nečas, L. Bilateral versus unilateral total knee replacement-comparison of clinical and functional results in two-year follow-up. *Rozhl. Chir.* **2022**, *101*, 278–283. [CrossRef]
20. Fabi, D.W.; Mohan, V.; Goldstein, W.M.; Dunn, J.H.; Murphy, B.P. Unilateral vs. bilateral total knee arthroplasty risk factors increasing morbidity. *J. Arthroplast.* **2011**, *26*, 668–673. [CrossRef]
21. Gill, S.D.; Hatton, A.; de Steiger, R.; Page, R.S. One-Surgeon vs. Two-Surgeon Single-Anesthetic Bilateral Total Knee Arthro-plasty: Revision and Mortality Rates From the Australian Orthopedic Association National Joint Replacement Regis-try. *J. Arthroplast.* **2020**, *35*, 1852–1856. [CrossRef] [PubMed]
22. Kazubski, K.; Tomczyk, Ł.; Ciszewski, M.; Witkowski, J.; Reichert, P.; Morasiewicz, P. The Symmetry and Predictive Factors in Two-Stage Bilateral Hip Replacement Procedures. *Symmetry* **2021**, *13*, 1472. [CrossRef]
23. De Luca, M.L.; Ciccarello, M.; Martorana, M.; Infantino, D.; Letizia Mauro, G.; Bonarelli, S.; Benedetti, M.G. Pain monitoring and management in a rehabilitation setting after total joint replacement. *Medicine* **2018**, *97*, e12484. [CrossRef] [PubMed]
24. Malik, A.T.; Mufarrih, S.H.; Ali, A.; Noordin, S. Predictors of an increased length of stay following Total Knee Arthroplasty-Survey Report. *J. Pak. Med. Assoc.* **2019**, *69*, 1159–1163. [PubMed]
25. Halawi, M.J.; Vovos, T.J.; Green, C.L.; Wellman, S.S.; Attarian, D.E.; Bolognesi, M.P. Preoperative predictors of extended hospital length of stay following total knee arthroplasty. *J. Arthroplast.* **2015**, *30*, 361–364. [CrossRef] [PubMed]
26. Song, X.; Xia, C.; Li, Q.; Yao, C.; Yao, Y.; Chen, D.; Jiang, Q. Perioperative predictors of prolonged length of hospital stay following total knee arthroplasty: A retrospective study from a single center in China. *BMC Musculoskelet. Disord.* **2020**, *21*, 62. [CrossRef] [PubMed]

Disclaimer/Publisher's Note: The statements, opinions and data contained in all publications are solely those of the individual author(s) and contributor(s) and not of MDPI and/or the editor(s). MDPI and/or the editor(s) disclaim responsibility for any injury to people or property resulting from any ideas, methods, instructions or products referred to in the content.

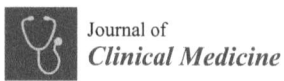

Article

Total Knee Arthroplasty in Haemophilia: Long-Term Results and Survival Rate of a Modern Knee Implant with an Oxidized Zirconium Femoral Component

Christian Carulli, Matteo Innocenti *, Rinaldo Tambasco, Alessandro Perrone and Roberto Civinini

Orthopaedic Clinic, University of Florence, 50139 Florence, Italy; christian.carulli@unifi.it (C.C.)
* Correspondence: matteo.innocenti@unifi.it; Tel.: +39-3389-361-528

Abstract: (1) Background: Total Knee Arthroplasty (TKA) in patient with haemophilia (PWH) has usually been performed with the use of cobalt-chrome femoral and titanium tibial components, coupled with standard polyethylene (PE) inserts. The aim of this retrospective study was to evaluate the long-term outcomes and survival rates of TKA in a series of consecutive PWH affected by severe knee arthropathy at a single institution. (2) Methods: We followed 65 patients undergoing 91 TKA, implanted using the same implant, characterized by an oxidized zirconium femoral component, coupled with a titanium tibial component, and a highly crosslinked PE. At 1, 6, and 12 months; then every year for 5 years; and finally, every other 3 years, all patients were scored for pain (VAS), function (HJHS; KSS), ROM, and radiographic changes. Kaplan–Meier survivorship curves were used to calculate the implant survival rates. (3) Results: The mean follow-up was 12.3 years (4.2–20.6). All clinical and functional scores improved significantly from preoperatively to the latest follow-up (VAS: from 6.9 to 1.3; HJHS: from 13.4 to 1.9; KSS: from 19.4 to 79; ROM: from 42.4° to 83.6°). The overall survivorship of the implants was 97.5% at the latest follow-up. (4) Conclusions: The present series showed a high survival rate of specific implants potentially linked to the choice of an oxidized zirconium coupled with a highly crosslinked PE. We promote the use of modern implants in these patients in order to ensure long-lasting positive outcomes.

Keywords: haemophilia; knee arthroplasty; inhibitors; loosening; oxidized zirconium; long-term results

Citation: Carulli, C.; Innocenti, M.; Tambasco, R.; Perrone, A.; Civinini, R. Total Knee Arthroplasty in Haemophilia: Long-Term Results and Survival Rate of a Modern Knee Implant with an Oxidized Zirconium Femoral Component. *J. Clin. Med.* **2023**, *12*, 4356. https://doi.org/10.3390/jcm12134356

Academic Editor: Hiroshi Horiuchi

Received: 30 March 2023
Revised: 17 June 2023
Accepted: 27 June 2023
Published: 28 June 2023

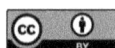

Copyright: © 2023 by the authors. Licensee MDPI, Basel, Switzerland. This article is an open access article distributed under the terms and conditions of the Creative Commons Attribution (CC BY) license (https://creativecommons.org/licenses/by/4.0/).

1. Introduction

Haemophilia is one of the most frequent rare diseases, consisting of a congenital lack of specific coagulative factors VIII (FVIII, haemophilia A) or IX (FIX, haemophilia B) through an inherited X-linked recessive condition. Each of these clotting factors plays a role in the intrinsic pathway of blood coagulation [1,2]. The prevalence of haemophilia is commonly reported as 1 in 5000 in the male population and 1 in 10,000 overall [3]. The prevalence of haemophilia A is approximately 1 in 5000 male live births, and that of haemophilia B is about 1 in 30,000 male live births [2,4]. Patients with haemophilia can have mild, moderate, or severe types of the condition, defined by plasma factor levels of 6–40%, 1–5%, or less than 1%, respectively [5]. Subjects with factor plasma levels less than 1 IU/dL are classified as severe haemophiliacs, whereas those with factor levels between 1 and 5 IU/dL and more than 5 IU/dL are affected by moderate and mild haemophilia [4]. However, the bleeding phenotype may be rather heterogeneous [6,7]. Patients with haemophilia (PWH), almost exclusively males, suffer from frequent haemorrhages and hemarthroses from childhood [8]. In the past, this rare disease was associated with high rates of mortality in the case of "noble" organ bleedings, but in modern times and thanks to early preventive haematological management (periodic administration of recombinant coagulative factors), PWH mostly complain of joint pain and impairment in the so-called "target joints" (TJ). TJ are generally synovial joints (knees, elbows, ankles; less frequently hips and shoulders) that develop synovitis and progressive deterioration on the basis of blood persistence in the articular space [9]. The cartilage is progressively damaged by iron deposition, lysosomal enzymes, and pro-inflammatory cytokines produced by the inflamed synovium, which eventually leads to subarticular bone cyst formation. Repeated hemarthroses are responsible for the development of synovial hyperplasia and angiogenesis, with further bleeding occurring in the friable and thickened synovium. Joint bleeding stretches the joint capsule and ligaments and leads to joint instability, which is worsened because reduced joint motility from pain causes peri-articular muscle weakness. In more advanced stages, the joint is grossly damaged by cartilage loss and subchondral bone sclerosis, which further limits movement and leads to crepitus and deformity. Soft-tissue swelling and effusions are rare, and joint contracture occurs from muscle retraction and bone ankylosis, particularly if the muscles are weak. The level of pain varies and fluctuates but may be severe [10]. Blood, in fact, induces a direct degenerative action on synovium and cartilage and, consequently, an indirect involvement of all intra-articular structures (capsule, ligaments, meniscus, labrum). The result is an early and severe specific arthritis, named "haemophilic arthropathy," that alters the physiological development of young subjects: the more the number of involved joints, the worst the quality of life of PWH from childhood. The haematological prophylaxis alone is not enough to prevent this joint disease, even if it is considered the most important strategy [11]. Association with other approaches is mandatory. Several conservative treatments have been reported during recent years with high rates of clinical success when indicated for early stages of arthropathy, namely muscle maintenance, braces, anti-inflammatory drugs (paracetamol, cox-1 inhibitors), intra-articular injections, and physical therapy [11–16]. For persistent synovitis, an arthroscopic treatment is often necessary, while for severe arthropathy, joint replacement is the gold standard [17–20]. However, even if joint replacement with total knee arthroplasty in PWH is an effective treatment, it is also a different procedure than TKA in patients with primary arthritis because the pathophysiology of both conditions is substantially different. The arthropathy in PWH is usually characterized by repeated intra-articular bleedings with intra-articular deposits of hemosiderin and iron, which leads to the upregulation of pro-inflammatory cytokines and, consequently, synovial hypertrophy. This process also happens after the implantation of a TKA, potentially leading to early aseptic loosening of the prosthesis components. Consequently, in patients with bleeding disorders, the results of TKA are expected to be inferior to those in patients without bleeding disorders [18,21–23]. Patients with haemophilia are at risk for complications following orthopaedic surgery for a number of reasons. The risk of bleeding may be increased because of inadequate coagulation factor replacement, the presence of coagulation factor inhibitors, and/or structural articular damage. A higher prevalence of comorbidities, such as human immunodeficiency virus (HIV) and hepatitis C virus (HCV) infection, may predispose patients with haemophilia to postoperative infection and delayed wound-healing. Indeed, previous studies have reported that patients with haemophilia who underwent orthopaedic surgery had high rates of postoperative bleeding (39%), infection (7%), and delayed wound-healing (2.2%) [24]. Historically, the results of this surgery in haemophilic patients have shown good rates of success despite the high risk of complications mostly related to intra- or postoperative bleedings (causing early septic or aseptic loosening) and coinfections (hepatitis, HIV) [18,21–23]. Indeed, the key to success in such complex patients is not just the surgery itself but also and foremost a multidisciplinary approach. It has already been reported in the literature that through a multidisciplinary approach, with appropriate pre-and postoperative management of bleeding, good clinical results and lower complication rates can be obtained. In particular, to achieve satisfactory mid/long-term clinical results, it is detrimental to treat PWH in dedicated haemophilia comprehensive care centres where modern haematological management can be employed. Nevertheless, in the majority of the dedicated haemophilia centres, joint replacements with total knee arthroplasty (TKA) have been performed using old-generation cemented or standard implants. Specifically, in most series reported in the literature, TKA in PWH has been performed using cobalt-chrome femoral and titanium tibial components, coupled with standard polyethylene (PE) inserts [25–34]. We believe that the use of more modern implants could enhance the already described beneficial action of modern haematological agents in order to obtain long-term implant survivorship in PWH.

The aim of this retrospective study is the evaluation of the long-term clinical outcomes and survival rate of TKA in a series of consecutive PWH affected by severe knee arthropathy at a single institution, performed using a single modern knee implant, which is characterized by an oxidized zirconium femoral component, coupled with a titanium tibial component, and a highly crosslinked PE.

2. Materials and Methods

The medical records of all PWH undergoing a TKA at the authors' institution in the period between 2001 and 2022 were evaluated, and a total of 124 procedures were found. The cohort flow diagram for patient selection (inclusion and exclusion) is shown in Figure 1. Inclusion criteria were subjects with Haemophilia A or B, having undergone a primary knee arthroplasty with a femoral component in oxidized zirconium, with a minimum follow-up of 4 years. Exclusion criteria were patients operated by a cobalt/chrome femoral component or other implants, patients operated by unicompartmental or revision surgery, patients with a follow-up of less than 4 years. The final study population consisted of 65 patients, undergoing a total of 91 TKA (52 right knees, 39 left knees; 13 bilateral TKA: 12 staged, 1 simultaneous), with a mean age at the time of surgery of 39.3 years (range: 23–64) and a mean BMI of 24.1 (range 21–29). All patients were male and were affected by Haemophilia A (52 patients) and B (13 patients). Overall, 20 patients had inhibitors (antibodies against recombinant factors). Four of them had a chronic human immunodeficiency virus (HIV) infection without related clinical issues, and 49 reported a previous hepatitis infection without complications. The Institutional Review Board of Azienda Ospedaliero Universitaria Careggi accepted the proposal of this retrospective study, and all selected patients were properly informed before surgery about the treatment and follow-up visits after discharge (cod. DCMT/ort12-m2-y01; date 12 February 2001).

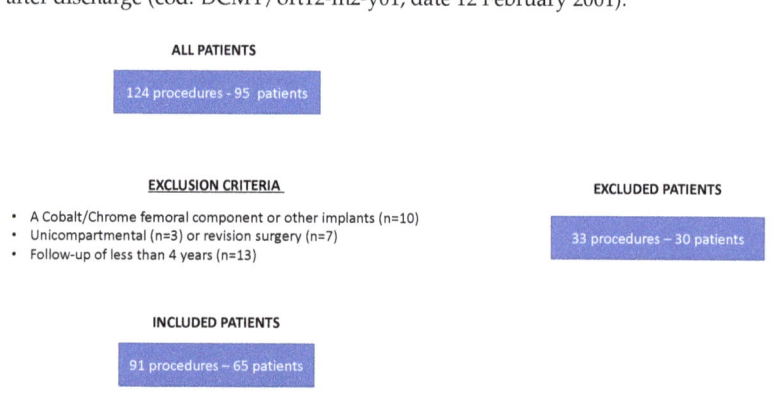

Figure 1. Cohort flow diagram of patient selection.

2.1. Surigical Technique

All patients were operated on by two surgeons over the years, with the same surgical technique, the same implant (Genesis II®, Smith & Nephew, Indianapolis, IN, USA), general anaesthesia, short-term antibiotic prophylaxis (preoperatively: 1 g of endovenus vancomycin and 2 g of endovenous cefazolin; postoperatively 1 g of ev vancomycin every 12 h and 1 g of ev cefazolin every 8 h for 24 h. In the case of B-lattamic allergy, only the vancomycin was administered; in the case of tailored haematological prophylaxis, depending on the type of haemophilia affecting the patients, infusive boli was provided 30 min before anaesthesia. A pneumatic tourniquet applied at the level of the upper thigh and inflated to about 250 mm Hg was used in all cases. The tourniquet was released after the cement had set, allowing haemostasis before wound closure.

A standard longitudinal midline incision with a medial parapatellar approach was used in all patients with no previous surgery. When present, previous scars were utilized with the normal rules adopted for total knee revision arthroplasties. An extensive removal of the anterior, posterior, lateral, and medial synovial membrane was performed. Anterior and posterior bone surfaces were left untouched in order to maintain stability in flexion. The Genesis II (Smith & Nephew, Indianapolis, IN, USA) total knee arthroplasty used is a modular implant whose main features are the presence of an asymmetrical tibial base plate to match the cut surface of the tibia and a femoral component to ensure flexion space filling without external rotation. The femoral component was specifically designed with a thicker postero-lateral femoral condyle compared to the postero-medial femoral condyle. The trochlear groove was designed to allow patellar tracking in a more anatomical manner.

All patients underwent the same rehabilitative protocol in the same facility and were discharged with planned periodic evaluations at the outpatient clinic (1, 6, 12 months; every year postoperatively for the following 5 years; then, every 3 years).

2.2. Clinical and Radiographic Evaluations

All patients underwent a clinical evaluation for pain (Visual Analogue Scale—VAS); function (Haemophilia Joint Health Score—HJHS; Knee Society Score—KSS) [35,36]; Forgotten Joint Score-12 (FJS-12) for joint awareness during activities of daily living [37]; Western Ontario and McMaster Universities Osteoarthritis Index (WOMAC osteoarthritis index) for a self-reported outcome measure about pain, stiffness and pain [38]; and Range of Motion (ROM) of the operated joint, as well as a standard radiologic study (weight-bearing full leg X-rays, weight-bearing antero-posterior and lateral views), to assess the severity of the arthropathy following the Pettersson score [39].

The Knee Society Rating System was used for patient evaluation. Two separate scores were assigned: one for walking, stair climbing, and the use of walking aids (functional score), and another for pain, range of motion, and stability (knee score). Knee scores greater than 90 points were considered as excellent, 80–89 as good, 70–79 as fair, and less than 69 as poor. The FJS-12 is composed of 12 items, measuring the patient's ability to forget the presence of an artificial joint in their daily life. For each item, there is a five-point Likert scale response. The raw results are converted to a 0–100-point scale. The highest score corresponds to a good outcome with the patient not being aware of the presence of the prosthesis [40]. The WOMAC score is used to determine the improvement following knee arthroplasty (KA). Its items are pain, stiffness, and physical function. The final score is from 12 to 96. [41,42].

VAS, HJHS, KSS, FSJ-12, and WOMAC scores were recorded at every follow-up visit, in particular at 1, 3, 6, 12, 24, and 48 months and then every 3–5 years after surgery.

Standard antero-posterior and lateral views weight-bearing X-rays were performed at 1, 12, and 48 months postoperatively, and then every 3–5 years.

The radiolucency results were documented in millimetres by the zone of the prosthesis in both the coronal and sagittal planes for the femur and tibia according to the method recommended by The Knee Society [43].

The frequency of hemarthrosis before and after knee replacement was documented.

2.3. Statistical Analysis

The statistical analysis was performed using the SPSS® statistics software (version 23.0 for Windows, IBM Corporation, Armonk, NY, USA).

Statistical analysis was first performed based on an a priori assumption of $p = 0.05$ and calculation of variance to justify that the population from which it was extracted was generally homogeneous. All data were tested for normal distribution using the Kolmogorov–Smirnov test. Finally, the Student's *t*-test was used both to compare preoperative and postoperative clinical scores. The non-parametric Kaplan-Meier estimator with 95% of confidence intervals was calculated using the Rothman formula; aseptic and septic loosening or instability requiring revision surgery were the endpoints. Survival tables were constructed using 12-month intervals. For each interval, the total number of TKAs entering the interval, the number of failures and withdrawals, the number at risk, the annual rates of failure and success, and the cumulative success rate were calculated.

3. Results

The mean follow-up was 12.3 years (range: 4.2–20.6 years). The mean Pettersson score at the time of surgery was 11.6 (range: 10–13). No early failures, no infections, and no intraoperative complications were documented. Three patients deceased during the years for clinical issues not related to TKA (11, 16, and 20 years after surgery, respectively). The mean surgical time was 68.4 min (range: 50–119). Only two patients needed blood transfusions (not related to vascular damage). All patients were able to begin the rehabilitation protocol starting within two days after surgery and performed continuous passive mobilization and weight-bearing exercises before discharge to the rehabilitative unit. At the time of discharge from the hospital, all patients were able to walk with full weight bearing, with two crutches. All clinical and functional scores improved significantly from pre-operation to the latest follow-up ($p < 0.05$). The mean preoperative HJHS score was 13.4 (range: 9–22); postoperatively, at the last follow-up, the mean score was 1.9 (range: 1–5). VAS scores improved from a mean preoperative value of 6.9 (range: 5–9) to a mean postoperative value of 1.3 (range: 0–3) at the latest follow-up. The mean preoperative ROM was 42.4° (range: 15–85°), and the mean post-operative value was 83.6° (range: 55–115°). Similarly, KSS scores improved from a mean value of 19.4 (range: 14–36) to a mean final score of 79.0 (range: 68–92). The WOMAC score improved from a mean value of 51.4 (range: 33–62) to a mean final score of 77.0 (range: 59–89). The FJS-12 score improved from a mean value of 49.3 (range: 35–59) to a mean final score of 61.0 (range: 53–81). Symptoms and functional impairments were improved in all cases, and most of the patients reported satisfaction with excellent outcomes. However, given the involvement of other target joints (mostly ipsilateral ankle and contralateral knee and/or ankle, one or both elbows) affecting the postoperative recovery, in 12 cases, the operated subjects referred to their outcomes rather as good.

From a radiological point of view, the preoperative alignment was, in all cases, in varus deviation, with a mean angle of 12.1° (range: 1–19°), reaching a mean value of 4.3° in valgus deviation (range: 0–7°) (Figure 2). No periarticular ossifications were found, and in the first 4 years postoperatively, no radiolucency or osteolysis was recorded. In 15 patients, radiolucency was observed with a low progression over time, and one case of osteolysis was found. There was a progression of these alterations in only three patients. In one patient with severe haemophilia A and inhibitors (alloantibodies against coagulative factors used for treatment), 4 years after the index operation, due to recurrent bleedings, an early mechanical loosening of both components was recorded. The patient underwent a revision with cementless stems and a higher constraint implant. In another patient, a heavy worker with severe haemophilia A, 13 years after TKA, a femoral aseptic loosening was recorded. The patient underwent a revision with an oxidized zirconium femoral component and a constrained implant with cementless stems and wedges (Figure 3). A third patient, 16 years after surgery, showed progressive radiolucency but without any mechanical symptoms, and he had still not been scheduled for surgery at the latest follow-up.

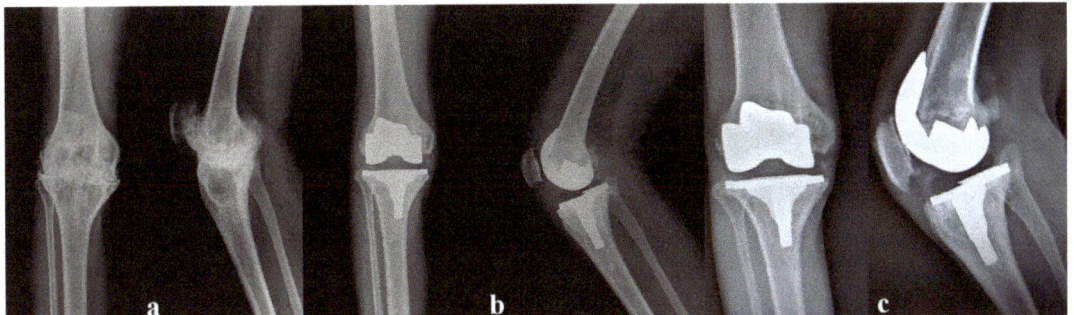

Figure 2. A 39-year-old patient with severe arthropathy of his left knee—Pettersson score 12 (**a**), undergoing a posterior stabilized TKA. X-rays at 1 year (**b**) and 16 years (**c**) after surgery. The implant was still in place without significant osteolysis or radiolucency. The patient was still satisfied, and his joint was well functioning.

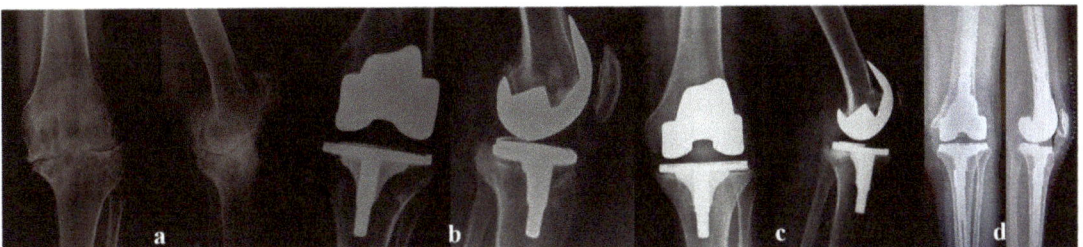

Figure 3. A 34-year-old and heavy worker patient with severe arthropathy of his right knee—Pettersson score 11 (**a**), undergoing a posterior stabilized TKA. X-rays at 1 year (**b**) and 13 years (**c**) after surgery. A symptomatic aseptic loosening was demonstrated, and the patient underwent a revision with an oxidized zirconium femoral component, titanium tibial component, and posterior stabilized high-flexion PE insert with cementless stems (**d**).

The overall survivorship of the implants was 97.5% at the latest follow-up (Figure 4).

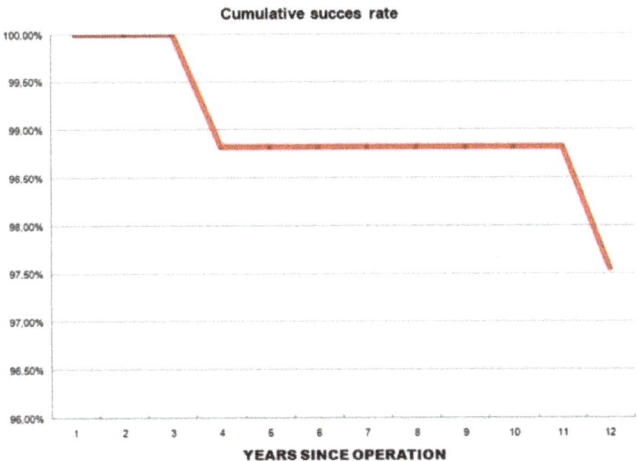

Figure 4. The Kaplan–Meier curve shows very good survival rates of the implants.

4. Discussion

Haemophilia is a haemorrhagic disease inducing damage to the joint and its structures, leading to a status of chronic synovitis and then severe arthropathy [1,8]. The result is a complete disruption of the shape and function of the involved joint in very young subjects. Therefore, TKA in such patients is often challenging due to a severely altered anatomy and bony deformity, bony defects, high levels of soft tissue contracture, and muscle atrophy, often leading to high rates of postoperative complications. However, TKA has shown positive outcomes when performed in dedicated centres, despite the higher rates of complications with respect to TKA performed for primary osteoarthritis [18,34,44]. Nonetheless, functional outcomes and survival rates of TKA in such patients have been generally reported as inferior to osteoarthritic patients. The majority of experiences reported in the literature involved the use of standard chrome-cobalt femoral components and titanium tibial plates; these materials are the same as those usually chosen for elderly patients worldwide. As mentioned, PWH typically need TKA at a young or adult age, when the choice of better-performing implants should be made. To date, the longest follow-up reported using conventional cr-co prosthesis was shown by Ernstbrunner et al. The authors reported 18 years (SD ± 4) of survivorship of 15 patients (21 knees) out of 30 consecutive patients (43 knees) undergoing TKA due to haemophilic arthropathy. In 13 (30%) of the 43 consecutive knees, revision surgery was necessary due to infection or aseptic loosening, among which eight (19%) occurred due to aseptic loosening and five (12%) occurred due to haematogenous infection. The 15- and 20-year survival rates were 78% and 59%, respectively. Moreover, the authors reported that all patients with the primary TKA in situ at the latest follow-up observed progressive radiolucent lines around the implants [45]. More recently, Song et al. described a 10-year survival rate of 97% using standard implants in 131 knees. The mid-term results of TKA in haemophilic arthropathy were satisfactory in pain relief, improved function, and decreased flexion contracture. The authors remarked the fact that bleeding and PJI continued to be major concerns for TKA in haemophilic arthropathy, and the risk of periprosthetic fracture should be always taken into account for patient education and appropriate prevention [46].

Only few experiences have been reported in the literature concerning materials with in vitro high-performing tribological properties compared to the standard ones [47–50]. Such series have mainly focused on the use of oxidized zirconium components for younger patients, as well as on metal hypersensitive subjects with survival rates ranging from 100–98.7% at 5–7 years to 97.8% at 10 years [51,52]. Oxidized zirconium is composed of Zr (97.5%) and niobium (2.5%). It is produced by submitting the alloy to heat in air to greater than 500 °C. Thermal oxidation occurs, and as the oxygen diffuses through the alloy, the immediate surface oxidizes into a Zr ceramic approximately 5 lm thick. The alloy immediately underlying the ceramic surface has a high oxygen concentration, and this gradually decreases until the alloy is just composed of the two base materials. This does not result in a coated surface treatment, but rather in a gradual transition of the material and its properties; the finished product is a stable monolithic crystalline structure. Thanks to those properties, the oxidized zirconium was one of the best-performing materials introduced during the last decades for the following rationale: the younger the patient, the lesser wear should be obtained, and the longer the survivorship has to be expected [47,53,54]. The reason for such use can be attributed to fact that the oxidized zirconium femoral component for TKA has shown promising results in some laboratory analyses, with better wear properties than CoCr when articulating with ultra-high molecular weight polyethylene causing a reduction of PE wear and secondary osteolysis and an improvement in long-term survival of knee joint arthroplasties [47,53,54].

The first report on the adoption of this material in haemorrhagic patients was proposed by Innocenti et al., obtaining very good outcomes and no failure at short- to mid-term follow-up in haemophilic subjects. The authors reported that at the final follow-up, the knee score improved from an average of 23 points (11 to 45) to 86 points (62 to 100; $p < 0.001$), the mean knee flexion contracture improved from 22 degrees (0 degrees to 45 degrees) to

3 degrees (0 degrees to 10 degrees; $p < 0.0001$), and the mean total flexion arc improved from 69 degrees (5 degrees to 130 degrees) to 92 degrees (80 degrees to 145 degrees $p < 0.001$) [55]. Later, Carulli et al. proposed a series of primary and revision TKA with the same modular implant but with a long-term follow-up. The authors reported a single failure (aseptic loosening) in a series with a median follow-up of 12.2 years (3–21) for a group of primary TKA, and 8.6 years (4–12) for a group of revision TKA with an overall survival rate of 94.7% at 15 years [56]. No other similar experiences have been reported. The most probable cause of this limited series is related to the high costs of an implant made with such materials [57]. However, in the authors' experience, higher costs are widely justified when performing a joint replacement in very young patients with a long life expectancy, undergoing surgery with more consistent costs related to the recombinant coagulative prophylaxis [58]. In the present study, we reported a 97.5% survival rate at 12-year with just three failures.

In our series, the mean postoperative hip-knee alignment was 4°. This result is related to the severe preoperative deformities and very low quality or defect of bone, both on the femoral and tibial sides. Obtaining a pure mechanical alignment using a modern implant with highly performing material and adopting the best available haematological prophylaxis, we obtained a high survival rate. It would be interesting to evaluate the outcomes of robotic-assisted TKA as reported by Song et al. in the future. In their series, the postoperative axis was mechanically neutral at 0° [46].

The present study has some limitations. The study population was not highly consistent, as haemophilia is a rare condition; however, it represents the most unique series to date reported with the use of a specific modern implant for a long-term period. No control group was considered since, from the beginning of our experience with the surgical treatment of PWH we, decided to adopt the single best-performing implant from a tribological point of view.

5. Conclusions

Knee arthroplasty in haemophilic patients is still the most performed surgery despite improvements related to modern haematological prophylaxis. This surgery has a high rate of success, but survivorship is still debated. One of the factors that the history of joint replacement has demonstrated is the quality of prosthetic materials and their tribology. The present series showed a high survival rate of the implants, surely due also to this choice of oxidized zirconium coupled with highly crosslinked PE. Thus, we promote the use of modern implants in these patients in order to ensure long-lasting positive outcomes.

Author Contributions: Conceptualization, C.C. and M.I.; methodology, C.C. and M.I.; software, R.T. and A.P.; validation, R.C., C.C. and M.I.; formal analysis, A.P.; investigation, R.T. and A.P.; resources, C.C. and R.C.; data curation, M.I.; writing—original draft preparation, C.C.; writing—review and editing, M.I. and R.C.; visualization, A.P.; supervision, C.C.; project administration, C.C. All authors have read and agreed to the published version of the manuscript.

Funding: This research received no external funding.

Institutional Review Board Statement: The study was conducted in accordance with the Declaration of Helsinki and approved by the Institutional Review Board (or Ethics Committee) of Azienda Ospedaliero Universitaria Careggi—AOUC (DCMT/ort12-m2-y01; date 12 February 2001).

Informed Consent Statement: All selected patients were properly informed before surgery about the treatment and follow-up visits after discharge.

Data Availability Statement: All data are available in clinical records of the hospital (on paper up to 2016, on electornic format from 2017).

Conflicts of Interest: The authors declare no conflict of interest.

References

1. Melchiorre, D.; Linari, S.; Matassi, F.; Castaman, G. Chapter 1 "Pathogenesis of the haemophilic arthropathy". In *The Management of Haemophilic Arthropathy*; Christian, C., Ed.; Bentham Ltd.: Karachi, Pakistan, 2017; Volume 2, pp. 1–8.
2. Franchini, M.; Mannucci, P.M. Past, present and future of hemophilia: A narrative review. *Orphanet J. Rare Dis.* **2012**, *7*, 24. [CrossRef]
3. Berntorp, E.; Shapiro, A.D. Modern haemophilia care. *Lancet* **2012**, *379*, 1447–1456. [CrossRef]
4. Bolton-Maggs, P.H.; Pasi, K.J. Haemophilias A and B. *Lancet* **2003**, *361*, 1801. [CrossRef]
5. Mannucci, P.M.; Tuddenham, E.G. The hemophilias—From royal genes to gene therapy. *N. Engl. J. Med.* **2001**, *344*, 1773. [CrossRef] [PubMed]
6. Jayandharan, G.R.; Srivastava, A. The phenotypic heterogeneity of severe hemophilia. *Semin. Thromb. Hemost.* **2008**, *34*, 128–141. [CrossRef] [PubMed]
7. Pavlova, A.; Oldenburg, J. Defining severity of hemophilia: More than factor levels. *Semin. Thromb. Hemost.* **2013**, *39*, 702–710. [CrossRef] [PubMed]
8. Mulder, K.; Llinás, A. The target joint. *Haemophilia* **2004**, *10* (Suppl. S4), 152–156. [CrossRef] [PubMed]
9. Manco-Johnson, M.J.; Abshire, T.C.; Shapiro, A.D.; Riske, B.; Hacker, M.R.; Kilcoyne, R.; Ingram, J.D.; Manco-Johnson, M.L.; Funk, S.; Jacobson, L.; et al. Prophylaxis versus Episodic Treatment to Prevent Joint Disease in Boys with Severe Hemophilia. *N. Engl. J. Med.* **2007**, *357*, 535–544. [CrossRef]
10. Arnold, W.D.; Hilgartner, M.W. Hemophilic arthropathy. Current concepts of pathogenesis and management. *J. Bone Joint Surg. Am.* **1977**, *59*, 287–305. [CrossRef]
11. Molho, P.; Verrier, P.; Stieltjes, N.; Schacher, J.-M.; Ounnoughène, N.; Vassilieff, D.; Menkes, C.-J.; Sultan, Y. A retrospective study on chemical and radioactive synovectomy in severe haemophilia patients with recurrent haemarthrosis. *Haemophilia* **1999**, *5*, 115–123. [CrossRef]
12. Athanassiou-Metaxa, M.; Koussi, A.; Economou, M.; Tsagias, I.; Badouraki, M.; Trachana, M.; Christodoulou, A. Chemical synoviorthesis with rifampicine and hyaluronic acid in haemophilic children. *Haemophilia* **2002**, *8*, 815–816. [CrossRef]
13. Carulli, C.; Civinini, R.; Martini, C.; Linari, S.; Morfini, M.; Tani, M.; Innocenti, M. Viscosupplementation in haemophilic arthropathy: A long-term follow-up study. *Haemophilia* **2012**, *18*, e210–e214. [CrossRef]
14. Carulli, C.; Matassi, F.; Civinini, R.; Morfini, M.; Tani, M.; Innocenti, M. Intra-articular injections of hyaluronic acid induce positive clinical effects in knees of patients affected by haemophilic arthropathy. *Knee* **2013**, *20*, 36–39. [CrossRef]
15. Carulli, C.; Rizzo, A.R.; Innocenti, M.; Civinini, R.; Castaman, G.C.; Innocenti, M. Viscosupplementation in symptomatic haemophilic arthropathy of the knee and ankle: Experience with a high molecular weight hyaluronic acid. *Haemophilia* **2020**, *26*, e198–e200. [CrossRef]
16. De Martis, F.; Tani, M. Chapter 9 "Lifestyle strategies and physical therapy". In *The Management of Haemophilic Arthropathy*; Christian, C., Ed.; Bentham Ltd.: Karachi, Pakistan, 2017; Volume 2, pp. 1–8.
17. Beeton, K.; Rodriguez Merchan, E.C.; Alltree, J. Total joint arthroplasty in haemophilia. *Haemophilia* **2000**, *6*, 474–481. [CrossRef]
18. Powell, D.L.; Whitener, C.J.; Dye, C.E.; Ballard, J.O.; Shaffer, M.L.; Eyster, M.E. Knee and hip arthroplasty infection rates in persons with haemophilia: A 27 year single center experience during the HIV epidemic. *Haemophilia* **2005**, *11*, 233–239. [CrossRef]
19. Goddard, N.J.; Rodriguez Merchan, E.C.; Wiedel, J.D. Total knee replacement in haemophilia. *Haemophilia* **2002**, *8*, 382–386. [CrossRef]
20. Carulli, C.; Felici, I.; Martini, C.; Civinini, R.; Linari, S.; Castaman, G.; Innocenti, M. Total Hip Arthroplasty in haemophilic patients with modern cementless implants. *J. Arthroplast.* **2015**, *30*, 1757–1760. [CrossRef]
21. Ragni, M.V.; Crossett, L.S.; Herndon, J.H. Postoperative infection following orthopaedic surgery in human immunodeficiency virus infected hemophiliacs with CD4 counts=200/mm^3. *J. Arthroplast.* **1995**, *10*, 716–721. [CrossRef]
22. Lehman, C.R.; Ries, M.D.; Paiement, G.D.; Davidson, A.B. Infection after total joint arthroplasty in patients with human immunodeficiency virus or intravenous drug use. *J. Arthroplast.* **2001**, *16*, 330–335. [CrossRef]
23. Hicks, J.L.; Ribbans, W.J.; Buzzard, B.; Kelley, S.S.; Toft, L.; Torri, G.; Wiedel, J.D.; York, J. Infected joint replacements in HIV-positive patients with haemophilia. *J. Bone Joint Surg. Br.* **2001**, *83-B*, 1050–1054. [CrossRef]
24. Hirose, J.; Takedani, H.; Nojima, M.; Koibuchi, T. Risk factors for postoperative complications of orthopedic surgery in patients with hemophilia: Second report. *J. Orthop.* **2018**, *15*, 558–562. [CrossRef] [PubMed]
25. Lachiewicz, P.F.; Inglis, A.E.; Insall, J.N.; Sculco, T.P.; Hilgartner, M.W.; Bussel, J.B. Total knee arthroplasty in hemophilia. *J. Bone Joint Surg. Am* **1985**, *67-A*, 1361–1366. [CrossRef]
26. Magone, J.B.; Dennis, D.A.; Weis, L.D. Total knee arthroplasty in chronic hemophilic arthropathy. *Orthopedics* **1986**, *9*, 653–657. [CrossRef]
27. Karthaus, R.P.; Novakova, I.R. Total knee replacement in haemophilic arthropathy. *J. Bone Joint Surg. Br.* **1988**, *70*, 382–385. [CrossRef]
28. Figgie, M.P.; Goldberg, V.M.; Figgie, H.E., III; Heiple, K.G.; Sobel, M. Total knee arthroplasty for the treatment of chronic hemophilic arthropathy. *Clin. Orthop.* **1989**, *248*, 98–107.
29. Teigland, J.C.; Tjonnfjord, G.E.; Evensen, S.A.; Charania, B. Knee arthroplasty in hemophilia. 5–12 year follow-up of 15 patients. *Acta Orthop. Scand.* **1993**, *64*, 153–156. [CrossRef]

30. Thomason, H.C., III; Wilson, F.C.; Lachiewicz, P.F.; Kelley, S.S. Knee arthroplasty in hemophilic arthropathy. *Clin. Orthop.* **1999**, *360*, 169–173. [CrossRef]
31. Norian, J.M.; Ries, M.D.; Karp, S.; Hambleton, J. Total knee arthroplasty in hemophilic arthropathy. *J. Bone Joint Surg. Am.* **2002**, *84-A*, 1138–1141. [CrossRef]
32. Sheth, D.S.; Oldfield, D.; Ambrose, C.; Clyburn, T. Total knee arthroplasty in hemophilic arthropathy. *J. Arthroplast.* **2004**, *19*, 56–60. [CrossRef]
33. Bae, D.K.; Yoon, K.H.; Kim, H.S.; Song, S.J. Total knee arthroplasty in hemophilic arthropathy of the knee. *J. Arthroplast.* **2005**, *20*, 664–668.
34. Silva, M.; Luck, J.V., Jr. Long-term results of primary total knee replacement in patients with hemophilia. *J. Bone Joint Surg. Am.* **2005**, *87-A*, 85–91.
35. Feldman, B.M.; Funk, S.M.; Bergstrom, B.M.; Zourikian, N.; Hilliard, P.; van der Net, J.; Engelbert, R.; Petrini, P.; van den Berg, H.M.; Manco-Johnson, M.J.; et al. Validation of a new pediatric joint scoring system from the International Hemophilia Prophylaxis Study Group: Validity of the hemophilia joint health score. *Arthritis Care Res.* **2011**, *63*, 223–230. [CrossRef]
36. Insall, J.N.; Dorr, L.D.; Scott, R.D.; Scott, W.N. Rationale of the Knee Society clinical rating system. *Clin. Orthop.* **1989**, *248*, 13–14. [CrossRef]
37. Giesinger, J.M.; Behrend, H.; Hamilton, D.F.; Kuster, M.S.; Giesinger, K. Normative Values for the Forgotten Joint Score-12 for the US General Population. *J. Arthroplast.* **2019**, *34*, 650–655. [CrossRef]
38. Walker, L.C.; Clement, N.D.; Deehan, D.J. Predicting the Outcome of Total Knee Arthroplasty Using the WOMAC Score: A Review of the Literature. *J. Knee Surg.* **2019**, *32*, 736–741. [CrossRef]
39. Petterson, H.; Ahlber, A.; Nilsson, I.M. A radiologic classification of hemophilic arthropathy. *Clin. Orthop.* **1980**, *149*, 153. [CrossRef]
40. Behrend, H.; Giesinger, K.; Giesinger, J.M.; Kuster, M.S. The forgotten joint as the ultimate goal n joint arthroplasty. Validation new patient-reported outcome measure. *J. Arthroplast.* **2012**, *27*, 430. [CrossRef]
41. Qadir, I.; Khan, L.; Mazari, J.; Ahmed, U.; Zaman, A.U.; Aziz, A. Comparison of functional outcome of simultaneous and staged bilateral total knee arthroplasty: Systematic review of literature. *Acta Orthop. Belg.* **2021**, *87*, 487–493. [CrossRef]
42. Küçükdeveci, A.A.; Elhan, A.H.; Erdoğan, B.D.; Kutlay, Ş.; Gökmen, D.; Ateş, C.; Yüksel, S.; Lundgren-Nilsson, A.; Escorpizo, R.; Stucki, G.; et al. Use and detailed metric properties of patient-reported outcome measures for rheumatoid arthritis: A systematic review covering two decades. *RMD Open* **2021**, *7*, e001707. [CrossRef]
43. Ewald, F.C. The Knee Society total knee arthroplasty roentgenographic evaluation and scoring system. *Clin. Orthop.* **1998**, *351*, 270–274. [CrossRef]
44. Solimeno, L.P.; Mancuso, M.E.; Pasta, G.; Santagostino, E.; Perfetto, S.; Mannucci, P.M. Factors influencing the long-term outcome of primary total knee replacement in haemophiliacs: A review of 116 procedures at a single institution. *Br. J. Haematol.* **2009**, *145*, 227–234. [CrossRef] [PubMed]
45. Ernstbrunner, L.; Hingsammer, A.; Catanzaro, S.; Sutter, R.; Brand, B.; Wieser, K.; Fucentese, S.F. Long-term results of total knee arthroplasty in haemophilic patients: An 18-year follow-up. *Knee Surg. Sports Traumatol. Arthrosc.* **2017**, *25*, 3431–3438. [CrossRef] [PubMed]
46. Song, S.J.; Bae, J.K.; Park, C.H.; Yoo, M.C.; Bae, D.K.; Kim, K.I. Mid-term outcomes and complications of total knee arthroplasty in haemophilic arthropathy: A review of consecutive 131 knees between 2006 and 2015 in a single institute. *Haemophilia* **2018**, *24*, 299–306. [CrossRef] [PubMed]
47. Laskin, R.S.; Davis, J. Total knee replacement using the Genesis II prosthesis: A 5-year follow up study of the first 100 consecutive cases. *Knee* **2005**, *12*, 163–167. [CrossRef]
48. Innocenti, M.; Matassi, F.; Carulli, C.; Nistri, L.; Civinini, R. Oxidized zirconium femoral component for TKA: A follow-up note of a previous report at a minimum of 10 years. *Knee* **2014**, *21*, 858–861. [CrossRef]
49. Glover, A.W.; Santini, A.J.A.; Davidson, J.S.; Pope, J.A. Mid- to long-term survivorship of oxidised zirconium total knee replacements performed in patients under 50years of age. *Knee* **2018**, *25*, 617–622. [CrossRef]
50. Papasoulis, E.; Karachalios, T. A 13- to 16-year clinical and radiological outcome study of the Genesis II cruciate retaining total knee arthroplasty with an oxidised zirconium femoral component. *Knee* **2019**, *26*, 492–499. [CrossRef]
51. Civinini, R.; Matassi, F.; Carulli, C.; Sirleo, L.; Lepri, A.C.; Innocenti, M. Clinical Results of Oxidized Zirconium Femoral Component in TKA. A Review of Long-Term Survival. *HSS J.* **2017**, *13*, 32–34. [CrossRef]
52. Innocenti, M.; Carulli, C.; Matassi, F.; Carossino, A.M.; Brandi, M.L.; Civinini, R. Total knee arthroplasty in patients with hypersensitivity to metals. *Int. Orthop.* **2014**, *38*, 329–333. [CrossRef]
53. Ezzet, K.A.; Hermida, J.C.; Colwell, C.W., Jr.; D'Lima, D.D. Oxidized zirconium femoral components reduce polyethylene wear in a knee wear simulator. *Clin. Orthop.* **2004**, *428*, 120–124. [CrossRef]
54. Matassi, F.; Paoli, T.; Civinini, R.; Carulli, C.; Innocenti, M. Oxidized zirconium versus cobalt-chromium against the native patella in total knee arthroplasty: Patellofemoral outcomes. *Knee* **2017**, *24*, 1160–1165. [CrossRef]
55. Innocenti, M.; Civinini, R.; Carulli, C.; Villano, M.; Linari, S.; Morfini, M. A modular total knee arthroplasty in haemophilic arthropathy. *Knee* **2007**, *14*, 264–268. [CrossRef]

56. Carulli, C.; Innocenti, M.; Linari, S.; Morfini, M.; Castman, G.; Innocenti, M. Joint replacement for the management of haemophilic arthropathy in patients with inhibitors: A long-term experience at a single Haemophilia centre. *Haemophilia* **2020**, *27*, e93–e101. [CrossRef]
57. Kim, Y.H.; Park, J.W.; Kim, J.S. The 2018 Mark Coventry, MD Award: Does a Ceramic Bearing Improve Pain, Function, Wear, or Survivorship of TKA in Patients Younger Than 55 Years of Age? A Randomized Trial. *Clin. Orthop. Relat. Res.* **2019**, *477*, 49–57. [CrossRef]
58. Messori, A.; Trippoli, S.; Innocenti, M.; Morfini, M. Risk-sharing approach for managing factor VIIa reimbursement in haemophilia patients with inhibitors. *Haemophilia* **2010**, *16*, 548–550. [CrossRef]

Disclaimer/Publisher's Note: The statements, opinions and data contained in all publications are solely those of the individual author(s) and contributor(s) and not of MDPI and/or the editor(s). MDPI and/or the editor(s) disclaim responsibility for any injury to people or property resulting from any ideas, methods, instructions or products referred to in the content.

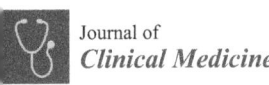

Article

Effectiveness of Robotic Arm-Assisted Total Knee Arthroplasty on Transfusion Rate in Staged Bilateral Surgery

Jong Hwa Lee [1], Ho Jung Jung [2], Byung Sun Choi [3], Du Hyun Ro [3] and Joong Il Kim [1,*]

1. Department of Orthopaedic Surgery, Kangnam Sacred Heart Hospital, Hallym University College of Medicine, 1 Singil-ro, Yeongdeungpo-gu, Seoul 07441, Republic of Korea; bigdawg@hallym.or.kr
2. Department of Orthopaedic Surgery, Chuncheon Sacred Heart Hospital, Hallym University College of Medicine, 77 Sakju-ro, Chuncheon 24253, Republic of Korea; hodge.jung@gmail.com
3. Department of Orthopaedic Surgery, Seoul National University Hospital, 101, Daehak-ro, Jongno-gu, Seoul 13620, Republic of Korea; cbsknee@gmail.com (B.S.C.); duhyunro@gmail.com (D.H.R.)
* Correspondence: jungil@hanmail.net; Tel.: +82-2829-5165

Citation: Lee, J.H.; Jung, H.J.; Choi, B.S.; Ro, D.H.; Kim, J.I. Effectiveness of Robotic Arm-Assisted Total Knee Arthroplasty on Transfusion Rate in Staged Bilateral Surgery. *J. Clin. Med.* **2023**, *12*, 4570. https://doi.org/10.3390/jcm12144570

Academic Editor: Christian Carulli

Received: 7 June 2023
Revised: 6 July 2023
Accepted: 7 July 2023
Published: 9 July 2023

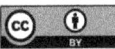

Copyright: © 2023 by the authors. Licensee MDPI, Basel, Switzerland. This article is an open access article distributed under the terms and conditions of the Creative Commons Attribution (CC BY) license (https://creativecommons.org/licenses/by/4.0/).

Abstract: The transfusion rate in staged bilateral total knee arthroplasty (TKA) remains high despite the application of blood management techniques. The potential of robotic arm-assisted TKA (R-TKA) in reducing the transfusion rate in staged bilateral surgery has not yet been investigated. Therefore, we aimed to evaluate the effectiveness of R-TKA on transfusion reduction compared with conventional TKA (C-TKA) in staged bilateral surgery. This retrospective study involved two groups of patients who underwent 1-week interval staged bilateral TKA—the C-TKA group and the R-TKA group—using MAKO SmartRobotics (Stryker, Kalamazoo, MI, USA). Each group comprised 53 patients after propensity score matching and was compared in terms of nadir hemoglobin (Hb) level and transfusion rate after each stage of surgery. Both groups showed no significant differences in the propensity-matched variables of age, sex, body mass index, American Society of Anesthesiologists physical status score, and preoperative Hb level. The R-TKA group showed a significantly higher nadir Hb level than the C-TKA group after the second TKA ($p = 0.002$). The transfusion rate was not significantly different between the two groups after the first TKA ($p = 0.558$). However, the R-TKA group showed a significantly lower transfusion rate in the TKA ($p = 0.030$) and overall period ($p = 0.023$) than the C-TKA group. Patients who undergo staged bilateral R-TKA have lower transfusion rate than those who undergo C-TKA. R-TKA may be effective in minimizing unnecessary allogeneic transfusions in staged bilateral surgery.

Keywords: robotic arm-assisted total knee arthroplasty; transfusion; total knee arthroplasty; staged bilateral total knee arthroplasty; perioperative blood management

1. Introduction

Total knee arthroplasty (TKA) is associated with substantial blood loss due to bone cuts and soft tissue dissection, often resulting in postoperative anemia and necessitating allogeneic blood transfusion [1–4]. However, allogeneic blood transfusions can increase risk of periprosthetic joint infection, immune-associated reactions, volume overload, and coagulopathy [5]. These conditions require additional medical care, leading to increased length of hospital stay and higher expenses [6,7].

To reduce transfusion rate, various blood management strategies have been applied, including preoperative hemoglobin (Hb) optimization through iron supplementation before surgery, use of a tourniquet with adequate pressure, preoperative or perioperative administration of tranexamic acid (TXA), and meticulous hemostasis before closing the knee capsule [8–12]. Recently, robot-assisted TKA has been used for accurate surgical planning, resulting in fewer bone cuts, requiring less soft tissue management [13], and leading to reduced blood loss [14]. The haptic technology of the robotic system reduces bleeding by preventing the operator from blindly damaging the posterior soft tissue when cutting through the far cortex of the femur and tibia [15]. Additionally, the three-dimensional array system enables the assessment of knee alignment without reaming the intramedullary (IM) canal, which can cause bone marrow damage and additional bleeding [16].

Previous studies have reported low transfusion rates for unilateral knee arthroplasty, with or without robotic assistance, owing to various perioperative blood management (PBM) strategies. Before the use of PBM, the transfusion rate after TKA was as high as 38% [17]. However, the transfusion rate has reduced significantly (as low as 1.9%) after PBM implementation [18]. This finding suggests that the current PBM strategy is sufficient for reducing the transfusion rate in patients undergoing unilateral TKA. In contrast, the transfusion rate for staged bilateral TKA (SBTKA) remains relatively high. Even with the implementation of PBM strategies, the transfusion rate after SBTKA ranges from 34.7% [19] to up to 96.5% [20]. This highlights the need for a new strategy to lower the transfusion rate after SBTKA. With the advantages of the robot arm-assisted system, the transfusion rate after SBTKA can be reduced by replacing the IM guide with bone pins, less bone resection, and less soft tissue damage. However, no study has compared the transfusion rates between staged bilateral robotic arm-assisted TKA (R-TKA) and conventional TKA (C-TKA).

The primary aim of this study was to evaluate the effectiveness of R-TKA on transfusion reduction compared with C-TKA in staged bilateral surgery. We hypothesized that the transfusion rate after the first TKA is not significantly different between the R-TKA and C-TKA groups but is significantly different after the second TKA.

2. Materials and Methods

2.1. Patients

This retrospective study included 167 consecutive patients from a single center who were treated by a single fellowship-trained arthroplasty surgeon. All patients underwent SBTKA 1 week after surgery by either C-TKA or R-TKA between 9 September 2019 and 31 December 2022. The first 112 consecutive patients underwent C-TKA; thereafter, 55 consecutive knees underwent R-TKA after installation of the MAKO Robotic Arm Interactive Orthopedic System (RIO; Stryker, Kalamazoo, MI, USA) in December 2021. Electronic medical records were reviewed to identify patients' age; body mass index (BMI); American Society of Anesthesiologists physical status (ASA-PS) score; preoperative Hb values; Hb values on postoperative days 0, 1, 2, 4, and 6; and largest decrease in Hb values from the preoperative stage to the postoperative stage (nadir Hb). Hb data after any transfusion were excluded from the statistical analysis because they could be potential outliers. Patients who received a transfusion after their first TKA were not included in the analysis for the second TKA, as the transfusion may have affected their preoperative hemoglobin levels prior to the second surgery. The operation times of the first and second TKAs were recorded. All patients who underwent primary TKA for degenerative or inflammatory arthritis were included in this study. We excluded (1) patients with a history of bleeding disorders with an increased bleeding tendency, (2) those who took anticoagulants for medical conditions, and (3) those who could not meet the preoperative Hb requirements (>10 g/dL) and required a preoperative transfusion. In total, 107 and 53 patients were included in the C-TKA and R-TKA groups, respectively (Figure 1). This study was approved by the institutional review board of our hospital (2023-04-023), and the requirement for informed consent was waived due to the retrospective nature of this study.

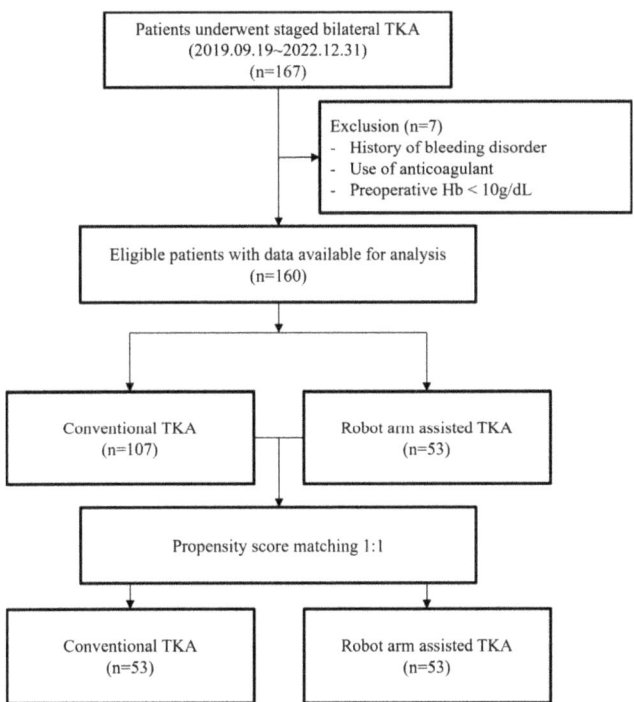

Figure 1. Flow diagram for the patients' enrollment.

2.2. Surgical Intervention

Both groups of patients underwent the same surgical protocol, with the only difference being the use of the Robotic Arm Interactive Orthopedic System in the R-TKA group. The medial parapatellar approach was used for all cases, and a tourniquet set at a pressure of 300 mmHg was applied. The tourniquet was inflated just prior to making the incision.

In cases of R-TKA, two pins were inserted into the femur and tibia, 10 cm away from the main skin incision. The femoral and tibial arrays were placed on the pins, and the bone surface was registered. After confirming the patient-specific computed tomography (CT)-based bone model using registered landmarks, the kinematic data were integrated to adjust the CT-based preoperative plan to achieve a balanced knee with functional alignment. Either posterior-stabilizing (PS) prosthesis or cruciate-retaining (CR) prosthesis (Triathlon®, Stryker, Kalamazoo, MI, USA) was implanted and final components were cemented in place.

For C-TKA, distal femur resection was performed with IM cutting guide, and proximal tibia resection was performed with extramedullary cutting guide. The femoral entry point was drilled slightly superior to the top of the femoral intercondylar notch. The tibial alignment guide was positioned parallel to the anatomical axis of tibia. Subsequently, it was adjusted to a target slope of 3° in the sagittal plane. The femoral component rotations were determined using a gap balancing technique controlled by the gravity traction method. The PS prosthesis was implanted for all cases and final components were cemented in place.

The tourniquet was deflated after the final fixation of the prosthesis, and the remaining bleeding focus was cauterized after manual compression through gauze packing at the surgical site. A closed suction drain was placed inside the joint, and the capsule was closed in a watertight manner. An intra-articular injection of 1 g of TXA mixed with 50 mL of normal saline was administered inside the capsule, and the solution was left in the joint with the drain clamped. After injection, the knee was moved throughout the range of motion to confirm the watertight closure of the capsule.

2.3. Postoperative Management

All drains were removed on postoperative day (POD) 1. From POD 2 to POD 6 of the first surgery, the patients were administered 10 mg rivaroxaban once a day as an anticoagulant to prevent deep vein thrombosis and switched to 100 mg aspirin once a day on POD 2 of the second TKA until POD 6. Range of motion exercises were started on POD 1 after each surgery, and walker ambulation was initiated on POD 2. Transfusion of allogeneic blood was indicated only when the Hb concentration decreased below 7 g/dL or 7–8 g/dL with symptoms of anemia, such as tachycardia and hypotension.

2.4. Statistical Analyses

Statistical analysis was performed using the Statistical Package for the Social Sciences software (version 28; IBM, Armonk, NY, USA). To minimize possible confounding factors, patients in both groups underwent 1:1 propensity score matching analysis. The matched variables included age, sex, BMI, ASA-PS score, preoperative Hb level, Kellgren–Lawrence grade (K–L grade), and hip–knee–ankle (HKA) angle. As the number of patients in the C-TKA group (n = 107) was larger than that in the R-TKA group (n = 53), every patient in the R-TKA group was matched to a patient in the C-TKA group. After propensity score adjustment, matched variables were not significantly different between two groups. For continuous data, independent t-tests were used to express results as means and 95% confidence intervals. Pearson's chi-squared and Fisher's exact tests were used to compare the percentages of binary data. A p-value less than 0.05 was considered statistically significant.

3. Results

Both groups showed no significant differences in the propensity-matched variables of age, sex, BMI, ASA-PS score, K–L grade, HKA angle, and preoperative Hb level (Table 1).

Table 1. Propensity score-matched data.

Characteristics	C-TKA (n = 53)	R-TKA (n = 53)	p Value *
Age, years	70.6 ± 7.5	72.3 ± 5.9	0.187 [a]
Sex (F:M)	42:11	45:8	0.447 [b]
BMI (kg/m^2)	27.2 ± 3.6	27.7 ± 3.4	0.459 [a]
ASA physical status score (1/2/3)	2/37/14	1/36/16	0.788 [b]
Preop Hb level	13.4 ± 1.4	13.1 ± 1.2	0.177 [a]
1st TKA			
HKA angle (°)	9.9 ± 5.3	8.6 ± 5.5	0.203 [a]
K–L grade (III/IV)	13/40	13/40	1.0 [b]
2nd TKA			
HKA angle (°)	7.3 ± 5.8	8.0 ± 4.1	0.473 [a]
K–L grade (III/IV)	22/31	21/32	1.0 [b]

* Statistically significant p-values are shown in bold. C-TKA, conventional total knee arthroplasty; R-TKA, robotic arm-assisted total knee arthroplasty; F:M, female–male; BMI, body mass index; ASA, American Society of Anesthesiologists; HKA, hip–knee–ankle; Hb, hemoglobin; K–L, Kellgren–Lawrence; TKA, total knee arthroplasty. [a] t-test. [b] Pearson's chi square Test.

The R-TKA group had a significantly higher nadir Hb level than the C-TKA group after the second TKA (R-TKA: 8.55 ± 0.50 g/dL; C-TKA: 8.11 ± 0.86 g/dL; $p < 0.05$). However, it was not significantly different after the first TKA (R-TKA: 9.80 ± 0.99 g/dL; C-TKA: 9.63 ± 1.06 g/dL; $p > 0.05$) (Table 2).

Table 2. Continuous Outcome Measures.

	C-TKA (n = 53)	R-TKA (n = 53)	p Value *
	Mean, std dev	Mean, std dev	
Preop Hb level (g/dL)	13.50 ± 1.44	13.15 ± 1.19	0.177 [a]
1st TKA POD 0	12.65 ± 1.36	12.96 ± 1.39	0.241 [a]
1st TKA POD 1	11.22 ± 1.19	11.12 ± 1.32	0.671 [a]
1st TKA POD 2	10.09 ± 1.12	10.13 ± 1.13	0.863 [a]
1st TKA POD 4	10.03 ± 1.09	10.18 ± 1.06	0.463 [a]
1st TKA POD 6	10.04 ± 0.97	10.40 ± 1.02	0.069 [a]
2nd TKA POD 0	10.32 ± 1.25	10.75 ± 1.20	0.078 [a]
2nd TKA POD 1	8.89 ± 1.05	9.27 ± 0.85	**0.044** [a]
2nd TKA POD 2	8.47 ± 1.01	8.74 ± 0.61	0.110 [a]
2nd TKA POD 4	9.13 ± 0.85	9.44 ± 0.88	**<0.001**
2nd TKA POD 6	9.41 ± 1.12	9.55 ± 0.71	0.487 [a]
Nadir Hb level after 1st TKA (g/dL)	9.63 ± 1.06	9.80 ± 0.99	0.405 [a]
Nadir Hb level after 2nd TKA (g/dL)	8.11 ± 0.86	8.55 ± 0.50	**0.002** [a]
1st TKA operation time (min)	90.3 ± 10.4	94.8 ± 14.6	0.068 [a]
2nd TKA operation time (min)	89.4 ± 18.5	93.8 ± 15.3	0.194 [a]

* Statistically significant p-values are shown in bold. Hb, hemoglobin; C-TKA, conventional total knee arthroplasty; R-TKA, robotic arm-assisted total knee arthroplasty; POD, postoperative day; TKA, total knee arthroplasty. [a] t-test.

No significant difference in the transfusion rate was noted between the two groups after the first TKA (R-TKA: 1.8%; C-TKA: 3.7%; $p > 0.05$). However, compared with the C-TKA group, the R-TKA group had a significantly lower transfusion rate in the second stage (R-TKA: 7.6%; C-TKA: 23.5%; $p < 0.05$) and overall period (R-TKA: 9.4%; C-TKA: 26.4%; $p < 0.05$) (Table 3).

Table 3. Binary Outcome Measures.

	C-TKA (n = 53)	R-TKA (n = 53)	p Value *
Transfusion rate after 1st TKA (%)	2/53 (3.8%)	1/53 (1.9%)	0.558 [b]
Transfusion rate after 2nd TKA (%)	12/51 (23.5%)	4/52 (7.7%)	**0.030** [b]
Overall transfusion (%)	14/53 (26.4%)	5/53 (9.4%)	**0.023** [b]

* Statistically significant p-values are shown in bold. TKA, total knee arthroplasty; C-TKA, conventional total knee arthroplasty; R-TKA, robotic arm-assisted total knee arthroplasty. [b] Pearson's chi square Test.

4. Discussion

Our study revealed no significant difference in the transfusion rate after the first TKA between the C-TKA and R-TKA groups. However, the R-TKA group had a significantly lower transfusion rate in the second TKA than the C-TKA group. The overall transfusion rate differed significantly between the two groups. Additionally, the R-TKA group had a significantly higher nadir Hb level than the C-TKA group after the second TKA procedure. To the best of our knowledge, this is the first clinical study to analyze the difference in postoperative transfusion rates after SBTKA with a 1-week interval between R-TKA and C-TKA.

Our study confirmed that robotic arm-assisted TKA procedures resulted in reduced blood loss and eventually reduced transfusion rate after the second TKA. The robotic system links preoperative CT data with intraoperative kinematic data to perform exact bone resection and execute precise implant positioning, requiring fewer bone cuts and soft tissue dissection. Moreover, the haptic boundary prevents the saw blade from cutting through the soft tissue behind the far cortex of the bone [21]. Kayani et al. [22] measured the extent of soft tissue injury based on key anatomical structures to propose a classification system (macroscopic soft tissue injury) and demonstrated that patients undergoing robot-arm-assisted TKA had decreased bone and periarticular soft tissue injuries compared with those undergoing C-TKA. Molloy et al. [23] demonstrated that soft tissue manipulation was associated with the amount of postoperative bleeding, indicating that iatrogenic tissue injury leads to increased perioperative and postoperative bleeding. Robotic arm-assisted TKA prevents iatrogenic tissue injury, leading to reduced bleeding [24,25].

Our study demonstrated that the transfusion rate after the first TKA was not significantly different between the two groups. TKA is a major surgery that is susceptible to substantial bleeding, leading to the need for allogeneic blood transfusion [26]. This led to the implementation of PBM [3,27]. Lee et al. [28] demonstrated that significant decrease in transfusion rate was achieved with oral iron supplement and tourniquet use. Similarly, Morais et al. [29] demonstrated that preoperative Hb optimization through IV iron injection, perioperative tourniquet use, and TXA injection resulted in a zero transfusion rate. This indicates that traditional PBM with additional TXA significantly reduces the transfusion rate. In our study, PBM was performed, using a tourniquet with an adequate pressure of 300 mmHg, intraoperative TXA injection, and meticulous hemostasis, before closing the knee capsule with deflation of the tourniquet. Although preoperative Hb optimization such as intravenous iron supplementation was not performed in our institution, patients with preoperative Hb levels < 10 mg/dL were excluded from our study. With these measures, the transfusion rate after the first TKA was low in both the R-TKA (1.8%) and C-TKA (3.7%) groups and was not significantly different between the two groups. This finding indicates that preoperative Hb optimization, tourniquet use, and TXA injections are sufficient to reduce the transfusion rate in unilateral TKA.

Our study also demonstrated that the transfusion rate after the second TKA differed significantly between the two groups. No study has compared the transfusion rates of SBTKA between the R-TKA and C-TKA groups before our study. In our study, the nadir Hb level after the first TKA was significantly higher than that after the second TKA. Chen et al. [30] demonstrated that Hb level continually decreased until POD 4 and started to recover on POD 5. The ongoing occult blood sequestration from the first TKA site accumulates and affects the second TKA. Recovery of Hb level continued on POD 6 but was still lower than the preoperative Hb level, and additional blood loss inflicted by the second TKA further lowered the Hb level. The preoperative Hb level before the second TKA was lower than that before the first TKA, and the value was closer to our transfusion indication of 8 g/dL, which indicates a higher likelihood of transfusion after the second TKA with even a slight drop in Hb level after the second surgery. All surgeries were performed using the same procedures and PBM with the only difference being the use of robotic system. This indicates that the procedural difference between the R-TKA and C-TKA groups is the primary factor in lowering the transfusion rate. This proves that precise bone cuts, less soft tissue injury, and use of bone pins instead of an IM guide maximize the reduction in unwanted bleeding and transfusion. However, it remains unclear which robot-arm-assisted TKA procedure contributes the most to reducing blood loss. Therefore, further studies are required.

Our study had a few limitations. First, this was a retrospective study, which is subject to a selection bias. To overcome this limitation, propensity score matching was used to match patients with similar demographic characteristics, physical status, and osteoarthritis severity. Second, the decision to perform transfusion was dependent on the surgeon's preference. In this study, restrictive transfusion thresholds were implemented, and transfusion was not administered until the Hb level reached 7 g/dL. However, in patients who were hemodynamically unstable or presented with anemic symptoms, such as tachycardia, transfusion was performed with a higher Hb level (7–8 g/dL) [3]. Depending on the operator, different decisions may be made regarding whether to observe a patient with an acute onset of anemic symptoms or to transfuse immediately. This may have led to a potential bias. Third, our study was conducted on patients who underwent SBTKA with a 1-week interval, but the results of this study could differ with varying time intervals. However, the optimal interval for SBTKA remains controversial [31–33]. Chen et al. [34] demonstrated that a second TKA performed > 90 days and < 270 days after first TKA had fewer complications. However, such a long interval requires re-admission of patients for second TKA surgery, and enduring pain and discomfort of contralateral knee until second surgery could be very difficult for patients. Johnson et al. [35] demonstrated that bilateral TKA staged at 1-week interval was safer than a longer time interval in terms of overall complication rate. In addition, 1-week interval between two surgeries was based on patients' needs of two surgeries within a single admission and surgeon's preference. Liu et al. [36] demonstrated in the meta-analyses that simultaneous bilateral TKA showed increased mortality, pulmonary embolism, and deep-vein thrombosis but lower risk of deep infection and respiratory complications compared to staged bilateral TKA. This indicates that both procedures have risks and benefits, and the surgeon's preference and experiences play huge a role in the decision of optimal timing. Further studies should be conducted to determine whether varying time intervals between bilateral surgeries result in different transfusion rates. Finally, some R-TKA cases with mild to moderate deformities were performed using the CR prosthesis type, whereas all C-TKA cases were performed using the PS prosthesis type. As the CR prosthesis type does not require box preparation, less bleeding can be expected [37]. However, Mähringer-Kunz et al. [38] demonstrated that the transfusion rate was not significantly different between the two groups. Therefore, we assumed that the effect of the difference between the two techniques was negligible.

5. Conclusions

Patients who undergo staged bilateral R-TKA have lower transfusion rate than those who undergo C-TKA. Therefore, R-TKA can be an effective strategy for minimizing unnecessary allogeneic transfusions in SBTKA.

Author Contributions: J.H.L. collected the data, performed the data collection and analysis, participated in the study design, and drafted the manuscript. H.J.J. collected the data, performed the data interpretation, and participated in the study design. B.S.C. collected the data and performed the data interpretation. D.H.R. revised the manuscript. J.I.K. designed the study, supervised the whole study process, and helped to draft and review the manuscript. All authors have read and agreed to the published version of the manuscript.

Funding: This research received no external funding.

Institutional Review Board Statement: The study was conducted in accordance with the Declaration of Helsinki and approved by the Institutional Review Board of Hallym University Kangnam Sacred Heart Hospital (No. 2023-04-023; approval date 12 May 2023).

Informed Consent Statement: The requirement for written informed consent was waived owing to the retrospective nature of the study. However, the opportunity to refuse participation through the opt-out method was guaranteed.

Data Availability Statement: The data presented in this study are available on request from the corresponding author. The data are not publicly available.

Acknowledgments: The authors thank the Medical Research Collaborating Centre of Hallym University for the support in statistical analysis.

Conflicts of Interest: The authors declare no conflict of interest.

References

1. Gascón, P.; Zoumbos, N.C.; Young, N.S. Immunologic abnormalities in patients receiving multiple blood transfusions. *Ann. Intern. Med.* **1984**, *100*, 173–177. [CrossRef] [PubMed]
2. Heddle, N.M.; Klama, L.N.; Griffith, L.; Roberts, R.; Shukla, G.; Kelton, J.G. A prospective study to identify the risk factors associated with acute reactions to platelet and red cell transfusions. *Transfusion* **1993**, *33*, 794–797. [CrossRef] [PubMed]
3. Lu, Q.; Peng, H.; Zhou, G.J.; Yin, D. Perioperative blood management strategies for total knee arthroplasty. *Orthop. Surg.* **2018**, *10*, 8–16. [CrossRef] [PubMed]
4. Schreiber, G.B.; Busch, M.P.; Kleinman, S.H.; Korelitz, J.J. The risk of transfusion-transmitted viral infections. The Retrovirus Epidemiology Donor Study. *N. Engl. J. Med.* **1996**, *334*, 1685–1690. [CrossRef] [PubMed]
5. Taneja, A.; El-Bakoury, A.; Khong, H.; Railton, P.; Sharma, R.; Johnston, K.D.; Puloski, S.; Smith, C.; Powell, J. Association between allogeneic blood transfusion and wound infection after total hip or knee arthroplasty: A retrospective case-control study. *J. Bone Jt. Infect.* **2019**, *4*, 99–105. [CrossRef]

6. Husted, H.; Hansen, H.C.; Holm, G.; Bach-Dal, C.; Rud, K.; Andersen, K.L.; Kehlet, H. What determines length of stay after total hip and knee arthroplasty? A nationwide study in Denmark. *Arch. Orthop. Trauma Surg.* 2010, *130*, 263–268. [CrossRef]
7. Husted, H.; Holm, G.; Jacobsen, S. Predictors of length of stay and patient satisfaction after hip and knee replacement surgery: Fast-track experience in 712 patients. *Acta Orthop.* 2008, *79*, 168–173. [CrossRef]
8. Good, L.; Peterson, E.; Lisander, B. Tranexamic acid decreases external blood loss but not hidden blood loss in total knee replacement. *Br. J. Anaesth.* 2003, *90*, 596–599. [CrossRef]
9. Palmer, A.; Chen, A.; Matsumoto, T.; Murphy, M.; Price, A. Blood management in total knee arthroplasty: State-of-the-art review. *J. ISAKOS* 2018, *3*, 358–366. [CrossRef]
10. Seo, J.G.; Moon, Y.W.; Park, S.H.; Kim, S.M.; Ko, K.R. The comparative efficacies of intra-articular and IV tranexamic acid for reducing blood loss during total knee arthroplasty. *Knee Surg. Sports Traumatol. Arthrosc.* 2013, *21*, 1869–1874. [CrossRef]
11. Xie, J.; Hu, Q.; Huang, Q.; Ma, J.; Lei, Y.; Pei, F. Comparison of intravenous *versus* topical tranexamic acid in primary total hip and knee arthroplasty: An updated meta-analysis. *Thromb. Res.* 2017, *153*, 28–36. [CrossRef] [PubMed]
12. Zufferey, P.; Merquiol, F.; Laporte, S.; Decousus, H.; Mismetti, P.; Auboyer, C.; Samama, C.M.; Molliex, S. Do antifibrinolytics reduce allogeneic blood transfusion in orthopedic surgery? *Anesthesiology* 2006, *105*, 1034–1046. [CrossRef] [PubMed]
13. Li, C.; Zhang, Z.; Wang, G.; Rong, C.; Zhu, W.; Lu, X.; Liu, Y.; Zhang, H. Accuracies of bone resection, implant position, and limb alignment in robotic-arm-assisted total knee arthroplasty: A prospective single-centre study. *J. Orthop. Surg. Res.* 2022, *17*, 61. [CrossRef] [PubMed]
14. Stimson, L.N.; Steelman, K.R.; Hamilton, D.A.; Chen, C.; Darwiche, H.F.; Mehaidli, A. Evaluation of blood loss in conventional vs MAKOplasty total knee arthroplasty. *Arthroplast. Today* 2022, *16*, 224–228. [CrossRef] [PubMed]
15. Khan, H.; Dhillon, K.; Mahapatra, P.; Popat, R.; Zakieh, O.; Kim, W.J.; Nathwani, D. Blood loss and transfusion risk in robotic-assisted knee arthroplasty: A retrospective analysis. *Int. J. Med. Robot.* 2021, *17*, e2308. [CrossRef] [PubMed]
16. St Mart, J.P.; Goh, E.L. The current state of robotics in total knee arthroplasty. *EFORT Open Rev.* 2021, *6*, 270–279. [CrossRef] [PubMed]
17. Cushner, F.D.; Friedman, R.J. Blood loss in total knee arthroplasty. *Clin. Orthop. Relat. Res.* 1991, *269*, 98–101. [CrossRef]
18. Chan, P.K.; Hwang, Y.Y.; Cheung, A.; Yan, C.H.; Fu, H.; Chan, T.; Fung, W.C.; Cheung, M.H.; Chan, V.W.K.; Chiu, K.Y. Blood transfusions in total knee arthroplasty: A retrospective analysis of a multimodal patient blood management programme. *Hong Kong Med. J.* 2020, *26*, 201–207. [CrossRef]
19. Vaish, A.; Belbase, R.J.; Vaishya, R. Is blood transfusion really required in simultaneous bilateral total knee replacement: A retrospective observational study. *J. Clin. Orthop. Trauma* 2020, *11* (Suppl. 2), S214–S218. [CrossRef]
20. Lee, S.S.; Lee, J.; Moon, Y.W. Efficacy of immediate postoperative intravenous iron supplementation after staged bilateral total knee arthroplasty. *BMC Musculoskelet. Disord.* 2023, *24*, 17. [CrossRef]
21. Van der List, J.P.; Chawla, H.; Pearle, A.D. Robotic-assisted knee arthroplasty: An overview. *Am. J. Orthop. (Belle Mead NJ)* 2016, *45*, 202–211. [PubMed]
22. Kayani, B.; Konan, S.; Pietrzak, J.R.T.; Haddad, F.S. Iatrogenic bone and soft tissue trauma in robotic-arm assisted total knee arthroplasty compared with conventional jig-based total knee arthroplasty: A prospective cohort study and validation of a new classification system. *J. Arthroplast.* 2018, *33*, 2496–2501. [CrossRef]
23. Molloy, D.O.; Mockford, B.J.; Wilson, R.K.; Beverland, D.E. Blood loss following soft tissue release in total knee arthroplasty of the valgus knee. *Orthop. Proc.* 2005, *87* (Supp_II), 156. [CrossRef]
24. Hampp, E.L.; Sodhi, N.; Scholl, L.; Deren, M.E.; Yenna, Z.; Westrich, G.; Mont, M.A. Less iatrogenic soft-tissue damage utilizing robotic-assisted total knee arthroplasty when compared with a manual approach: A blinded assessment. *Bone Jt. Res.* 2019, *8*, 495–501. [CrossRef] [PubMed]
25. Lei, K.; Liu, L.M.; Guo, L. Robotic systems in total knee arthroplasty: Current surgical trauma perspectives. *Burn. Trauma* 2022, *10*, tkac049. [CrossRef] [PubMed]
26. Hu, Y.; Li, Q.; Wei, B.G.; Zhang, X.S.; Torsha, T.T.; Xiao, J.; Shi, Z.J. Blood loss of total knee arthroplasty in osteoarthritis: An analysis of influential factors. *J. Orthop. Surg. Res.* 2018, *13*, 325. [CrossRef] [PubMed]
27. Liu, D.; Dan, M.; Martinez Martos, S.; Beller, E. Blood management strategies in total knee arthroplasty. *Knee Surg. Relat. Res.* 2016, *28*, 179–187. [CrossRef]
28. Lee, Q.J.; Mak, W.P.; Yeung, S.T.; Wong, Y.C.; Wai, Y.L. Blood management protocol for total knee arthroplasty to reduce blood wastage and unnecessary transfusion. *J. Orthop. Surg.* 2015, *23*, 66–70. [CrossRef]
29. Moráis, S.; Ortega-Andreu, M.; Rodríguez-Merchán, E.C.; Padilla-Eguiluz, N.G.; Pérez-Chrzanowska, H.; Figueredo-Zalve, R.; Gómez-Barrena, E. Blood transfusion after primary total knee arthroplasty can be significantly minimised through a multimodal blood-loss prevention approach. *Int. Orthop.* 2014, *38*, 347–354. [CrossRef]
30. Chen, Z.Y.; Wu, H.Z.; Zhu, P.; Feng, X.B. Postoperative changes in hemoglobin and hematocrit in patients undergoing primary total hip and knee arthroplasty. *Chin. Med. J.* 2015, *128*, 1977–1979. [CrossRef]
31. Makaram, N.S.; Roberts, S.B.; Macpherson, G.J. Simultaneous bilateral total knee arthroplasty is associated with shorter length of stay but increased mortality compared with staged bilateral total knee arthroplasty: A systematic review and meta-analysis. *J. Arthroplast.* 2021, *36*, 2227–2238. [CrossRef] [PubMed]
32. Tsay, E.L.; Grace, T.R.; Vail, T.; Ward, D. Bilateral simultaneous vs staged total knee arthroplasty: Minimal difference in perioperative risks. *J. Arthroplast.* 2019, *34*, 2944–2949.e1. [CrossRef] [PubMed]

33. Abdelaal, M.S.; Calem, D.; Sherman, M.B.; Sharkey, P.F. Short interval staged bilateral total knee arthroplasty: Safety compared to simultaneous and later staged bilateral total knee arthroplasty. *J. Arthroplast.* **2021**, *36*, 3901–3908. [CrossRef] [PubMed]
34. Chen, A.F.; Rasouli, M.R.; Vegari, D.N.; Huang, R.C.; Maltenfort, M.G.; Parvizi, J. Staged bilateral total knee arthroplasty: Time of the second side. *J. Knee Surg.* **2015**, *28*, 311–314. [CrossRef]
35. Johnson, M.A.; Barchick, S.R.; Kerbel, Y.E.; DeAngelis, R.D.; Velasco, B.; Nelson, C.L.; Israelite, C.L. No difference in perioperative complications for bilateral total knee arthroplasty staged at 1 week compared with delayed staging. *J. Am. Acad. Orthop. Surg.* **2022**, *30*, 992–998. [CrossRef] [PubMed]
36. Liu, L.; Liu, H.; Zhang, H.; Song, J.; Zhang, L. Bilateral total knee arthroplasty: Simultaneous or staged? A systematic review and meta-analysis. *Medicine* **2019**, *98*, e15931. [CrossRef] [PubMed]
37. Cankaya, D.; Ozkurt, B.; Aydin, C.; Tabak, A.Y. No difference in blood loss between posterior-cruciate-ligament-retaining and posterior-cruciate-ligament-stabilized total knee arthroplasties. *Knee Surg. Sports Traumatol. Arthrosc.* **2014**, *22*, 1865–1869. [CrossRef] [PubMed]
38. Mähringer-Kunz, A.; Efe, T.; Fuchs-Winkelmann, S.; Schüttler, K.F.; Paletta, J.R.; Heyse, T.J. Bleeding in TKA: Posterior stabilized vs. cruciate retaining. *Arch. Orthop. Trauma Surg.* **2015**, *135*, 867–870. [CrossRef]

Disclaimer/Publisher's Note: The statements, opinions and data contained in all publications are solely those of the individual author(s) and contributor(s) and not of MDPI and/or the editor(s). MDPI and/or the editor(s) disclaim responsibility for any injury to people or property resulting from any ideas, methods, instructions or products referred to in the content.

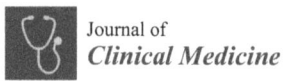

Article

Characteristics of Preoperative Arteriosclerosis Evaluated by Cardio-Ankle Vascular Index in Patients with Osteoarthritis before Total Knee Arthroplasty

Yoshinori Ishii [1,*], Hideo Noguchi [1], Junko Sato [1], Ikuko Takahashi [1], Hana Ishii [2], Ryo Ishii [3], Kei Ishii [4], Kai Ishii [5] and Shin-ichi Toyabe [6]

1. Ishii Orthopaedic & Rehabilitation Clinic, Saitama 361-0037, Japan; hid_166super@mac.com (H.N.); jun-sato@hotmail.co.jp (J.S.); itakahashi110@gmail.com (I.T.)
2. School of Plastic Surgery, Kanazawa Medical University, Ishikawa 920-0253, Japan; hanamed12@gmail.com
3. Shinshu University Hospital, Nagano 390-8621, Japan; kmuyakyu@gmail.com
4. Iwate Prefectural Chuo Hospital, Iwate 020-0066, Japan; kei141.0852@gmail.com
5. Kouseiren Takaoka Hospital, Toyama 933-8555, Japan; kai.nd1209@live.com
6. Niigata University Crisis Management Office, Niigata University Hospital, Niigata University Graduate School of Medical and Dental Sciences, Niigata 951-8520, Japan; toyabe@med.niigata-u.ac.jp
* Correspondence: ishii@sakitama.or.jp; Tel.: +81-11-81-485-55-3519; Fax: +81-11-81-485-55-3520

Abstract: Purpose: Cardiovascular disease (CVD) is a major risk factor for mortality in patients with osteoarthritis, and comorbidities increase postoperative complications after total knee arthroplasty (TKA). Arteriosclerosis plays a main role in hemodynamic dysfunction and CVD; however, arteriosclerosis has not been preoperatively evaluated before TKA using the cardio-ankle vascular index (CAVI). In this study, we evaluated the degree of preoperative arteriosclerosis using the CAVI in patients undergoing TKA, as well as its correlations with several preoperative patient factors. Methods: Arteriosclerosis was evaluated in 209 consecutive patients (251 knees) with osteoarthritis who underwent TKA at our institution between May 2011 and June 2022. The CAVI was measured in the supine position 1 day before TKA, and the correlations between the CAVI and several clinical factors were analyzed. Results: The CAVI was normal in 62 knees (25%), borderline in 71 knees (28%), and abnormal in 118 knees (47%). Univariate analysis revealed a moderate positive correlation between preoperative CAVI and age ($r = 0.451$, $p < 0.001$) and a weak negative correlation between preoperative CAVI and body weight ($r = -0.306$, $p < 0.001$) and body mass index (BMI) ($r = -0.319$, $p < 0.001$). Multivariate analysis showed that age ($\beta = 0.349$, $p < 0.001$) and BMI ($\beta = -0.235$, $p < 0.001$) were significantly correlated with preoperative CAVI. Conclusion: Arteriosclerosis should be carefully managed intraoperatively and postoperatively in patients with osteoarthritis undergoing TKA, particularly in older patients and patients with a low BMI.

Keywords: osteoarthritis; arteriosclerosis; cardio-ankle vascular index; total knee arthroplasty; age; body mass index

Citation: Ishii, Y.; Noguchi, H.; Sato, J.; Takahashi, I.; Ishii, H.; Ishii, R.; Ishii, K.; Ishii, K.; Toyabe, S.-i. Characteristics of Preoperative Arteriosclerosis Evaluated by Cardio-Ankle Vascular Index in Patients with Osteoarthritis before Total Knee Arthroplasty. *J. Clin. Med.* 2023, 12, 4685. https://doi.org/10.3390/jcm12144685

Academic Editor: Christian Carulli

Received: 20 June 2023
Revised: 8 July 2023
Accepted: 11 July 2023
Published: 14 July 2023

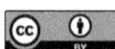

Copyright: © 2023 by the authors. Licensee MDPI, Basel, Switzerland. This article is an open access article distributed under the terms and conditions of the Creative Commons Attribution (CC BY) license (https://creativecommons.org/licenses/by/4.0/).

1. Introduction

Patients with osteoarthritis experience walking difficulty due to swelling, pain, or stiffness in the affected joints [1]. This leads to decreased mobility, which is a cardiovascular (CV) risk factor [2]. Kendzerska et al. [2] concluded that increased attention to the management of osteoarthritis with the aim of improving mobility may lead to a reduction in CV events. Patients with osteoarthritis of the hip and knee have a higher risk of mortality than does the general population [3], and major risk factors reported by Nüesch et al. [3] include pre-existing diabetes, cancer, CV disease (CVD), and gait disturbance. The authors concluded that the management of patients with osteoarthritis and gait disturbance should focus not only on increasing physical activity but also on the effective treatment of CV risk factors and comorbidities. Arteriosclerosis (AS) plays a main role in hemodynamic dysfunction characterized by excessive pulsation, i.e., CVD [4]. Therefore, it is important to verify the progression of AS in patients with osteoarthritis. Although no studies to date have provided conclusive results, several systematic multicenter analyses have revealed correlations between AS and osteoarthritis [5–7]. The cardio-ankle vascular index (CAVI) is a marker of arterial stiffness based on stiffness parameter β and was developed in 2004 [8]. Measurement of the CAVI is simple and well-standardized, and its reproducibility and accuracy are acceptable [4]. Thus, the CAVI is a promising diagnostic tool for evaluating arterial stiffness [9]. In addition, a recent meta-analysis of the Asian population confirmed that the CAVI is an independent risk factor for CVD [10].

Total knee arthroplasty (TKA) is a reliable procedure for pain relief and functional improvement in patients with knee osteoarthritis [11–13]. Comorbidities, rather than age, are responsible for the increase in postoperative morbidity after TKA, and preoperative risk assessment should be optimized to reduce complications [14]. To the authors' knowledge, however, the preoperative evaluation of AS (one of the comorbidities in patients undergoing TKA) using the CAVI has not been performed. The preoperative assessment of the severity of AS in patients with osteoarthritis is beneficial to verify the correlations between AS and osteoarthritis and to take measures against AS during the TKA procedure and in the early postoperative period.

Therefore, the purpose of the present study was to evaluate the CAVI in patients with osteoarthritis before TKA and to identify influential factors. The clinical significance of this study is that it will clarify the correlation between knee osteoarthritis requiring TKA and the degree of preoperative AS while identifying those patients for whom AS interventions are necessary before TKA.

2. Materials and Methods

This prospective study was conducted at our institute from May 2011 to June 2022. Informed consent was obtained from all patients after a discussion of the study, which included a description of the protocol and possible CAVI measurement-related complications. The institutional review board approved the study before commencement. In total, 209 consecutive patients (251 knees) undergoing TKA were investigated. The preoperative diagnosis indicating TKA was primary osteoarthritis. Patients who had undergone revision arthroplasties or previous tibial osteotomies and patients with rheumatoid arthritis were excluded.

The following preoperative factors were analyzed: sex, age, body mass index (BMI), body weight (BW), blood cholesterol level, blood triglyceride level, smoking history, diabetes mellitus, hypertension (all of which have been previously reported to affect the CAVI [15–19]), body height, American Society of Anesthesiologists (ASA) grade [20], Kellgren–Lawrence (KL) classification [21], Hospital for Special Surgery (HSS) knee score [22], and knee range of motion. The severity of knee osteoarthritis was radiographically scaled using the KL grading system as follows: very mild (grade I), mild (grade II), moderate (grade III), and severe (grade IV) [21]. All TKAs were evaluated using the HSS knee score [22], which is not a patient-derived score but a physician-derived score. The HSS knee score is divided into seven categories: pain, function, range of motion, muscle strength, flexion deformity, instability, and subtraction.

2.1. Measurement of CAVI

The CAVI was measured by the standardized method using a noninvasive blood pressure-independent device (VaSera VS-1 3000; Fukuda Denshi, Tokyo, Japan) [23] at 1 day before surgery. The examination was performed in a room in which a standard temperature was maintained. In brief, the CAVI measurements were performed in the supine position. Cuffs were applied bilaterally to the upper arms and lower legs superior to the ankles. Electrocardiogram electrodes and a microphone were placed on both wrists, both ankles, and the sternum. An electrocardiogram, blood pressure, and waveforms of the brachial and ankle arteries were measured (Figure 1). The pulse wave velocity (PWV) was calculated by measuring the time between the closing sound of the aortic valve, the notch of the brachial pulse wave, and the ankle pulse wave. Using this value, the CAVI was calculated by the following equation: CAVI = $2\rho/$(systolic blood pressure − diastolic blood pressure) × (ln systolic blood pressure/diastolic blood pressure) × PWV^2, where ρ = blood viscosity. The CAVI cutoff values of 8 and 9 were proposed by the Japan Society for Vascular Failure (<8, normal; 8 to <9, borderline; and ≥9, abnormal) [24].

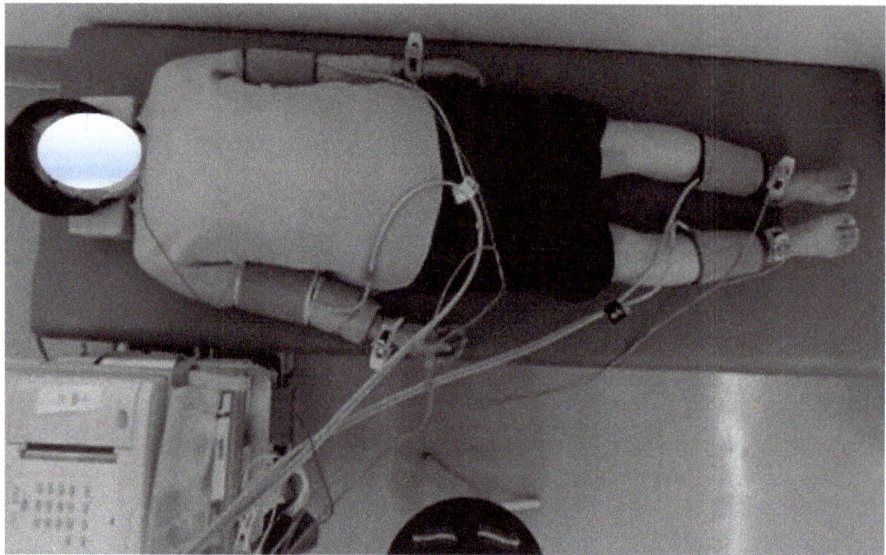

Figure 1. Measurement of the cardio-ankle vascular index (CAVI). First, the distance from the origin of the aorta to the ankle was measured with the patient lying in the supine position on a bed at rest. Next, cuffs used to measure blood pressure were wrapped around the right and left upper arms as well as the right and left ankle joints, and a microphone that detects heart sounds was attached to the chest. At the flip of a switch, the instrument automatically measured the pulse wave and blood pressure and calculated the CAVI. The entire measurement took about 15 min, and the test was painless.

2.2. Reproducibility

To eliminate interobserver variability, all tests were performed by the same observer. Test–retest reliability was assessed using intraclass correlation coefficients, which were performed by the same observer on 30 patients at 1-month intervals. The intraclass correlation coefficient was calculated to be 0.788 (0.603–0.898).

2.3. Statistical Analysis

Because data for certain variables did not pass the Kolmogorov–Smirnov normality test or Shapiro–Wilk normality test, we used the non-parametric Wilcoxon rank sum test and Spearman's rank correlation test. Univariate and multivariate analyses were performed to examine factors related to the preoperative CAVI. Spearman's rank correlation coefficient was used to investigate the association between the preoperative CAVI and each variable. The strength of the correlation of the rank coefficients was defined as strong (0.70–1.00), moderate (0.40–0.69), or weak (0.20–0.39). The Wilcoxon rank sum test was used to determine differences in the CAVI between two groups. Multiple linear regression analysis was performed to identify variables significantly associated with the preoperative CAVI. Multiple linear regression models were constructed by entering all variables shown in Table 1, and variables significantly associated with the preoperative CAVI were selected using the stepwise selection method. In all tests, a p value of <0.05 was considered significant. All statistical analyses were performed using IBM SPSS Statistics version 23 (IBM Japan, Tokyo, Japan). The values are expressed as median (25th percentile, 75th percentile) (minimum–maximum).

Table 1. Patients' backgrounds.

Variables (Patients/Knees)	209/251
Sex (male vs. female)	42/209
Body height (cm)	150 (146, 155)
Body weight (kg)	59 (53, 67)
Body mass index (kg/m^2)	26 (24, 28)
Age (years)	74 (69, 79), M; 76 (70, 81), F; 73 (69, 78)
Smoking history (yes/no)	12/239
Diabetes mellitus (yes/no)	35/216
Hypertension (yes/no)	164/87
Preop. blood cholesterol level (mg/dL)	205 (185, 234)
Preop. blood triglyceride level (mg/dL)	132 (101, 175)
Knee flexion (Preop) (°)	115 (100, 125)
Knee extension (Preop) (°)	−10.0 (−15, −5)
Knee range of motion (Preop) (°)	100 (90, 120)
HSS score [22]	45 (37, 52)
Kellgren–Laurence classification [21]	I 0, II 0, III 10, IV 241
ASA grade [20]	I 34, II 217

Data are presented as n or median (25th percentile, 75th percentile). M, male; F, female; Preop, preoperative; HSS, Hospital for Special Surgery; ASA, American Society of Anesthesiologists.

3. Results

The patients' clinical backgrounds are summarized in Table 1. The preoperative CAVIs in the operative and contralateral knee were 8.9 (8.0, 9.7) (3.1–12.0) and 8.9 (8.0, 9.7) (3.1–13.2), respectively. In accordance with the cutoff values of the CAVI, the CAVI was defined as normal in 62 (25%) knees, borderline in 71 (28%), and abnormal in 118 (47%) (Figures 2 and 3).

According to the univariate analyses using Spearman's correlation coefficient for continuous variables, there was a moderate positive correlation between age and the preoperative CAVI (r = 0.451, $p < 0.001$) (Figure 2) and a weak negative correlation between BW/BMI and the CAVI (r = −0.306/−0.319, $p < 0.001/p < 0.001$) (Table 2) (Figure 3). However, the other study variables (both continuous and discrete) showed no significant correlations (Tables 2 and 3).

Table 2. Correlations between preoperative CAVI and study variables by Spearman's rank correlation coefficient.

Variables	r	p
Pre CAVI (contra-lateral)	0.901	$p < 0.001$
Age	0.451	$p < 0.001$
Body height	−0.049	0.442
Body weight	**−0.307**	**$p < 0.001$**
Body mass index	**−0.322**	**$p < 0.001$**
HSS score [22]	−0.089	$p = 0.160$
Flexion	0.069	0.275
Extension	−0.096	0.130
ROM	0.024	0.700
Cholesterol	0.025	0.695
Triglyceride	0.044	0.484

Values in bold indicate statistically significant values. CAVI, cardio-ankle vascular index; HSS, Hospital for Special Surgery; ROM, range of motion.

Table 3. Comparison of preoperative CAVI in discrete study variables by Wilcoxon rank sum test.

Variables Knees (Patients)	Median (Interquartile) Range		p
Sex: male/female 42 (36) (17%)/209 (173) (83%)	Male; 9.1 (8.4, 9.7) 6.4–11.9	Female; 8.8 (7.8, 9.6) 3.1–12.0	0.223
KL [21]: III 10 (4%), IV 241 (96%)	III; 9.1 (8.0, 9.4) 6.9–10.6	IV; 8.8 (8.0, 9.7) 3.1–12.0	0.950
ASA [20]: I 34 (14%), II 217 (86%)	I; 8.9 (7.8, 9.9) 6.2–11.6	II; 8.9 (8.0, 9.6) 3.1–12	0.691
Smoking history: yes 12 (5%)	Yes; 8.8 (8.5, 9.3) 6.7–10.4	No; 8.9 (8.0, 9.7) 3.1–12.0	0.987
Hypertension: yes 164 (65%)	Yes; 9.0 (8.1, 9.7) 3.1–12.0	No; 8.7 (7.7, 9.6) 6.2–11.7	0.078
Diabetes mellitus: yes 35 (14%)	Yes; 8.9 (8.0, 9.5) 7.0–11.6	No; 8.8 (8.0, 9.7) 3.1–12.0	0.962

Data are presented as n or median (25th percentile, 75th percentile) (minimum–maximum). CAVI, cardio-ankle vascular index; KL, Kellgren–Lawrence classification; ASA, American Society of Anesthesiologists.

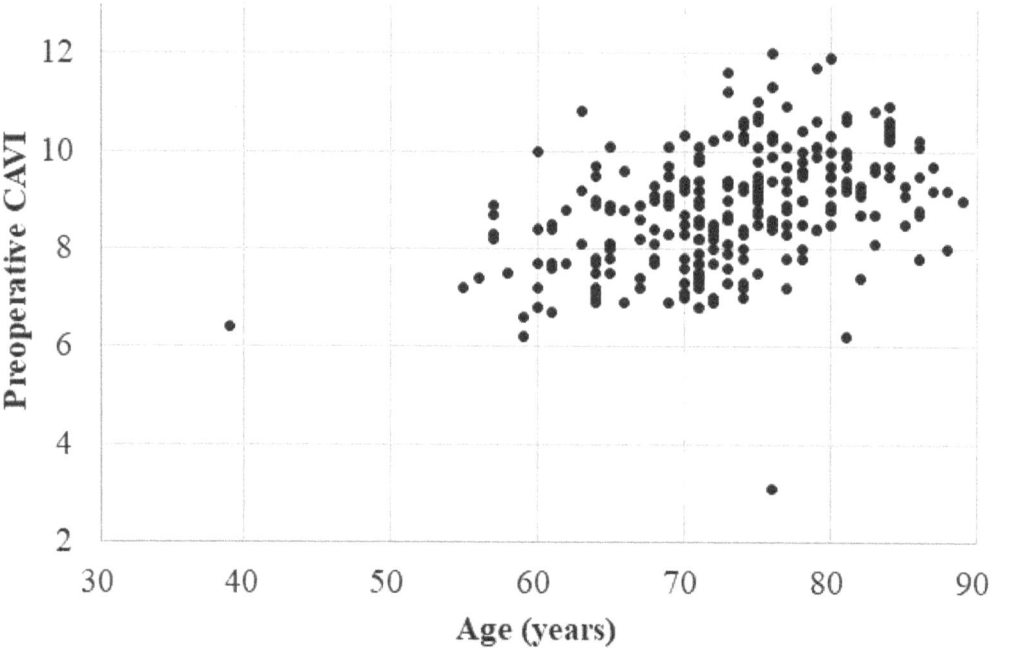

Figure 2. Scatterplot of preoperative CAVI and age. The horizontal axis indicates patient age, and the vertical axis indicates the preoperative CAVI. Correlation equation: CAVI = 4.064 + 0.065 × AGE. CAVI, cardio-ankle vascular index.

Finally, based on the multivariate analyses using multiple linear regression analysis with stepwise variable selection, the age and BMI were significantly correlated with the preoperative CAVI (β = 0.349, p < 0.001 and β = −0.235, p < 0.001, respectively) (Table 4).

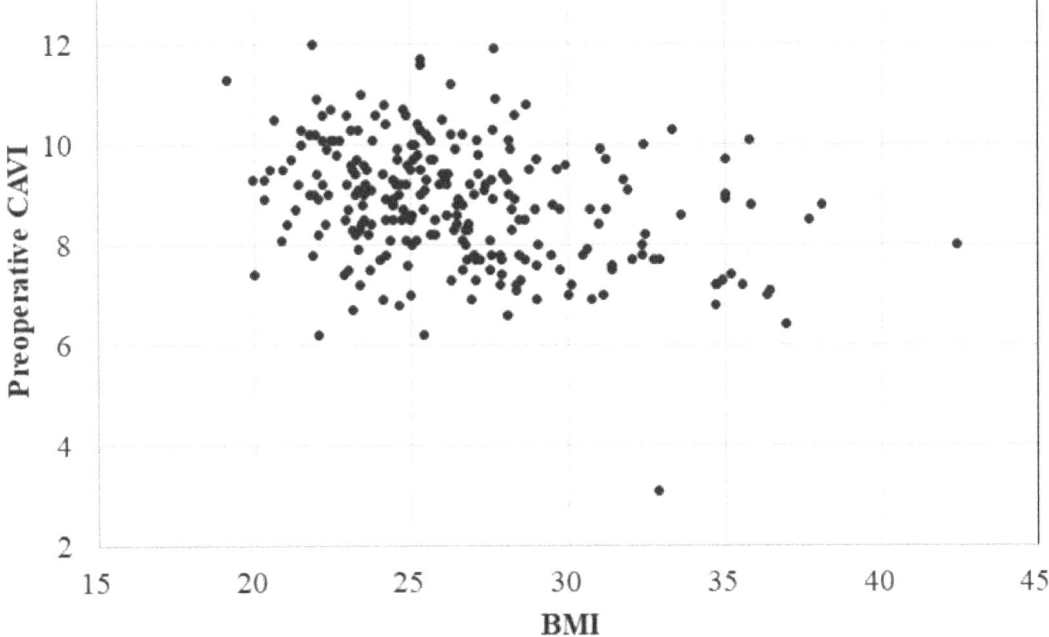

Figure 3. Scatterplot of preoperative CAVI and BMI. The horizontal axis indicates the BMI, and the vertical axis indicates the preoperative CAVI. Correlation equation: CAVI = 11.445 − 0.099 × BMI, CAVI, cardio-ankle vascular index; BMI, body mass index.

Table 4. Results of multiple regression analysis using stepwise variable selection.

	B	S.E.	β	Sig.	95% CI	
(Constant)	6.699	0.920		<0.001	4.887	8.512
Age	0.055	0.009	0.349	<0.001	0.035	0.073
BMI	−0.072	0.015	−0.235	<0.001	−0.107	−0.037

BMI, body mass index; S.E., standard error; Sig., significance; CI, confidence interval.

4. Discussion

This study produced two important findings. First, we found a positive correlation of the preoperative CAVI (or AS) with age and a negative correlation of the CAVI with BMI and BW. Second, there were no correlations between AS and factors previously reported to impact AS, such as sex [15–17], hypertension [15–17], diabetes mellitus [15,16], the triglyceride level [17,18], the cholesterol level [16,17], and smoking [15,19].

Shirai et al. [23] reported that worsening of the CAVI with age occurs at a rate of 0.5 per decade in the Japanese general population according to the linear regression equation. If we calculate the CAVI using the same linear regression equation (5.43 + 0.053x age for males and CAVI = 5.34 + 0.049x age for females) in the general population, the equation performed separately for males and females in the present study would yield a CAVI of 9.5 for males because they were 76 years old and 8.9 for females because they were 73 years old. Thus, the median CAVI of 8.9 at the age of 74 years, including both males and females with end-stage osteoarthritis in this study, is comparable to that in the general population. Finally, the multivariate analysis showed that age was the strongest factor affecting AS in patients with osteoarthritis.

Another finding of this study is that the BW and BMI were negatively correlated with CAVI, suggesting that some muscle mass and fat are necessary for maintenance of the

CAVI or prevention of its deterioration. Two previous studies support our results. Park et al. [25] stated that low muscle mass is independently and significantly associated with an increased CAVI and should be considered when assessing the risk of atherosclerosis in asymptomatic patients. Nagayama et al. [16] speculated that systemic accumulation of adipose tissue may itself lead to a linear reduction in arterial stiffness in non-obese and obese patients without metabolic disorders. The significant correlation of the BMI with the CAVI in the present study also suggests that proper muscle mass and moderate adipose tissue may have a positive effect on AS. Thus, the present study may suggest that the patient characteristic that warrants caution regarding AS during and immediately after TKA is a lean body habitus (low BMI) in patients of advanced age.

In the present analysis, the CAVI was not correlated with factors other than age, BW, and BMI, as previously reported [15–19]. This result does not mean that preoperative complications and comorbidities do not impact the CAVI, but the fact that all patients in this study had an ASA of I or II suggests that their clinical condition had little impact on the CAVI or that they were successfully treated. This is a reasonable assumption given that a preoperative ASA score of ≥ 3 has been reported to be an independent risk factor for serious adverse events after TKA [26]. The finding that less than half of the patients (47%) had a preoperative CAVI of ≥ 9.0 and were judged abnormal [23] seems to corroborate the conclusion that preoperative comorbidities were not severe in this study.

Finally, there was no correlation between the preoperative CAVI and the degree of osteoarthritis by the KL classification [21] or HSS knee score [22], suggesting that increased pain and decreased walking ability in association with the severity of osteoarthritis may not play a major role in the progression of the CAVI or AS. However, considering previous reports of higher all-cause mortality in patients with osteoarthritis than in the general population [3] and reports that the severity of osteoarthritis-related disability is associated with significantly increased all-cause mortality and serious CVD events [27] (also demonstrating the association between osteoarthritis and comorbidities, including AS), osteoarthritis may play a supporting role in amplifying AS-aggravating factors such as diabetes, hypertension, and hyperlipidemia.

This study had three limitations. First, this study was conducted at a single institution; thus, the distribution of the patients was skewed, with a disproportionate number of males and females and only mild comorbidity in patients with ASA classifications of I and II. Future studies should analyze patients with various backgrounds at multiple centers. Second, the analysis was limited to Japanese patients. Interestingly, several studies have suggested differences in the mean CAVI among countries [28–30]. Therefore, multinational studies should be performed to verify the validity of our results. Third, the HSS clinical scores, including activity assessment [22], were evaluated prior to TKA surgery, but specific measures of activity, such as the number of steps, were not evaluated. Specific step counts are generally confirmed using pedometers. Despite these limitations, the main strength of this study is that it is the first report of AS evaluation using the CAVI with a focus on patients with osteoarthritis. Furthermore, not only do the results of this study clarify the patient population that is likely to require AS countermeasures intraoperatively and immediately postoperatively, but the results also make it possible to confirm the spillover effects of TKA on AS if CAVI trends after TKA surgery are observed over the middle to long term.

5. Conclusions

The results of this study suggest the following:

1. The patient characteristics that warrant special attention to AS intraoperatively and immediately postoperatively are a lean body habitus (low BMI) and advanced age.
2. Future studies based on the accumulation of preoperative CAVI data in patients with osteoarthritis who have various backgrounds, including patients with an ASA score of $\geq$III, are essential to more practically evaluate the impact of end-stage osteoarthritis on AS.

Author Contributions: Y.I. contributed to the study conception and design, drafted the article, and ensured the accuracy of the data and analysis. H.N., J.S. and I.T. contributed to the study conception and design and to the analysis and interpretation of the data. H.I., R.I., K.I. (Kei Ishii) and K.I. (Kai Ishii) contributed to the data collection. S.-i.T. provided statistical expertise and contributed to ensuring the accuracy of the data and analysis. All authors have read and agreed to the published version of the manuscript.

Funding: This research received no external funding.

Institutional Review Board Statement: The study was conducted in accordance with the Declaration of Helsinki, and the local institutional review board approved this study. Approval for this study was obtained from the Research Board of Healthcare Corporation Ashinokai, Gyoda, Saitama, Japan (ID number: 2022-6). All patients provided informed consent.

Informed Consent Statement: All patients provided informed consent.

Data Availability Statement: The datasets used and/or analyzed during the current study are available from the corresponding author on reasonable request.

Acknowledgments: We thank Shohei Yoshizawa RN for his contributions in gathering the data.

Conflicts of Interest: The authors declare that they have no competing interest. Each author certifies that he or she has no commercial associations (e.g., consultancies, stock ownership, equity interest, patent/licensing arrangements, etc.) that might pose a conflict of interest in connection with the submitted article.

References

1. King, L.K.; Kendzerska, T.; Waugh, E.J.; Hawker, G.A. Impact of osteoarthritis on difficulty walking: A population-based study. *Arthritis Care Res.* **2018**, *70*, 71–79. [CrossRef] [PubMed]
2. Kendzerska, T.; Jüni, P.; King, L.K.; Croxford, R.; Stanaitis, I.; Hawker, G.A. The longitudinal relationship between hand, hip and knee osteoarthritis and cardiovascular events: A population-based cohort study. *Osteoarthr. Cartil.* **2017**, *25*, 1771–1780. [CrossRef] [PubMed]
3. Nüesch, E.; Dieppe, P.; Reichenbach, S.; Williams, S.; Iff, S.; Jüni, P. All cause and disease specific mortality in patients with knee or hip osteoarthritis: Population based cohort study. *BMJ* **2011**, *342*, d1165. [CrossRef]
4. Miyoshi, T.; Ito, H. Arterial stiffness in health and disease: The role of cardio-ankle vascular index. *J. Cardiol.* **2021**, *78*, 493–501. [CrossRef]
5. Bierma-Zeinstra, S.M.A.; Waarsing, J.H. The role of atherosclerosis in osteoarthritis. *Best Pract. Res. Clin. Rheumatol.* **2017**, *31*, 613–633. [CrossRef]
6. Hussain, S.M.; Dawson, C.; Wang, Y.; Tonkin, A.M.; Chou, L.; Wluka, A.E.; Cicuttini, F.M. Vascular pathology and osteoarthritis: A systematic review. *J. Rheumatol.* **2020**, *47*, 748–760. [CrossRef]
7. Macêdo, M.B.; Santos, V.M.O.S.; Pereira, R.M.R.; Fuller, R. Association between osteoarthritis and atherosclerosis: A systematic review and meta-analysis. *Exp. Gerontol.* **2022**, *161*, 111734. [CrossRef]
8. Shirai, K.; Utino, J.; Otsuka, K.; Takata, M. A novel blood pressure-independent arterial wall stiffness parameter; cardio-ankle vascular index (CAVI). *J. Atheroscler. Thromb.* **2006**, *13*, 101–107. [CrossRef] [PubMed]
9. Namba, T.; Masaki, N.; Takase, B.; Adachi, T. Arterial stiffness assessed by cardio-ankle vascular index. *Int. J. Mol. Sci.* **2019**, *20*, 3664. [CrossRef]
10. Matsushita, K.; Ding, N.; Kim, E.D.; Budoff, M.; Chirinos, J.A.; Fernhall, B.; Hamburg, N.M.; Kario, K.; Miyoshi, T.; Tanaka, H.; et al. Cardio-ankle vascular index and cardiovascular disease: Systematic review and meta-analysis of prospective and cross-sectional studies. *J. Clin. Hypertens.* **2019**, *21*, 16–24. [CrossRef]
11. Goh, G.S.; Liow, M.H.; Bin Abd Razak, H.R.; Tay, D.K.; Lo, N.N.; Yeo, S.J. Patient-reported outcomes, quality of life, and satisfaction rates in young patients aged 50 years or younger after total knee arthroplasty. *J. Arthroplast.* **2017**, *32*, 419–425. [CrossRef]
12. Kim, Y.H.; Park, J.W.; Jang, Y.S. Long-term (up to 27 Years) prospective, randomized study of mobile-bearing and fixed-bearing total knee arthroplasties in patients < 60 years of age with osteoarthritis. *J. Arthroplast.* **2021**, *36*, 1330–1335.
13. Kremers, H.M.; Sierra, R.J.; Schleck, C.D.; Berry, D.J.; Cabanela, M.E.; Hanssen, A.D.; Pagnano, M.W.; Trousdale, R.T.; Lewallen, D.G. Comparative survivorship of different tibial designs in primary total knee arthroplasty. *J. Bone Jt. Surg. Am.* **2014**, *96*, e121. [CrossRef] [PubMed]
14. Andreozzi, V.; Conteduca, F.; Iorio, R.; Di Stasio, E.; Mazza, D.; Drogo, P.; Annibaldi, A.; Ferretti, A. Comorbidities rather than age affect medium-term outcome in octogenarian patients after total knee arthroplasty. *Knee Surg. Sports Traumatol. Arthrosc.* **2020**, *28*, 3142–3148. [CrossRef] [PubMed]

15. Alghamdi, Y.A.; Al-Shahrani, F.S.; Alanazi, S.S.; Alshammari, F.A.; Alkhudair, A.M.; Jatoi, N.A. The Association of blood glucose levels and arterial stiffness (Cardio-ankle vascular index) in patients with type 2 diabetes mellitus. *Cureus* **2021**, *13*, e20408. [CrossRef] [PubMed]
16. Nagayama, D.; Imamura, H.; Sato, Y.; Yamaguchi, T.; Ban, N.; Kawana, H.; Nagumo, A.; Shirai, K.; Tatsuno, I. Inverse relationship of cardioankle vascular index with BMI in healthy Japanese subjects: A cross-sectional study. *Vasc. Health Risk Manag.* **2016**, *13*, 1–9. [CrossRef] [PubMed]
17. Pavlovska, I.; Kunzova, S.; Jakubik, J.; Hruskova, J.; Skladana, M.; Rivas-Serna, I.M.; Medina-Inojosa, J.R.; Lopez-Jimenez, F.; Vysoky, R.; Geda, Y.E.; et al. Associations between high triglycerides and arterial stiffness in a population-based sample: Kardiovize Brno 2030 study. *Lipids Health Dis.* **2020**, *19*, 170. [CrossRef] [PubMed]
18. Dobsak, P.; Soska, V.; Sochor, O.; Jarkovsky, J.; Novakova, M.; Homolka, M.; Soucek, M.; Palanova, P.; Lopez-Jimenez, F.; Shirai, K. Increased cardio-ankle vascular index in hyper-lipidemic patients without diabetes or hypertension. *J. Atheroscler. Thromb.* **2015**, *22*, 272–283. [CrossRef]
19. Kubozono, T.; Miyata, M.; Ueyama, K.; Hamasaki, S.; Kusano, K.; Kubozono, O.; Tei, C. Acute and chronic effects of smoking on arterial stiffness. *Circ. J.* **2011**, *75*, 698–702. [CrossRef]
20. Anonymous. American Society of Anaesthesiologists Physical Status Classification System. Available online: http://www.asahq.org/resources/clinical-information/asa-physical-statusclassification-system (accessed on 24 March 2023).
21. Kellgren, J.H.; Lawrence, J.S. Radiographical assessment of osteo-arthrosis. *Ann. Rheum. Dis.* **1957**, *16*, 494–502. [CrossRef]
22. Alicea, J. Scoring systems and their validation for the arthritic knee. In *Surgery of the Knee*, 3rd ed.; Insall, J.N., Scott, W.N., Eds.; Churchill Livingstone: New York, NY, USA, 2001; Volume 2, pp. 1507–1515.
23. Shirai, K.; Hiruta, N.; Song, M.; Kurosu, T.; Suzuki, J.; Tomaru, T.; Miyashita, Y.; Saiki, A.; Takahashi, M.; Suzuki, K.; et al. Cardioankle vascular index (CAVI) as a novel indicator of arterial stiffness: Theory, evidence and perspectives. *J. Atheroscler. Thromb.* **2011**, *18*, 924–938. [CrossRef] [PubMed]
24. Tanaka, A.; Tomiyama, H.; Maruhashi, T.; Matsuzawa, Y.; Miyoshi, T.; Kabutoya, T.; Kario, K.; Sugiyama, S.; Munakata, M.; Ito, H.; et al. Physiological diagnostic criteria for vascular failure. *Hypertension* **2018**, *72*, 1060–1071. [CrossRef] [PubMed]
25. Park, H.E.; Chung, G.E.; Lee, H.; Kim, M.J.; Choi, S.Y.; Lee, W.; Yoon, J.W. Significance of Low Muscle mass on arterial stiffness as measured by cardio-ankle vascular index. *Front. Cardiovasc. Med.* **2022**, *9*, 857871. [CrossRef] [PubMed]
26. Bovonratwet, P.; Fu, M.C.; Tyagi, V.; Gu, A.; Sculco, P.K.; Grauer, J.N. Is discharge within a day total knee arthroplasty safe in the octogenarian population? *J. Arthroplast.* **2019**, *34*, 235–241. [CrossRef]
27. Hawker, G.A.; Croxford, R.; Bierman, A.S.; Harvey, P.J.; Ravi, B.; Stanaitis, I.; Lipscombe, L.L. All-cause mortality and serious cardiovascular events in people with hip and knee osteoarthritis: A population based cohort study. *PLoS ONE* **2014**, *9*, e91286. [CrossRef]
28. Uurtuya, S.; Taniguchi, N.; Kotani, K.; Yamada, T.; Kawano, M.; Khurelbaatar, N.; Itoh, K.; Lkhagvasuren, T. Comparative study of the cardio-ankle vascular index and ankle–brachial index between young Japanese and Mongolian subjects. *Hypertens. Res.* **2009**, *32*, 140–144. [CrossRef]
29. Yingchoncharoen, T.; Sritara, P. Cardio-ankle vascular index in a Thai population. *Pulse* **2017**, *4* (Suppl. S1), 8–10. [CrossRef]
30. Wang, H.; Shirai, K.; Liu, J.; Lu, N.; Wang, M.; Zhao, J.; Xie, J.; Yu, X.; Fu, X.; Shi, H.; et al. Comparative study of cardio-ankle vascular index between Chinese and Japanese healthy subjects. *Clin. Exp. Hypertens.* **2014**, *36*, 596–601. [CrossRef]

Disclaimer/Publisher's Note: The statements, opinions and data contained in all publications are solely those of the individual author(s) and contributor(s) and not of MDPI and/or the editor(s). MDPI and/or the editor(s) disclaim responsibility for any injury to people or property resulting from any ideas, methods, instructions or products referred to in the content.

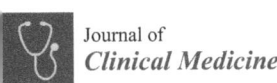

Article

Large Osteophytes over 10 mm at Posterior Medial Femoral Condyle Can Lead to Asymmetric Extension Gap Following Bony Resection in Robotic Arm–Assisted Total Knee Arthroplasty with Pre-Resection Gap Balancing

Jong Hwa Lee [1], Ho Jung Jung [2], Joon Kyu Lee [3], Ji Hyo Hwang [1] and Joong Il Kim [1,*]

[1] Department of Orthopaedic Surgery, Kangnam Sacred Heart Hospital, Hallym University College of Medicine, Seoul 07441, Republic of Korea; bigdawg@hallym.or.kr (J.H.L.); hwangjihyo7309@gmail.com (J.H.H.)
[2] Department of Orthopaedic Surgery, Chuncheon Sacred Heart Hospital, Hallym University College of Medicine, Chuncheon 24253, Republic of Korea; hodge.jung@gmail.com
[3] Department of Orthopaedic Surgery, Konkuk University Medical Center, Konkuk University School of Medicine, Seoul 05030, Republic of Korea; ndfi@naver.com
* Correspondence: jungil@hanmail.net; Tel.: +82-2829-5165

Abstract: Robotic arm–assisted total knee arthroplasty (TKA) involves a pre-resection gap balancing technique to obtain the desired gap. However, the expected gap may change owing to the soft-tissue release effect of unreachable osteophytes. This study evaluated the effect of unreachable osteophytes of the posterior medial femoral condyle on gap changes following bony resection. We retrospectively analysed 129 robotic arm–assisted TKAs performed for varus knee osteoarthritis. Knees were classified according to the size of osteophytes on the posterior medial femoral condyle using preoperative computed tomography measurement. After the removal of reachable osteophytes, the robotic system measured pre- and post-resection medial extension (ME), lateral extension (LE), medial flexion (MF), and lateral flexion (LF) gaps. No extension gap changes were observed for 25 (19.4%), and no flexion gap changes were observed 41 (31.8%) knees, following bone cuts. ME, LE, MF, and LF gaps increased with the osteophyte size ($p < 0.05$). For osteophytes <10 mm, all the gaps increased symmetrically. However, for osteophytes >10 mm, the ME gap increased asymmetrically more than LE, MF, and LF gaps ($p < 0.05$). The gap changes due to bony resection were correlated to the osteophyte sizes of the posterior medial femoral condyle. Surgeons should plan a slightly tight medial extension gap to attain the desired gaps for >10 mm osteophytes.

Keywords: robotic arm–assisted total knee arthroplasty; total knee arthroplasty; osteophytes; gap balancing

1. Introduction

Precise extension and flexion gap balancing represent critical objectives in achieving favourable short- and long-term outcomes for total knee arthroplasty (TKA) [1]. Traditionally, proper soft-tissue balance has been characterised by equivalent and symmetrical flexion and extension gaps [2,3]. Studies have demonstrated that attaining this balance can effectively reduce postoperative instability and stiffness, thereby decreasing the need for revision surgeries and substantially enhancing patient-reported outcomes [4,5].

Robotic arm–assisted TKA (R-TKA) was developed to increase the accuracy of gap balancing and bone cutting through the incorporation of preoperative computed tomography (CT) planning and intraoperative kinematic data [6]. Furthermore, the final ligament balance can be objectively quantified using the robot-assisted system [7]. Since the introduction of these systems, multiple studies have shown that certain robotic arm–assisted systems are more accurate and efficient at balancing gaps than manual systems [8–10].

In R-TKA, following the removal of reachable osteophytes and preliminary soft-tissue release, pre-resection gap balancing is performed by modifying the implant position according to the intraoperative gaps verified by the robot system. However, once balanced, these gaps can change following bone resection. Cutting of the femoral and tibial bones can loosen the collateral ligament and joint capsule, and unreachable osteophytes of the posterior femur that cannot be completely removed before bone cutting may affect gaps by eliminating the tenting effect [11,12]. If the gap increases asymmetrically following bone cuts, additional procedures for ligament balancing and bone recutting must be performed to match the mediolateral flexion–extension gaps. These issues negate the advantages of robotic systems, which emphasise precise bone cutting and reduced soft-tissue release [13].

The primary objectives of this study were to (1) quantitatively assess the accuracy of predicting the post-resection gap in R-TKA and (2) investigate the influence of unreachable osteophytes of the posterior medial femoral condyle, with specific reference to changes in gaps following bone resection. We hypothesised that there would be a discernible difference between the predicted and actual post-resection gaps and that this difference would be more pronounced in patients with larger osteophytes. The results of this study should provide valuable insights into improving soft-tissue balance during TKA procedures and contribute to enhancing the overall success and outcomes of surgical intervention.

2. Materials and Methods

2.1. Patients

In this analysis, 129 varus knees that underwent TKA for primary osteoarthritis between November 2019 and February 2023 were included. Patients with a history of femoral or tibial fractures, valgus knee deformity, osteotomy, rheumatoid arthritis, post-traumatic arthritis, or pyogenic arthritis of the knee joints were excluded. For the TKA procedures, posterior-stabilising prostheses (Triathlon®; Stryker, Kalamazoo, MI, USA) were implanted using the MAKO Robotic Arm Interactive Orthopaedic System (Stryker, Kalamazoo, MI, USA). The robotic system enabled the precise measurement of the medial and lateral gaps in flexion and extension before and after femoral bone cutting. The study protocol was approved by the institutional review board.

2.2. Surgical Techniques

All surgical procedures were performed by a single experienced surgeon (J.I.K.) using the medial parapatellar approach. Two pins were inserted into the femur and tibia and positioned approximately 10 cm from the main skin incision, and the femoral and tibial sensor arrays were then fixed onto the pins. Patient-specific CT-based bone models were confirmed using registered landmarks, and kinematic data were integrated to adjust the preoperative plan based on CT scans, with the goal of achieving optimal knee balance. After removing the anterior and posterior cruciate ligaments and accessible femoral osteophytes, the extension gap at 10° of flexion, or up to 25° if a flexion contracture was present, and the flexion gap at 90° of flexion were recorded with the robot system. Maximal manual varus and valgus stresses were applied to tension the collateral ligaments in the knee extension state to measure pre-resection extension mediolateral gaps. Gaps at 90° of flexion were measured using maximal-size spacer spoons in the medial and lateral compartments (gap in planning). Following the distal, anterior, and posterior femoral and tibial bone cuts, the trial components were inserted, and the resulting extension mediolateral gaps and flexion mediolateral gaps were recorded with the robot system (gap after cutting).

2.3. Radiographic Measurement

Leie et al. [11] devised an assessment of osteophytes of the posterior femoral condyle using plain radiographs and classified them into four different categories. As all patients who undergo R-TKA require CT scans for preoperative planning, we utilised the method described by Leie et al. to measure the size of the osteophytes using CT scans for optimal accuracy. The sagittal view of the CT scan was carefully assessed to obtain measurements of osteophyte size. Since the size of the osteophytes on the medial femoral condyle was thicker than on the lateral femoral condyle in all cases, we assumed that assessing the size of the osteophytes on the posterior medial femoral condyle reflected the overall amount of osteophyte.

Using a Picture Archiving and Communication System workstation, the largest sagittal size was measured in the sagittal view of the CT scans. The following standardised technique was employed to ensure accuracy. First, a mid-sagittal section of the knee displaying a clearly visible Blumensaat line was selected. Subsequently, a reference line (Line A; Figure 1a) was drawn on the Blumensaat line, extending from the anterior to the most posterior aspect of the femoral cortex. The sagittal section was medially moved to identify the largest posterior condylar osteophyte. The second line (Line B) was drawn perpendicular to Line A, copied from the mid-sagittal section on the most posterior aspect of the femoral cortex (Figure 1b). Finally, a third line (Line C), parallel to Line B, was drawn on the most posterior edge of the osteophyte. The distance between Lines B and C was recorded as the size of osteophytes. The obtained size measurements were subsequently categorised into four groups based on a classification system – the absence of osteophytes (group A), <5 mm (group B), 5–10 mm (group C), and >10 mm (group D) – to facilitate the comprehensive assessment and analysis of osteophyte size in the study population.

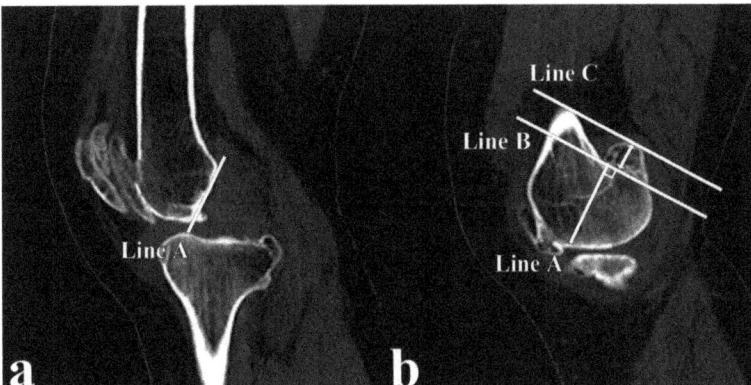

Figure 1. Technique of osteophyte size measurement. (**a**) Midsagittal section of CT: A line is drawn on the Blumensaat line extending from the anterior to the posterior-most aspect of the femoral cortex (Line A). (**b**) Sagittal section of CT with largest osteophytes: Line A is copied to sagittal section of CT with largest osteophytes, and second line (Line B) is drawn on the most posterior aspect of femoral cortex, perpendicular to Line A. A third line (Line C) is drawn parallel to line B and on the most posterior edge of osteophyte. The distance between Line B and Line C (yellow double-headed arrow) is recorded as the osteophyte size. CT: computed tomography.

2.4. Statistical Analysis

All statistical analyses were performed using SPSS for Windows (version 19.0; IBM Corp., Armonk, NY, USA). Statistical significance was set at $p < 0.05$. All measured values are expressed as the mean ± standard deviation. All data were tested for normal distribution using the Kolmogorov–Smirnov test. If the differences showed a normal distribution, a paired t-test was used to compare the gap changes measured using the robotic system before and after bone cutting. In the subgroup analysis of osteophyte size, a one-way analysis of variance for continuous variables was used to compare the four subgroups. In addition, a post hoc Bonferroni test was used to compare pairs of subgroups.

3. Results

The demographic characteristics of the study population are presented in Table 1.

Table 1. Patient demographics.

Characteristics	Values
Gender (male:female)	97:32
Left:right	79:50
K-L grade (III:IV)	27:102

	Mean ± SD
Age (years)	69.4 ± 5.52
BMI (kg/m^2)	25.84 ± 3.89
Mean HKA angle (°) [a]	6.43 ± 2.87
Size of osteophyte on posterior medial femoral condyle (mm)	
Group B	3.25 ± 1.03
Group C	6.93 ± 1.36
Group D	11.96 ± 1.09

[a] A positive value denotes varus alignment; SD: standard deviation; BMI: body mass index; K-L: Kellgren–Lawrence; HKA: hip–knee–ankle.

Of the 129 knees analysed, 25 knees (19.4%) showed no extension gap changes, and 41 knees (31.8%) showed no flexion gap changes, respectively, after bone cuts (Table 2). Overall, the gaps in medial extension (ME), lateral extension (LE), medial flexion (MF), and lateral flexion (LF) increased significantly after bone cuts (Table 3).

Table 2. Percentage of gap change following bone cutting.

	Extension Gap Change after Cutting				
Lateral Gap Δ	Medial Gap Δ	≥2 mm	1 mm	0 mm	Number of Knees (%)
	≥2 mm	15 (11.6)	14 (10.9)	0 (0.0)	29 (22.5)
	1 mm	21 (16.3)	37 (28.7)	9 (7.0)	67 (51.9)
	0 mm	2 (1.6)	6 (4.7)	25 (19.4)	33 (25.6)
	Number of knees (%)	38 (29.5)	57 (44.2)	34 (26.4)	129 (100)
	Flexion Gap Change after Cutting				
Lateral gap Δ	Medial Gap Δ	≥2 mm	1 mm	0 mm	Number of Knees (%)
	≥2 mm	6 (4.7)	4 (3.1)	1 (0.8)	11 (8.5)
	1 mm	9 (7.0)	47 (36.4)	5 (3.9)	61 (47.3)
	0 mm	4 (3.1)	12 (9.3)	41 (31.8)	57 (44.2)
	Number of knees (%)	19 (14.7)	63 (48.8)	47 (36.4)	129 (100)

Δ: change.

Table 3. Gap changes after bone cutting.

	Gap Changes (mm)			
	Gap in Planning	Gap after Cutting	Δ	p-Value
	Mean ± SD	Mean ± SD	Mean ± SD	
ME	18.68 ± 0.78	19.77 ± 0.95	1.10 ± 0.85	<0.01 *
LE	18.30 ± 0.76	19.28 ± 0.78	0.98 ± 0.72	<0.01 *
MF	18.93 ± 0.85	19.59 ± 0.91	0.79 ± 0.69	<0.01 *
LF	18.62 ± 0.72	19.42 ± 0.71	0.66 ± 0.68	<0.01 *

* paired t-test. Δ: change; SD: standard deviation; ME: medial extension; LE: lateral extension; MF: medial flexion; LF: lateral flexion.

The ME ($p = 0.001$), LE ($p = 0.001$), MF ($p = 0.002$), and LF ($p = 0.001$) gaps increased with the osteophyte size. For osteophytes <10 mm (groups A, B, and C), the increased gaps in ME, LE, MF, and LF were not significantly different, indicating symmetrical gap changes. However, for osteophytes >10 mm (group D), ME, LE, MF, and LF were significantly different, and post hoc analysis showed that the ME gap change was significantly higher than the other gaps, indicating asymmetrical gap changes (Table 4).

Table 4. Gap changes according to size of osteophytes on the posterior medial femoral condyle.

Δ	Size of Osteophytes and Effects on Gaps from Initial to Trialing				p-Value
	No Osteophytes (Group A) (n = 25) Mean ± SD	<5 mm (Group B) (n = 36) Mean ± SD	5–10 mm (Group C) (n = 51) Mean ± SD	>10 mm (Group D) (n = 17) Mean ± SD	
ME	0.53 ± 0.62	0.71 ± 0.69	1.28 ± 0.81	2.11 ± 0.70	<0.01 *
LE	0.59 ± 0.79	0.71 ± 0.62	1.21 ± 0.64	1.32 ± 0.52	<0.01 *
MF	0.52 ± 0.71	0.50 ± 0.59	0.97 ± 0.67	1.13 ± 0.35	<0.01 *
LF	0.35 ± 0.49	0.42 ± 0.50	0.82 ± 0.75	1.00 ± 0.53	<0.01 *
p	ns *	ns *	ns *	<0.01 *	

* One-way analysis of variance; SD: standard deviation; ME: medial extension; LE: lateral extension; MF: medial flexion; LF: lateral flexion; ns: not significant; Δ: change.

4. Discussion

Our results show a positive correlation between the size of the unreachable osteophytes of the posterior medial femoral condyle and the extension and flexion gaps. Of all the knees that underwent R-TKA, 80.6% exhibited an increased extension gap after bone cuts, whereas approximately 68.2% showed an increased flexion gap. When the size of the osteophyte was <10 mm, symmetrical increases in both the extension and flexion gaps were observed. In contrast, for osteophyte size exceeding 10 mm, a significant increase in the ME gap was observed compared to the LE, MF, and LF gaps, leading to an asymmetrical mediolateral extension gap.

In this study, all gaps (ME, LE, MF, and LF) increased after bone cutting, and this trend was also observed in the no-osteophytes group. These findings suggest that, regardless of the presence of osteophytes, the routine bone-cutting process leads to changes in the extension and flexion gaps. A prior study conducted by Sugama et al. [14] demonstrated that the initial ME gap measured by a tensioning device after cutting the distal femur and tibia increased by approximately 2.5 mm following the preparation of the flexion gap. Because the final extension gap was determined without a trial implant, and the impact of the femoral implant's condylar volume was not considered, the gap change was larger than that in our study. Kakuta et al. [15] reported a similar outcome. In this study, the joint gaps were measured at three stages: posterior femoral condylar resection, posterior osteophyte removal, and femoral component placement. This demonstrated the occurrence of a significant increase in the ME gap following femoral bone cutting. Thereafter, the ME gap was reduced by 0.6 mm following femoral component placement. Seo et al. [16] demonstrated similar results, with the bone-cutting process resulting in an increase in the extension gap by 1 mm. We can assume that the adhesion of the posterior capsule and the periarticular ligament structure surrounding the femoral condyle was released after the bone cuts.

Based on the observation that the size of the medial posterior femoral condyle osteophyte increases, we assumed that the tenting effect of the posterior capsule also increases, resulting in a widening of the gap. Theoretically, only the ME gap should be affected by medial osteophytes; however, in practice, the LE, MF, and LF gaps also increased, which agrees with the results of previous studies. In a study by Baldini et al. [17], the extension and flexion gaps were measured using a tension device, and a symmetrical gap increase was noted in the flexion and extension gaps after posterior condylar osteophyte removal. Sriphirom et al. [18] reported similar results, showing that the presence of a posterior condylar osteophyte in the femur resulted in an increase in both the extension and flexion gaps measured using a computer-assisted system. Unlike our study, these two studies showed that removal caused a greater increase in the flexion gap, while neither of these studies analysed the results according to osteophyte size. Gustke et al. [19] demonstrated the effect of posterior osteophytes on the size and location by measuring gaps using a robot-assisted system. In contrast to previous studies, no significant differences were observed, regardless of the presence of osteophytes.

In our study, for osteophytes <10 mm in size, the ME, LE, MF, and LF gaps increased symmetrically. However, for osteophytes >10 mm, the ME gap increased more asymmetrically than the LE, MF, and LF gaps ($p < 0.05$). Holst et al. [20] conducted a cadaveric study to evaluate the effects of 10 mm and 15 mm 3D-printed osteophyte-mimicking blocks on the medial and lateral contact forces using Verasense (OrthoSensor-Dania Beach, FL, USA). Although there were no significant differences between the 10 mm and 15 mm blocks on the medial contact forces, the presence of blocks caused an asymmetric contact force between the ME and LE. This indicates that the formation of a large osteophyte over time results in asymmetrical tightness of the medial side of the joint. However, if symmetric bone cutting is performed without considering this osteophyte effect, the posterior capsule, tightened by the osteophytes, would loosen again, resulting in an unexpected increase in the asymmetric gap. In cases where the osteophyte size is <10 mm, symmetrical gap changes can be expected, and the insertion of a thicker polyethylene insert can effectively address the issue without additional soft-tissue release and bone-cutting measures; however, when dealing with osteophytes thicker than 10 mm, performing symmetrical gap planning prior to bone cutting may result in an asymmetrical extension gap. Additional bone cuts and soft-tissue release are necessary to achieve a balanced mediolateral extension gap. Moreover, once the lateral extension gap matches the medial extension gap, resolving the mismatch between the extension and flexion gaps becomes a challenge. Therefore, for patients with osteophytes measuring >10 mm, it is advisable to plan for a slightly tighter medial extension gap by reducing the medial distal femoral resection by 2 mm. For patients with osteophytes measuring <10 mm, a symmetrical gap increase of up to 1 mm is negligible, and no additional measures need to be taken.

Our study has several limitations. First, we focused solely on varus osteoarthritic patients. Therefore, the observed changes in joint gaps may vary in valgus knees or varus knees with a predominant lateral femoral osteophyte because of differences in knee structures between the medial and lateral aspects. Second, gap recordings may be subjective. Herein, the extension and flexion medial gaps were measured by applying manual varus and valgus forces to the knee joints; consequently, the recorded values could vary based on the applied stress forces. However, this study was conducted by a single highly experienced surgeon with a high volume of cases, ensuring consistency in the application of stress forces.

5. Conclusions

Bony resection resulted in various changes in the flexion and extension gaps linked to the size of the osteophytes of the posterior medial femoral condyle. When patients have posterior osteophytes >10 mm, surgeons should expect an asymmetrical extension gap after bony resection; therefore, a slightly tight medial extension gap should be planned to achieve the desired gaps using the pre-resection gap balancing technique.

Author Contributions: J.I.K. and J.H.H. contributed to the study conception and design. Literature search, material preparation, and data collection were performed by J.K.L. and H.J.J. The first draft of the manuscript was written by J.H.L. and H.J.J.; J.I.K. and J.H.L. revised the manuscript. All authors have read and agreed to the published version of the manuscript.

Funding: This research received no external funding.

Institutional Review Board Statement: The study was conducted in accordance with the Declaration of Helsinki and approved by the Institutional Review Board of Hallym University Kangnam Sacred Heart Hospital (No. 2023-07-008; approval date 12 May 2023).

Informed Consent Statement: The requirement for written informed consent was waived owing to the retrospective nature of the study. However, the opportunity to refuse participation through the opt-out method was guaranteed.

Data Availability Statement: The data presented in this study are available on request from the corresponding author. The data are not publicly available.

Conflicts of Interest: The authors declare no conflict of interest.

References

1. Dennis, D.A.; Komistek, R.D.; Kim, R.H.; Sharma, A. Gap Balancing Versus Measured Resection Technique for Total Knee Arthroplasty. *Clin. Orthop. Relat. Res.* **2010**, *468*, 102–107. [CrossRef] [PubMed]
2. Lustig, S.; Bruderer, J.; Servien, E.; Neyret, P. The Bone Cuts and Ligament Balance in Total Knee Arthroplasty: The Third Way Using Computer Assisted Surgery. *Knee* **2009**, *16*, 91. [CrossRef]
3. Risitano, S.; Indelli, P.F. Is 'Symmetric' Gap Balancing Still the Gold Standard in Primary Total Knee Arthroplasty? *Ann. Transl. Med.* **2017**, *5*, 325. [CrossRef] [PubMed]
4. Babazadeh, S.; Stoney, J.D.; Lim, K.; Choong, P.F. The Relevance of Ligament Balancing in Total Knee Arthroplasty: How Important Is It? A Systematic Review of the Literature. *Orthop. Rev.* **2009**, *1*, e26. [CrossRef]
5. Matsuda, S.; Ito, H. Ligament Balancing in Total Knee Arthroplasty-Medial Stabilizing Technique. *Asia Pac. J. Sports Med. Arthrosc. Rehabil. Technol.* **2015**, *2*, 108–113. [CrossRef] [PubMed]
6. Sires, J.D.; Craik, J.D.; Wilson, C.J. Accuracy of Bone Resection in MAKO Total Knee Robotic-Assisted Surgery. *J. Knee Surg.* **2021**, *34*, 745–748. [CrossRef] [PubMed]
7. Mahoney, O.; Kinsey, T.; Sodhi, N.; Mont, M.A.; Chen, A.F.; Orozco, F.; Hozack, W. Improved Component Placement Accuracy with Robotic-Arm Assisted Total Knee Arthroplasty. *J. Knee Surg.* **2022**, *35*, 337–344. [CrossRef] [PubMed]
8. Hampp, E.L.; Chughtai, M.; Scholl, L.Y.; Sodhi, N.; Bhowmik-Stoker, M.; Jacofsky, D.J.; Mont, M.A. Robotic-Arm Assisted Total Knee Arthroplasty Demonstrated Greater Accuracy and Precision to Plan Compared with Manual Techniques. *J. Knee Surg.* **2019**, *32*, 239–250. [CrossRef] [PubMed]
9. Li, C.; Zhang, Z.; Wang, G.; Rong, C.; Zhu, W.; Lu, X.; Liu, Y.; Zhang, H. Accuracies of Bone Resection, Implant Position, and Limb Alignment in Robotic-Arm-Assisted Total Knee Arthroplasty: A Prospective Single-Centre Study. *J. Orthop. Surg. Res.* **2022**, *17*, 61. [CrossRef] [PubMed]
10. Parratte, S.; Price, A.J.; Jeys, L.M.; Jackson, W.F.; Clarke, H.D. Accuracy of a New Robotically Assisted Technique for Total Knee Arthroplasty: A Cadaveric Study. *J. Arthroplast.* **2019**, *34*, 2799–2803. [CrossRef] [PubMed]
11. Leie, M.A.; Klasan, A.; Oshima, T.; Putnis, S.E.; Yeo, W.W.; Luk, L.; Coolican, M. Large Osteophyte Removal from the Posterior Femoral Condyle Significantly Improves Extension at the Time of Surgery in a Total Knee Arthroplasty. *J. Orthop.* **2020**, *19*, 76–83. [CrossRef] [PubMed]
12. Yagishita, K.; Muneta, T.; Ikeda, H. Step-by-Step Measurements of Soft Tissue Balancing During Total Knee Arthroplasty for Patients with Varus Knees. *J. Arthroplast.* **2003**, *18*, 313–320. [CrossRef] [PubMed]
13. Mancino, F.; Cacciola, G.; Malahias, M.A.; De Filippis, R.; De Marco, D.; Di Matteo, V.; Gu, A.; Sculco, P.K.; Maccauro, G.; De Martino, I. What Are the Benefits of Robotic-Assisted Total Knee Arthroplasty over Conventional Manual Total Knee Arthroplasty? A Systematic Review of Comparative Studies. *Orthop. Rev.* **2020**, *12*, 8657. [CrossRef] [PubMed]
14. Sugama, R.; Kadoya, Y.; Kobayashi, A.; Takaoka, K. Preparation of the Flexion Gap Affects the Extension Gap in Total Knee Arthroplasty. *J. Arthroplast.* **2005**, *20*, 602–607. [CrossRef] [PubMed]
15. Kakuta, A.; Ikeda, R.; Takeshita, B.; Takamatsu, T.; Otani, T.; Saito, M. Intraoperative Changes in Medial Joint Gap After Posterior Femoral Condylar Resection, Posterior Osteophyte Removal, and Femoral Component Placement During Primary Total Knee Arthroplasty. *Knee* **2022**, *39*, 1–9. [CrossRef] [PubMed]
16. Seo, S.S.; Kim, C.W.; Seo, J.H.; Kim, D.H.; Kim, O.G.; Lee, C.R. Effects of Resection of Posterior Condyles of Femur on Extension Gap of Knee Joint in Total Knee Arthroplasty. *J. Arthroplast.* **2017**, *32*, 1819–1823. [CrossRef] [PubMed]
17. Baldini, A.; Scuderi, G.R.; Aglietti, P.; Chalnick, D.; Insall, J.N. Flexion-Extension Gap Changes During Total Knee Arthroplasty: Effect of Posterior Cruciate Ligament and Posterior Osteophytes Removal. *J. Knee Surg.* **2004**, *17*, 69–72. [CrossRef] [PubMed]
18. Sriphirom, P.; Siramanakul, C.; Chanopas, B.; Boonruksa, S. Effects of Posterior Condylar Osteophytes on Gap Balancing in Computer-Assisted Total Knee Arthroplasty with Posterior Cruciate Ligament Sacrifice. *Eur. J. Orthop. Surg. Traumatol.* **2018**, *28*, 677–681. [CrossRef] [PubMed]
19. Gustke, K.A.; Cherian, J.J.; Simon, P.; Morrison, T.A. Effect of Posterior Osteophytes on Total Knee Arthroplasty Coronal Soft Tissue Balance: Do They Matter? *J. Arthroplast.* **2022**, *37*, S226–S230. [CrossRef] [PubMed]
20. Holst, D.C.; Doan, G.W.; Angerame, M.R.; Roche, M.W.; Clary, C.W.; Dennis, D.A. What Is the Effect of Posterior Osteophytes on Flexion and Extension Gaps in Total Knee Arthroplasty? A Cadaveric Study. *Arthroplast. Today* **2021**, *11*, 127–133. [CrossRef] [PubMed]

Disclaimer/Publisher's Note: The statements, opinions and data contained in all publications are solely those of the individual author(s) and contributor(s) and not of MDPI and/or the editor(s). MDPI and/or the editor(s) disclaim responsibility for any injury to people or property resulting from any ideas, methods, instructions or products referred to in the content.

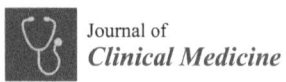

Article

The Correlation between Objective Ligament Laxity and the Clinical Outcome of Mechanically Aligned TKA

Stefano Campi [1,2], Rocco Papalia [1,2], Carlo Esposito [2], Vincenzo Candela [1,2], Andrea Gambineri [2] and Umile Giuseppe Longo [1,2,*]

1. Orthopaedic and Trauma Surgery, Fondazione Policlinico Universitario Campus Bio-Medico, Via Alvaro del Portillo 200, 00128 Rome, Italy; s.campi@policlinicocampus.it (S.C.); r.papalia@policlinicocampus.it (R.P.); v.candela@policlinicocampus.it (V.C.)
2. Research Unit of Orthopaedic and Trauma Surgery, Department of Medicine and Surgery, Università Campus Bio-Medico di Roma, Via Alvaro del Portillo 21, 00128 Rome, Italy; c.esposito@unicampus.it (C.E.); a.gambineri@unicampus.it (A.G.)
* Correspondence: g.longo@policlinicocampus.it

Abstract: Instability is one of the causes of failure in total knee arthroplasty (TKA). The aim of this study was to analyze the correlation between objective ligament laxity and the clinical outcome of mechanically aligned TKA. Fifty-one knees in 47 patients were evaluated at a minimum follow-up of 6 months. The correlation between the angular displacement and functional scores (Knee Society Score and Knee Injury and Osteoarthritis Score) was analyzed. A negative correlation (p-value < 0.05) was observed between medial laxity $\geq 5°$ at 0, 30, 60, and 90° of flexion and the outcome measures. Lateral laxity did not correlate with the clinical outcome. At 30° of knee flexion, a total varus and valgus laxity $\geq 10°$ was related to poorer outcomes. The same amount of angular displacement did not influence the outcome in the other flexion angles. There was no difference in single-radius vs multi-radius implants in terms of medial and lateral laxity and clinical outcome. A valgus displacement $\geq 5°$ measured at 0, 30, 60, and 90 degrees of flexion correlated with an inferior clinical outcome. In contrast, the same amount of displacement measured on the lateral compartment did not influence the clinical outcome after TKA.

Keywords: knee; arthroplasty; instability; of medial laxity; lateral laxity

Citation: Campi, S.; Papalia, R.; Esposito, C.; Candela, V.; Gambineri, A.; Longo, U.G. The Correlation between Objective Ligament Laxity and the Clinical Outcome of Mechanically Aligned TKA. J. Clin. Med. **2023**, 12, 6007. https://doi.org/10.3390/jcm12186007

Academic Editor: Hiroshi Horiuchi

Received: 25 July 2023
Revised: 5 September 2023
Accepted: 11 September 2023
Published: 16 September 2023

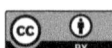

Copyright: © 2023 by the authors. Licensee MDPI, Basel, Switzerland. This article is an open access article distributed under the terms and conditions of the Creative Commons Attribution (CC BY) license (https://creativecommons.org/licenses/by/4.0/).

1. Introduction

Instability following primary total knee arthroplasty (TKA) is one of the major failure mechanisms leading to revision surgery [1]. However, the difference between "physiological" and "pathological" ligament laxity after mechanically aligned TKA remains unclear. Soft-tissue balancing is critical for successful TKA, providing stability and driving knee kinematics. However, the ideal range of medial and lateral ligament laxity of mechanically aligned TKA remains unclear, mainly because of the difficulty in achieving reliable measurements and the high heterogeneity among individuals.

In TKA practice, surgeons assess knee laxity both intraoperatively and at follow-up. Ligament balancing is based on bone resection and soft-tissue management, on patient's native phenotype and deformity, and implant design.

Different surgical techniques for ligament balancing have been developed [2,3], but in most cases soft-tissue balance is not based on an objective evaluation, depending mainly on surgeons' experience and preferences. Furthermore, the ligament laxity assessed with trial implants may vary when compared to the final implant [4] and change over time after the operation.

Several methods for measuring knee laxity during the clinical evaluation are available, but a gold standard has not yet been established.

Measuring medial and lateral laxity in the operating room throughout the range of motion is very difficult using conventional instruments. New technologies, such as navigation and robotic devices, have allowed to objectively measure tibio-femoral gaps in real time and to provide a better understanding of the effects of implant alignment on joint laxity before bone resections. However, these technologies are available but not incorporated in clinical practice on a large scale.

Medial, lateral, and sagittal joint stability have been reported to influence postoperative outcome [5,6]. However, the correlation between coronal and sagittal ligament laxity and patient-reported outcomes is controversial [7,8]. Only few studies have evaluated both the coronal and sagittal ligament laxity [9–11].

Similarly, studies on the influence of the curvature radius of the femoral component on mid-flexion stability have proved to be contradictory. Several studies have shown increased stability at 30° degrees of flexion in single-radius (SR) prostheses without, however, significant differences in outcomes between single-radius vs multi-radius groups [12]. Other studies have found no significant differences in varus–valgus stability between multi-radius (MR) and SRimplants, suggesting that the instability may be the result of unrecognized ligament laxity or technical errors during surgery rather than a factor intrinsic to the prosthetic implant [13].

The aim of our study is to investigate (1) the relationship between laxity in varus and valgus stress at 0°, 30°, 60°, and 90° knee flexion, anteroposterior translation measured at 90°, and the clinical outcome scores (Knee Injury and Osteoarthritis Outcome Score–KOOS and Knee Society Score–KSS); (2) the correlation between the use of single or multi-radius implants, laxity in varus–valgus, and clinical outcome.

2. Materials and Methods

A prospective evaluation of patients who underwent TKA surgery at the Campus Bio-Medico Hospital in Rome between October 2019 and July 2021 was performed. Data of the enrolled patients were subsequently collected between May 2021 and September 2021.

2.1. Patients' Selection

Patients who underwent primary TKA with minimum 6-month follow-up were considered eligible for the study.

Inclusion criteria were patients who underwent primary TKA at Campus Bio-Medico Hospital of Rome, minimum follow-up of 6 months, absence of intraoperative complications, absence of preoperative varus deformity >20°, absence of preoperative valgus deformity >15°, absence of preoperative flexion deformity >20°, absence of previous surgery, and infection of fractures on the knee.

Exclusion criteria were presence of a semi-constrained or constrained prosthetic implant, preoperative varus deformity >20° and valgus >15°, preoperative flexion deformity >20°, ligamentous or intraoperative iatrogenic tendon injuries, intraoperative fractures, previous tibial or femoral osteotomy, previous knee fractures, severe extra-articular deformities, inflammatory and autoimmune rheumatological diseases, history of previous prosthetic infection, neuropathies, and neuromuscular pathologies.

An experienced orthopedic knee surgeon who had more than 10 years of experience in knee surgery examined participants for inclusion and exclusion. To avoid selection bias and errors, included patients were then assessed by the Senior Author.

2.2. Surgical Technique

All procedures were performed through a central skin incision and a medial parapatellar arthrotomy. The anterior cruciate ligament was removed in all cases, while the posterior cruciate ligament was preserved or resected based on the type of prosthetic implant used. The type of prosthetic alignment performed is mechanical alignment. The distal femoral cut was made perpendicular to its mechanical axis in the coronal plane as measured on preoperative standing hip–knee–ankle (HKA) radiographs with the use of an intramedullary guide. The proximal tibial cut was then performed perpendicular to its mechanical axis in the coronal plane and with a 3–7° posterior tibial slope in the sagittal plane using extramedullary guide. Verification of the correct balance of the femoral and tibial cuts was carried out in extension. In order to reach the correct balance in extension, after selecting the correct size of the femoral component with an anterior or posterior reference system, the oblique, posterior condylar, and anterior cortical cuts of the femur were performed. Rotation of the femoral component was established by drawing the transepicondylar axis and the Whiteside line with 3–5° external rotation from the posterior condylar line.

Ligament releases were performed to achieve adequate balance. The prosthetic components were fixed without (6 knees) and with cementation (45 knees). Patella prosthesis was performed in eight cases. All surgeries were performed with tourniquet insufflation. Full weight bearing, quadriceps muscle setting, and range of motion exercises were started the day after surgery.

2.3. Laxity Measurements

Knee laxity was clinically evaluated both in the coronal and sagittal planes. To assess coronal laxity, a varus stress and a valgus stress were applied in full extension (Figure 1: valgus stress performed in full extension applying a standard force of 10 kg through the use of a dynamometer) and 30° (Figure 2: varus stress performed at 30° of knee flexion applying a standard force of 10 kg through the use of a dynamometer), 60°, and 90° knee flexion, applying a standard force of 10 kg through the use of a dynamometer (Salter Little Samson Dynamometer, Brecknell Fairmont, MN 56031-1439 USA) attached to an ankle in order to reduce the rotational forces that could have affected the results. The degree of opening in varus and valgus stress was measured clinically with an orthopedic goniometer [14].

The ROM (range of motion) was also measured with a goniometer (Shahe, China) [15]. The sagittal laxity at 90° knee flexion was measured with the drawer test (Figure 3: sagittal laxity at 90° knee flexion measured with the drawer test performed with the knee flexed at 90° with the quadriceps relaxed and the foot free), performed with the knee flexed at 90° with the quadriceps relaxed and the foot free [16–18].

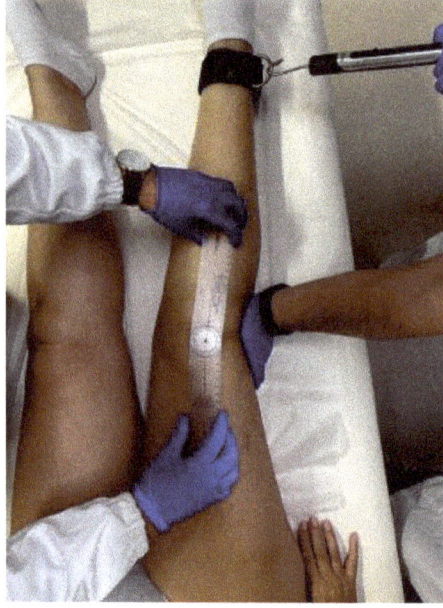

Figure 1. Valgus stress performed in full extension applying a standard force of 10 kg through the use of a dynamometer.

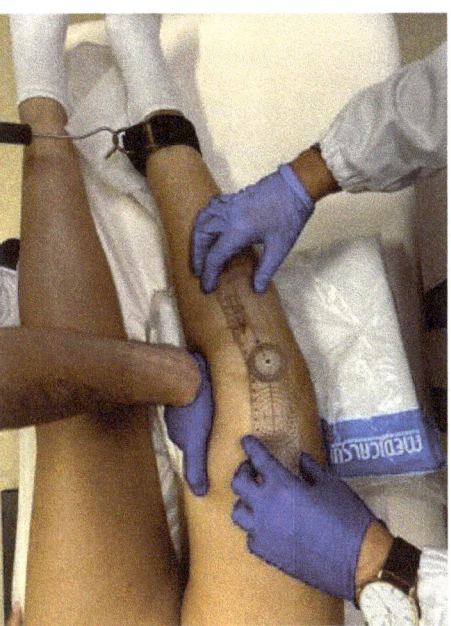

Figure 2. Varus stress performed at 30° of knee flexion applying a standard force of 10 kg through the use of a dynamometer.

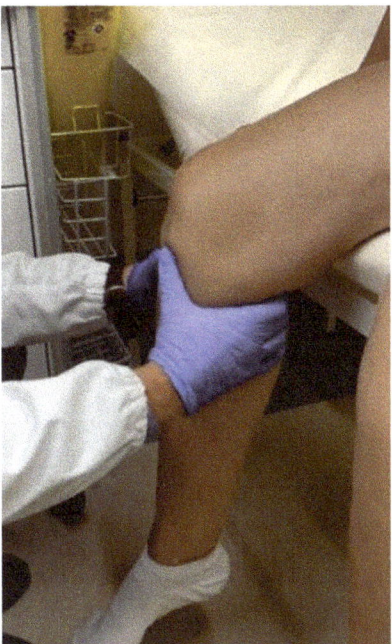

Figure 3. Sagittal laxity at 90° knee flexion measured with the drawer test performed with the knee flexed at 90° with the quadriceps relaxed and the foot free.

The Intraobserver reliability of the testing procedure was assessed in a preliminary study. In this preliminary study on 10 patients, the same test was performed twice by the same orthopedic knee surgeons. Intraobserver reliability was 0.83.

2.4. Clinical Outcome

The evaluation of clinical outcomes was carried out with the Knee Injury and Osteoarthritis Outcome Score (KOOS) [19,20] and the Knee Society Clinical Rating System (KSS) [21] at minimum follow-up of 6 months follow-up.

KOOS is a knee-specific subjective questionnaire consisting of forty-two questions, divided into five sections: subscales for pain, other symptoms and stiffness, activities of daily living (ADLs), function in sport and recreation, and knee-related quality of life (QOL). The KSS consists of two sections, "Knee Score" (KSS) and "Functional Score" (KSS-F), and provides us with an objective assessment of the functional prosthetic outcome. The self-administered questionnaires were completed by the patient alone.

2.5. Statistical Analysis

Data were summarized using mean and standard deviation (Mean ± SD). The normal distribution of the variables was verified by means of the Shapiro–Wilk test. Spearman's correlation was used to evaluate the correlation between laxity and scores. The Mann–Whitney U Test was used to evaluate statistically significant differences between total laxity (varus + valgus) <10° vs. ≥10°, varus laxity <5° vs. ≥5°, valgus laxity <5° vs. ≥5°, anteroposterior translation "<5 mm" vs. "≥5 mm" group, and "Single radius" group vs. "multi-radius" group in the various scores. The level of statistical significance was set $p < 0.05$. Correlation values: <0.3 low; [0.3–0.39] moderate; [0.4–0.69] high; >0.70 very strong. The post hoc power analysis made by using G power 3.1 for the correlation between medial laxity and KKS showed that the power of the study is 0.8 for a mean correlation (r), 0.38 for an alpha value of 0.05, and a sample size of 51.

3. Results

This study included 51 knees (20 right knees and 31 left knees) in a total of 47 patients (31 females and 16 males) with a mean age of 69.6 ± 8.3 years. Clinical outcomes were assessed at a mean follow-up of 7.2 months (SD 2.64, range 6–18).

A single-radius TKA was used in 19 cases and a multi-radius in 32 cases. The following implants were used in the single-radius group: GMK® Sphere Medacta, Triathlon® CR Stryker, Triathlon® PS Stryker, and Triathlon® CS (cruciate-substituting) Stryker. The following implants were used in the multi-radius group: Persona® PS Zimmer-Biomet, Persona® MC (medial congruent bearing) Zimmer-Biomet, Nexgen® PS Zimmer-Biomet, and Journey® II CR Smith & Nephew (Table 1).

Table 1. Single-radius and multi-radius implants and relative number.

Single-Radius	n 19	Multi-Radius	n 32
GMK Sphere	6	Persona PS	19
Triathlon CR	8	Persona MC	10
Thriatlon PS	3	Nexgen PS	1
Thriatlon CS	2	Journey II CR	2

The mean lateral and medial laxity measurement is reported in Table 2.

Table 2. Mean medial and lateral laxity (SD) at 0°, 30°, 60°, and 90° of knee flexion.

	Lateral Laxity (°)	Medial Laxity (°)
0°	1.5 (0.83)	1.6 (1.02)
30°	3.6 (1.82)	2.9 (2.14)
60°	4.6 (2.41)	3.6 (2.36)
90°	3.3 (1.81)	2.9 (2.19)

3.1. Coronal Laxity and Clinical Outcomes

There was a significant negative correlation between medial laxity at 0° and KOOS (r −0.304, p 0.03), K-Symptoms and Stiffness (r −0.43, p 0.002), K-Pain (r 0.29, p 0.04), K-Quality of Life (r −0.34, p 0.01), KSS (r −0.33, p 0.02), and KSS-Function (r −0.47, p < 0.001).

A high negative correlation was observed between increased medial laxity at 30° of flexion and KOOS (r −0.502, p < 0.001), K-Symptoms and Stiffness (r −0.415, p 0.002), K-Sports (r −0.415, p 0.002), K-Function Daily Living (r −0.407, p 0.003), K-Quality of Life (r −0.471, p < 0.001), KSS (r −0.455, p 0.001), and KSS-f (r −0.521, p < 0.001).

At 60° of flexion, we found a low negative correlation between medial laxity and KOOS (r −0.286, p 0.042) and K-Quality of Life (r −0.298, p 0.034) and a moderate negative correlation between medial laxity and K-Symptoms and Stiffness (r −0.365, p 0.008), KSS (r −0.306, p 0.029), and KSS-F (r −0.364, p 0.009).

Finally, medial laxity at 90° of flexion showed a low negative correlation with KOOS (r −0.294, p 0.036) and KSS (r −0.299, p 0.033) and a moderate negative correlation with K-Symptoms and Stiffness (r −0.349, p 0.012), K-Quality of Life (r −0.325, p 0.020), and KSS-F (r −0.337, p 0.016).

Lateral laxity showed no significant correlation with the reported outcome measures at 0°, 30°, 60°, and 90° of flexion, with some minor exceptions: a low positive correlation with K-Pain at 30° of flexion (r 0.289, p 0.040), a moderate positive correlation with ROM Max at 30° of flexion (r 0.305, p 0.029), a moderate positive correlation with K-Pain (rho = 0.303, p = 0.031), KSS-F (rho = 0.307, p = 0.028), and ROM Max (rho = 0.311, p = 0.026) at 60° flexion (Table 3).

Table 3. Correlation between coronary laxity at 0°, 30°, 60°, and 90° knee flexion and clinical outcomes.

			KOOS	K-Symptoms and Stifness	K-Pain	K-Function Daily Living	K-Sports	K-Quality of Life	KSS	KSS-F	ROM Max
0°	LATERAL	rho	−0.185	−0.294	−0.129	−0.137	−0.001	−0.128	−0.251	−0.076	0.119
		P	0.194	0.036	0.365	0.338	0.993	0.369	0.075	0.598	0.406
	MEDIAL	rho	−0.304	−0.425	−0.287	−0.171	−0.161	−0.344	−0.335	−0.471	−0.263
		P	0.030	0.002	0.041	0.229	0.259	0.013	0.016	<0.001	0.062
30°	LATERAL	rho	0.144	0.134	0.289	0.083	0.006	0.174	0.114	0.241	0.305
		P	0.312	0.348	0.040	0.562	0.964	0.222	0.427	0.088	0.029
	MEDIAL	rho	−0.502	−0.415	−0.391	−0.407	−0.415	−0.471	−0.455	−0.521	−0.168
		P	0.000	0.002	0.005	0.003	0.002	0.000	0.001	0.000	0.240
60°	LATERAL	rho	0.145	0.214	0.303	0.085	−0.008	0.158	0.062	0.307	0.311
		P	0.309	0.131	0.031	0.555	0.957	0.267	0.667	0.028	0.026
	MEDIAL	rho	−0.286	−0.365	−0.256	−0.203	−0.194	−0.298	−0.306	−0.364	−0.179
		P	0.042	0.008	0.070	0.153	0.172	0.034	0.029	0.009	0.209
90°	LATERAL	rho	0.002	0.101	0.086	−0.015	−0.084	0.030	−0.084	0.186	0.242
		P	0.991	0.480	0.548	0.915	0.558	0.836	0.558	0.191	0.087
	MEDIAL	rho	−0.294	−0.349	−0.249	−0.229	−0.258	−0.325	−0.299	−0.337	−0.179
		P	0.036	0.012	0.078	0.106	0.068	0.020	0.033	0.016	0.209

Patients with a medial laxity greater that 5° at 0, 30, 60, and 90 degrees of flexion reported significantly lower outcome measures when compared with patients with less than 5° of laxity (Table 4).

Table 4. Comparison of clinical outcome for patients with a medial laxity >5° versus patients with medial laxity <5°.

		<5°	>5°	p-Value
0°	Knees	0	0	
30°	Knees	40	11	
	KOOS	77.67 ± 11.91	55.55 ± 18.12	0.001
	KSS	88.83 ± 8.16	73.82 ± 13.14	0.001
	KSS-F	81.75 ± 15.17	57.73 ± 9.32	<0.001
60°	Knees	34	17	
	KOOS	78.42 ± 11.42	61.84 ± 18.72	0.002
	KSS	88.59 ± 8.62	79.59 ± 13.45	0.013
	KSS-F	82.65 ± 14.63	64.41 ± 15.80	<0.001
90°	Knees	38	13	
	KOOS	78.11 ± 11.65	57.67 ± 18.18	0.001
	KSS	88.95 ± 8.29	75.77 ± 13.03	0.001
	KSS-F	81.58 ± 14.43	61.92 ± 16.78	<0.001

There was no significant difference between patients with a lateral laxity greater than 5° versus lower than 5° at any flexion degree (Table 5).

Table 5. Comparison of clinical outcome for patients with a lateral laxity >5° versus patients with lateral laxity <5°. (NS: not significant).

		<5°	>5°	p-Value
0°	Knees	0	0	
30°	Knees	36	15	
	KOOS	72.33 ± 15.59	74.25 ± 17.90	NS
	KSS	85.47 ± 11.36	85.87 ± 11.16	NS
	KSS-F	74.58 ± 17.38	81.33 ± 16.42	NS
60°	Knees	22	29	
	KOOS	72.10 ± 17.89	73.50 ± 14.99	NS
	KSS	84.77 ± 11.06	86.21 ± 11.45	NS
	KSS-F	71.59 ± 19.72	80.34 ± 14.26	NS
90°	Knees	36	15	
	KOOS	72.81 ± 17.56	73.10 ± 12.65	NS
	KSS	85.69 ± 10.96	85.33 ± 12.13	NS
	KSS-F	74.86 ± 18.34	80.67 ± 13.87	NS

Patients with more than 10° of overall laxity (medial + lateral) showed a statistically significant decrease in the KOOS score, K-Symptoms and Stiffness, K-Pain, K-Function daily living, K-sports, K-quality of life, KSS, and KSS-F at 30° of flexion when compared with patients with less than 10° of overall laxity (Table 6).

Table 6. Comparison of clinical outcome for patients with an overall laxity >10° versus <10°.

		<10	>10	p-Value
0°	Knees	0	0	
30°	Knees	46	5	
	KOOS	74.96 ± 15.21	53.94 ± 12.56	0.005
	KSS	86.91 ± 10.14	73.40 ± 14.28	0.015
	KSS-F	78.15 ± 17.24	62.00 ± 8.37	0.038
60°	Knees	34	17	
	KOOS	73.95 ± 15.68	70.79 ± 17.33	0.562
	KSS	87.03 ± 10.65	82.71 ± 12.01	0.141
	KSS-F	79.12 ± 16.21	71.47 ± 18.52	0.144
90°	Knees	43	8	
	KOOS	74.64 ± 14.94	63.50 ± 20.09	0.125
	KSS	86.53 ± 10.75	80.50 ± 12.91	0.139
	KSS-F	78.95 ± 16.39	63.75 ± 16.85	0.021

3.2. Sagittal Laxity and Clinical Outcomes

No statistically significant differences in clinical outcome were found between patients with an anteroposterior translation <5 mm or >5 mm at 90° flexion (Table 7).

Table 7. Comparison of patients with antero-posterior translation >5 mm vs. <5 mm at 90° of flexion.

	<5 mm (n = 34)	>5 mm (n = 17)	p-Value
KOOS	73.45 ± 16.57	71.79 ± 15.69	0.660
K-Symptoms and Stiffness	75.42 ± 17.56	76.26 ± 15.57	0.992
K-Pain	79.09 ± 18.24	79.58 ± 13.64	0.771
K-Function Daily Living	80.80 ± 16.86	77.86 ± 15.32	0.395
K-Sports	43.97 ± 28.39	38.53 ± 30.76	0.609
K-Quality of Life	60.48 ± 25.41	63.97 ± 24.76	0.630
KSS	86.38 ± 10.44	84.00 ± 12.75	0.603
KSS-F	76.32 ± 17.29	77.06 ± 17.59	0.879
ROM Max	112.5 ± 7.2	114.4 ± 10.6	0.162

3.3. Single-Radius vs. Multi-Radius Implant

No statistically significant differences were found in terms of clinical outcomes and coronal laxity measured at 30°, 60°, and 90° between single-radius and multi-radius implants (Table 8).

Table 8. Comparison of single-radius vs multi-radius implants.

	Single Radius (n = 19)	Multradius (n = 32)	p-Value
KOOS	71.08 ± 13.80	73.97 ± 17.51	0.424
K-Symptoms and Stiffness	72.18 ± 16.13	77.78 ± 17.04	0.138
K-Pain	76.32 ± 15.83	80.99 ± 17.21	0.171
K-Function Daily Living	79.64 ± 13.76	79.92 ± 17.81	0.598
K-Sports	41.05 ± 24.81	42.81 ± 31.60	0.876

Table 8. Cont.

	Single Radius (n = 19)	Multradius (n = 32)	p-Value
K-Quality of Life	58.88 ± 22.76	63.28 ± 26.46	0.557
KSS	84.37 ± 11.63	86.31 ± 11.05	0.551
KSS-F	72.89 ± 18.66	78.75 ± 16.21	0.290
Varus 0°	1.42 ± 0.51	1.56 ± 0.98	0.991
Valgus 0°	1.47 ± 0.84	1.66 ± 1.12	0.544
Varus 30°	3.21 ± 1.23	3.78 ± 2.09	0.315
Valgus 30°	2.79 ± 2.10	2.91 ± 2.19	0.770
Varus 60°	3.84 ± 1.89	5.09 ± 2.58	0.069
Valgus 60°	3.11 ± 2.26	3.81 ± 2.42	0.177
Varus 90°	2.84 ± 1.50	3.56 ± 1.95	0.157
Valgus 90°	2.42 ± 1.95	3.13 ± 2.31	0.267
ROM Max	112.89 ± 7.69	113.28 ± 8.95	0.710

4. Discussion

The results of this study suggest that an increase in medial laxity at 0, 30, 60, and 90 degrees of flexion is correlated with poorer postoperative outcome of mechanically aligned TKA. Lateral laxity does not affect the clinical scores. There was no difference in the incidence of postoperative laxity and in the clinical outcome between single-radius vs. multi-radius implants.

These results are in line with previous studies demonstrating that medial stability is essential for an adequate functioning of the implant, while a lateral laxity does not negatively affect the clinical outcome. Indeed, a medial laxity induces non-physiological kinematics of the knee, while a lateral laxity has little effect on the kinematics [22,23] being physiological in the native knee both in extension and flexion. Okazaki et al. [24] analyzed 50 healthy knees with varus–valgus stress radiographs in extension and flexion and reported the following mean coronal laxity values as physiological: 4.9° and 2.4° of lateral and medial laxity in extension and 4.8° and 1.7° of lateral and medial flexion laxity, respectively.

Previous studies reported similar results. Tsukiyama et al. [6] found that knees with medial joint laxity during flexion resulted in an inferior postoperative outcome, while lateral joint laxity did not influence patient satisfaction or function. Aunan et al. [25] analyzed the association between ligamentous laxity measured intraoperatively and clinical outcome at one year of follow-up in 108 patients with TKR. Medial and lateral laxity were measured in extension and 90° knee flexion. They found a worsening of postoperative pain and knee function directly proportional to the increase in medial laxity both in extension and 90° of flexion. Watanabe et al. [11] found that lateral laxity was greater than the medial one both in extension and at 80° of flexion in all knees; the value of 3.6° was also defined as the ideal value of medial laxity in extension and at 80° of flexion, with a worsening of the overall satisfaction and pain scores due to increases in medial laxity above this threshold. Tanaka et al. [26] found that an asymmetrical coronal balance in extension and 90° knee flexion has no effect on postoperative ROM and on the subscales of the modified KSS and that a relative increase in lateral laxity does not lead to a worsening of clinical symptoms and function of the operated knees. Nakano et al. [27] reported an increase in ROM Max with increasing lateral laxity measured at 90° knee flexion. Seah et al. [28] evaluated the relationship between coronal stability measured at 30° knee flexion and clinical outcome. Better scores were associated with total laxity (varus + valgus) <5°. Matsuda et al. [29] studied the overall effects of varus–valgus laxity measured exclusively in extension on the ROM Max at one year of follow-up. The results obtained showed a significant increase in ROM in patients with a difference in laxity <2° and a concomitant increase in ROM in patients with a total laxity (varus + valgus) between 6–10°. Similar results were obtained by Yoshihara et al. [30] who analyzed coronal laxity in extension and 90° knee flexion. The results obtained identified as acceptable coronal laxity values <5° in valgus or varus and determined that a total laxity <10 ° in both extension and flexion did not determine either a worsening of the clinical outcome, calculated with KSS, or an increase in the prosthetic failure rate.

In the present study, the sagittal laxity at 90° knee flexion was evaluated and correlated with the clinical outcome. No statistically significant differences in clinical scores were found between patients with values <5 mm and values >5 mm. However, all patients had translational values <10 mm.

Jones et al. [31] observed in 97 knees undergoing CR TKR a decrease in maximum ROM and KSS in patients with AP translation >10 mm at 75° knee flexion compared to patients with an AP translation between 5–10 mm, concluding that the latter was the optimal range of sagittal stability. Watanabe et al. [11] indicated that adequate values of AP translation measured at 75° knee flexion were those in the range 5–10 mm. Warren et al. [32] in a comparative study on sagittal laxity among PS, CR, and double cruciate retention prostheses observed an increase in ROM max in patients with AP translation >5 mm, regardless of the type of prosthetic implant used, but did not identify a pathological upper limit of translation. Matsumoto et al. [33,34], evaluated in 110 knees undergoing PS TKR the association between sagittal laxity at 30°, 60°, and 90° knee flexion and functional outcomes and observed a significant decrease in the K-pain score with increasing AP translation at 60° knee flexion.

Finally, no statistically significant differences emerged regarding clinical outcomes and coronal laxity measured at 0, 30, 60, and 90 degrees of flexion between groups single-radius vs multi-radius implants.

Some studies have shown that the transition from a longer to a shorter radius in MR prostheses causes temporary instability during knee flexion between 30° and 45° due to a probable loss of tension in the collateral ligaments [35–38]. In contrast, some studies have shown increased stability at 30° of flexion in SR prostheses without, however, significant differences in outcomes between the two groups [12]. Other studies have found no significant differences in varus–valgus stability between MR and SR implants, suggesting that the instability may be the result of unrecognized ligament laxity during surgery rather than a factor dependent on intrinsic characteristics of the implant [13,39,40].

Several limitations of this study should be acknowledged. The main limitation concerns the method of measuring laxity. Both coronal laxity and sagittal laxity were measured clinically through the use of a dynamometer and a goniometer for the assessment of medial-lateral laxity in varus–valgus stress. The evaluation of sagittal laxity was conducted with the execution of the drawer test. The choice of the goniometer and dynamometer has proven to be more reliable from the comparison with the current literature: at present, there is no instrument that allows to measure laxity precisely in a clinical setting. Since the measurements were only taken clinically, it was equally difficult to accurately identify and distinguish the subtle changes in degrees of laxity. The choice to perform radiographic measurements of the degree of laxity, as was conducted by some of the studies cited in the text, would have significantly improved the significance of our results. However, the difficulty in carrying out further radiographic investigations must be taken into consideration, both at a more strictly hospital level and due to the poor compliance of the patients enrolled. The radiographic investigation flanked by advanced computer-assisted navigation systems, similar to those already used in surgical practice, could further improve the overall assessment of instabilities [41,42].

The number of patients enrolled in our study is relatively small when compared with similar studies in the literature. We tried to include only patients undergoing more recent prosthetic implants in the study to ensure that the surgical technique and postoperative rehabilitation did not differ significantly.

We were unable to calculate the preoperative laxity because it is not possible to objectively quantify the preoperative medial or lateral bone loss and how it can affect ligamentous stability. A possible significant correlation between preoperative and postoperative gap balances, both in extension and flexion, could influence our results. This aspect could be the subject of future studies.

In our study, we did not check if the medial-lateral laxity measured for the CR- and PS-TKAs revealed statistically significant differences over the studied flexion arc for the two versions of TKA. Excision of the PCL results in an increased flexion gap, which should increase varus–valgus laxity of the knee with increasing flexion. Our results could be influenced by the heterogeneity of the experimental group.

Moreover, clinical laxity was assessed by a single experienced orthopedic knee surgeon. The Intraobserver reliability of the testing procedure was assessed in a preliminary study to guarantee the accuracy of the measurement. However, the interobserver reliability was not assessed. Although a reproducible method was used for clinical measurements, the absence of an interobserver reliability evaluation could be a limitation of the study.

Finally, the selected patients were not stratified by homogeneous classes of preoperative deformity (varus and valgus) with consequent differences in the preoperative ligament structure [43,44].

Patient satisfaction after TKA is generally lower than after total hip arthroplasty. Several preoperative and intraoperative factors could affect the postoperative outcome. Among these factors, ligament balance could be associated with the subjective and functional results of patients. Few studies have analyzed the relationship between ligament balancing and patient-reported outcomes. The results of this study suggest that an increase in medial laxity at 0, 30, 60, and 90 degrees of flexion is correlated with poorer postoperative outcome of mechanically aligned TKA. These data could drive surgeons to focus on the relevance of medial stability of total knee arthroplasty. Future research is needed with the greatest and more homogeneous populations to obtain high-quality evidence on this topic.

5. Conclusions

The results of this study suggest that an increase in medial laxity at 0, 30, 60, and 90 degrees of flexion is correlated with poorer postoperative outcome of mechanically aligned TKA, while lateral laxity does not affect the clinical scores. An overall laxity (medial + lateral) of more than >10° at 30° of flexion leads to a lower clinical outcome. There was no difference in the incidence of postoperative laxity and in the clinical outcome between single-radius vs. multi-radius implants. Finally, an anteroposterior translation lower than 10 mm at 90 degrees of flexion does not influence the results of TKA.

Author Contributions: Conceptualization, U.G.L. and S.C.; methodology, C.E. and V.C.; software, A.G.; validation, U.G.L. and R.P.; formal analysis, S.C.; investigation, V.C.; resources, A.G.; data curation, V.C.; writing—original draft preparation, S.C.; writing—review and editing, U.G.L.; visualization, A.G.; supervision, R.P.; project administration, R.P.; funding acquisition, U.G.L. All authors have read and agreed to the published version of the manuscript.

Funding: This research received no external funding.

Institutional Review Board Statement: The study was conducted according to the guidelines of the Declaration of Helsinki and was approved by the Institutional Review Board of Campus Bio-Medico University of Rome (COSMO study, Protocol number: 78/18 OSS ComEt CBM, 16 October 18).

Informed Consent Statement: Informed consent was obtained from all subjects involved in the study.

Data Availability Statement: The datasets used and/or analyzed during the current study are available from the corresponding author on reasonable request.

Conflicts of Interest: The authors declare no conflict of interest.

References

1. Vince, K.G. Why knees fail. *J. Arthroplast.* **2003**, *18*, 39–44. [CrossRef] [PubMed]
2. Mihalko, W.M.; Saleh, K.J.; Krackow, K.A.; Whiteside, L.A. Soft-tissue balancing during total knee arthroplasty in the varus knee. *J. Am. Acad. Orthop. Surg.* **2009**, *17*, 766–774. [CrossRef] [PubMed]
3. Babazadeh, S.; Stoney, J.D.; Lim, K.; Choong, P.F. The relevance of ligament balancing in total knee arthroplasty: How important is it? A systematic review of the literature. *Orthop. Rev.* **2009**, *1*, e26. [CrossRef]
4. Nodzo, S.R.; Franceschini, V.; Gonzalez Della Valle, A. Intraoperative Load-Sensing Variability During Cemented, Posterior-Stabilized Total Knee Arthroplasty. *J. Arthroplast.* **2017**, *32*, 66–70. [CrossRef] [PubMed]
5. Kamenaga, T.; Muratsu, H.; Kanda, Y.; Miya, H.; Kuroda, R.; Matsumoto, T. The Influence of Postoperative Knee Stability on Patient Satisfaction in Cruciate-Retaining Total Knee Arthroplasty. *J. Arthroplast.* **2018**, *33*, 2475–2479. [CrossRef] [PubMed]
6. Tsukiyama, H.; Kuriyama, S.; Kobayashi, M.; Nakamura, S.; Furu, M.; Ito, H.; Matsuda, S. Medial rather than lateral knee instability correlates with inferior patient satisfaction and knee function after total knee arthroplasty. *Knee* **2017**, *24*, 1478–1484. [CrossRef] [PubMed]
7. Nakahara, H.; Okazaki, K.; Hamai, S.; Okamoto, S.; Kuwashima, U.; Higaki, H.; Iwamoto, Y. Does knee stability in the coronal plane in extension affect function and outcome after total knee arthroplasty? *Knee Surg. Sports Traumatol. Arthrosc.* **2015**, *23*, 1693–1698. [CrossRef] [PubMed]
8. Ishii, Y.; Noguchi, H.; Takeda, M.; Sato, J.; Sakurai, T.; Toyabe, S. In vivo anteroposterior translation after meniscal-bearing total knee arthroplasty: Effects of soft tissue conditions and flexion angle. *Eur. J. Orthop. Surg. Traumatol.* **2014**, *24*, 967–971. [CrossRef]
9. Dejour, D.; Deschamps, G.; Garotta, L.; Dejour, H. Laxity in posterior cruciate sparing and posterior stabilized total knee prostheses. *Clin. Orthop. Relat. Res.* **1999**, *364*, 182–193. [CrossRef]
10. Yamakado, K.; Kitaoka, K.; Yamada, H.; Hashiba, K.; Nakamura, R.; Tomita, K. Influence of stability on range of motion after cruciate-retaining TKA. *Arch. Orthop. Trauma. Surg.* **2003**, *123*, 1–4. [CrossRef]
11. Watanabe, T.; Koga, H.; Katagiri, H.; Otabe, K.; Nakagawa, Y.; Muneta, T.; Sekiya, I.; Jinno, T. Coronal and sagittal laxity affects clinical outcomes in posterior-stabilized total knee arthroplasty: Assessment of well-functioning knees. *Knee Surg. Sports Traumatol. Arthrosc.* **2020**, *28*, 1400–1409. [CrossRef] [PubMed]
12. Jo, A.R.; Song, E.K.; Lee, K.B.; Seo, H.Y.; Kim, S.K.; Seon, J.K. A comparison of stability and clinical outcomes in single-radius versus multi-radius femoral design for total knee arthroplasty. *J. Arthroplast.* **2014**, *29*, 2402–2406. [CrossRef] [PubMed]
13. Stoddard, J.E.; Deehan, D.J.; Bull, A.M.; McCaskie, A.W.; Amis, A.A. The kinematics and stability of single-radius versus multi-radius femoral components related to mid-range instability after TKA. *J. Orthop. Res.* **2013**, *31*, 53–58. [CrossRef] [PubMed]
14. Clarke, J.V.; Wilson, W.T.; Wearing, S.C.; Picard, F.; Riches, P.E.; Deakin, A.H. Standardising the clinical assessment of coronal knee laxity. *Proc. Inst. Mech. Eng. H.* **2012**, *226*, 699–708. [CrossRef] [PubMed]
15. Watkins, M.A.; Riddle, D.L.; Lamb, R.L.; Personius, W.J. Reliability of goniometric measurements and visual estimates of knee range of motion obtained in a clinical setting. *Phys. Ther.* **1991**, *71*, 90–96; discussion 96–97. [CrossRef] [PubMed]
16. Stambough, J.B.; Edwards, P.K.; Mannen, E.M.; Barnes, C.L.; Mears, S.C. Flexion Instability after Total Knee Arthroplasty. *J. Am. Acad. Orthop. Surg.* **2019**, *27*, 642–651. [CrossRef] [PubMed]
17. Schwab, J.H.; Haidukewych, G.J.; Hanssen, A.D.; Jacofsky, D.J.; Pagnano, M.W. Flexion instability without dislocation after posterior stabilized total knees. *Clin. Orthop. Relat. Res.* **2005**, *440*, 96–100. [CrossRef] [PubMed]
18. Abdel, M.P.; Pulido, L.; Severson, E.P.; Hanssen, A.D. Stepwise surgical correction of instability in flexion after total knee replacement. *Bone Joint J.* **2014**, *96-B*, 1644–1648. [CrossRef]
19. Monticone, M.; Ferrante, S.; Salvaderi, S.; Rocca, B.; Totti, V.; Foti, C.; Roi, G.S. Development of the Italian version of the knee injury and osteoarthritis outcome score for patients with knee injuries: Cross-cultural adaptation, dimensionality, reliability, and validity. *Osteoarthr. Cartil.* **2012**, *20*, 330–335. [CrossRef]
20. Vaquero, J.; Longo, U.G.; Forriol, F.; Martinelli, N.; Vethencourt, R.; Denaro, V. Reliability, validity and responsiveness of the Spanish version of the Knee Injury and Osteoarthritis Outcome Score (KOOS) in patients with chondral lesion of the knee. *Knee Surg. Sports Traumatol. Arthrosc.* **2014**, *22*, 104–108. [CrossRef]
21. Insall, J.N.; Dorr, L.D.; Scott, R.D.; Scott, W.N. Rationale of the Knee Society clinical rating system. *Clin. Orthop. Relat. Res.* **1989**, *248*, 13–14. [CrossRef]
22. Nakamura, S.; Ito, H.; Yoshitomi, H.; Kuriyama, S.; Komistek, R.D.; Matsuda, S. Analysis of the Flexion Gap on In Vivo Knee Kinematics Using Fluoroscopy. *J. Arthroplast.* **2015**, *30*, 1237–1242. [CrossRef] [PubMed]
23. Longo, U.G.; Ciuffreda, M.; Mannering, N.; D'Andrea, V.; Locher, J.; Salvatore, G.; Denaro, V. Outcomes of Posterior-Stabilized Compared with Cruciate-Retaining Total Knee Arthroplasty. *J. Knee Surg.* **2018**, *31*, 321–340. [CrossRef] [PubMed]
24. Okazaki, K.; Miura, H.; Matsuda, S.; Takeuchi, N.; Mawatari, T.; Hashizume, M.; Iwamoto, Y. Asymmetry of mediolateral laxity of the normal knee. *J. Orthop. Sci.* **2006**, *11*, 264–266. [CrossRef]
25. Aunan, E.; Kibsgård, T.J.; Diep, L.M.; Röhrl, S.M. Intraoperative ligament laxity influences functional outcome 1 year after total knee arthroplasty. *Knee Surg. Sports Traumatol. Arthrosc.* **2015**, *23*, 1684–1692. [CrossRef] [PubMed]
26. Tanaka, Y.; Nakamura, S.; Kuriyama, S.; Nishitani, K.; Ito, H.; Lyman, S.; Matsuda, S. Intraoperative physiological lateral laxity in extension and flexion for varus knees did not affect short-term clinical outcomes and patient satisfaction. *Knee Surg. Sports Traumatol. Arthrosc.* **2020**, *28*, 3888–3898. [CrossRef] [PubMed]

27. Nakano, N.; Matsumoto, T.; Muratsu, H.; Takayama, K.; Kuroda, R.; Kurosaka, M. Postoperative Knee Flexion Angle Is Affected by Lateral Laxity in Cruciate-Retaining Total Knee Arthroplasty. *J. Arthroplast.* **2016**, *31*, 401–405. [CrossRef] [PubMed]
28. Seah, R.B.; Yeo, S.J.; Chin, P.L.; Yew, A.K.; Chong, H.C.; Lo, N.N. Evaluation of medial-lateral stability and functional outcome following total knee arthroplasty: Results of a single hospital joint registry. *J. Arthroplast.* **2014**, *29*, 2276–2279. [CrossRef]
29. Matsuda, Y.; Ishii, Y.; Noguchi, H.; Ishii, R. Varus-valgus balance and range of movement after total knee arthroplasty. *J. Bone Joint Surg. Br.* **2005**, *87*, 804–808. [CrossRef]
30. Yoshihara, Y.; Arai, Y.; Nakagawa, S.; Inoue, H.; Ueshima, K.; Fujiwara, H.; Oda, R.; Taniguchi, D.; Kubo, T. Assessing coronal laxity in extension and flexion at a minimum of 10 years after primary total knee arthroplasty. *Knee Surg. Sports Traumatol. Arthrosc.* **2016**, *24*, 2512–2516. [CrossRef]
31. Jones, D.P.; Locke, C.; Pennington, J.; Theis, J.C. The effect of sagittal laxity on function after posterior cruciate-retaining total knee replacement. *J. Arthroplast.* **2006**, *21*, 719–723. [CrossRef] [PubMed]
32. Warren, P.J.; Olanlokun, T.K.; Cobb, A.G.; Walker, P.S.; Iverson, B.F. Laxity and function in knee replacements. A comparative study of three prosthetic designs. *Clin. Orthop. Relat. Res.* **1994**, *305*, 200–208. [CrossRef]
33. Matsumoto, K.; Ogawa, H.; Yoshioka, H.; Akiyama, H. Postoperative Anteroposterior Laxity Influences Subjective Outcome After Total Knee Arthroplasty. *J. Arthroplast.* **2017**, *32*, 1845–1849. [CrossRef] [PubMed]
34. Bravi, M.; Longo, U.G.; Laurito, A.; Greco, A.; Marino, M.; Maselli, M.; Sterzi, S.; Santacaterina, F. Supervised versus unsupervised rehabilitation following total knee arthroplasty: A systematic review and meta-analysis. *Knee* **2023**, *40*, 71–89. [CrossRef] [PubMed]
35. Wang, X.H.; Song, D.Y.; Dong, X.; Suguro, T.; Cheng, C.K. Motion type and knee articular conformity influenced mid-flexion stability of a single radius knee prosthesis. *Knee Surg. Sports Traumatol. Arthrosc.* **2019**, *27*, 1595–1603. [CrossRef] [PubMed]
36. Wang, H.; Simpson, K.J.; Ferrara, M.S.; Chamnongkich, S.; Kinsey, T.; Mahoney, O.M. Biomechanical differences exhibited during sit-to-stand between total knee arthroplasty designs of varying radii. *J. Arthroplast.* **2006**, *21*, 1193–1199. [CrossRef] [PubMed]
37. Kessler, O.; Dürselen, L.; Banks, S.; Mannel, H.; Marin, F. Sagittal curvature of total knee replacements predicts in vivo kinematics. *Clin. Biomech.* **2007**, *22*, 52–58. [CrossRef]
38. Clary, C.W.; Fitzpatrick, C.K.; Maletsky, L.P.; Rullkoetter, P.J. The influence of total knee arthroplasty geometry on mid-flexion stability: An experimental and finite element study. *J. Biomech.* **2013**, *46*, 1351–1357. [CrossRef]
39. Longo, U.G.; Loppini, M.; Trovato, U.; Rizzello, G.; Maffulli, N.; Denaro, V. No difference between unicompartmental versus total knee arthroplasty for the management of medial osteoarthritis of the knee in the same patient: A systematic review and pooling data analysis. *Br. Med. Bull.* **2015**, *114*, 65–73. [CrossRef]
40. Longo, U.G.; Candela, V.; Pirato, F.; Hirschmann, M.T.; Becker, R.; Denaro, V. Midflexion instability in total knee arthroplasty: A systematic review. *Knee Surg. Sports Traumatol. Arthrosc.* **2021**, *29*, 370–380. [CrossRef]
41. Barbotte, F.; Delord, M.; Pujol, N. Coronal knee alignment measurements differ on long-standing radiographs vs. by navigation. *Orthop. Traumatol. Surg. Res.* **2022**, *108*, 103112. [CrossRef]
42. Longo, U.G.; Ciuffreda, M.; D'Andrea, V.; Mannering, N.; Locher, J.; Denaro, V. All-polyethylene versus metal-backed tibial component in total knee arthroplasty. *Knee Surg. Sports Traumatol. Arthrosc.* **2017**, *25*, 3620–3636. [CrossRef]
43. Sasaki, S.; Sasaki, E.; Kimura, Y.; Tsukada, H.; Otsuka, H.; Yamamoto, Y.; Tsuda, E.; Ishibashi, Y. Effect of medial collateral ligament release and osteophyte resection on medial laxity in total knee arthroplasty. *Knee Surg. Sports Traumatol. Arthrosc.* **2021**, *29*, 3418–3425. [CrossRef]
44. Marchand, R.C.; Scholl, L.; Bhowmik-Stoker, M.; Taylor, K.B.; Marchand, K.B.; Chen, Z.; Mont, M.A. Total Knee Arthroplasty in the Valgus Knee: Can New Operative Technologies Affect Surgical Technique and Outcomes? *Surg. Technol. Int.* **2021**, *39*, 389–393. [CrossRef]

Disclaimer/Publisher's Note: The statements, opinions and data contained in all publications are solely those of the individual author(s) and contributor(s) and not of MDPI and/or the editor(s). MDPI and/or the editor(s) disclaim responsibility for any injury to people or property resulting from any ideas, methods, instructions or products referred to in the content.

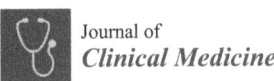

Article

Implant Preference and Clinical Outcomes of Patients with Staged Bilateral Total Knee Arthroplasty: All-Polyethylene and Contralateral Metal-Backed Tibial Components

Luboš Nachtnebl [1,2,†], Vasileios Apostolopoulos [1,2,†], Michal Mahdal [1,2], Lukáš Pazourek [1,2], Pavel Brančík [1,2], Tomáš Valoušek [1,2], Petr Boháč [3] and Tomáš Tomáš [1,2,*]

[1] First Department of Orthopaedic Surgery, St. Anne's University Hospital, 602 00 Brno, Czech Republic; lubos.nachtnebl@fnusa.cz (L.N.); vasileios.apostolopoulos@fnusa.cz (V.A.); michal.mahdal@fnusa.cz (M.M.); lukas.pazourek@fnusa.cz (L.P.); pavel.brancik@fnusa.cz (P.B.); tomas.valousek@fnusa.cz (T.V.)
[2] Faculty of Medicine, Masaryk University, 625 00 Brno, Czech Republic
[3] Institute of Solid Mechanics, Mechatronics and Biomechanics, Faculty of Mechanical Engineering, Brno University of Technology, 601 90 Brno, Czech Republic; 201394@vutbr.cz
* Correspondence: tomas.tomas@fnusa.cz; Tel.: +420-737391662
† These authors contributed equally to this work.

Abstract: Numerous studies have compared metal-backed components (MBTs) and all-polyethylene tibial components (APTs), but none of them specifically analysed the clinical results and the overall patient preference in patients who had undergone a staged bilateral knee replacement. The purpose of this study is to compare clinical results, perceived range of motion, and overall implant preference among patients who had undergone staged bilateral knee replacement with an APT and contralateral knee replacement with MBTs. A dataset of 62 patients from a single centre who underwent staged bilateral TKA between 2009 and 2022 was selected and retrospectively analysed. Tibial component removal was performed in three knees overall, all of which had MBTs. The mean measured Knee Score (KS) of knees with APTs was 78.37 and that of contralateral knees with MBTs was 77.4. The mean measured Function (FS) of knees with APTs was 78.22, and that of contralateral knees with MBs was 76.29. The mean flexion angle of knees with APTs was 103.8 and that for knees with MBTs was 101.04 degrees. A total of 54.8% of the patients preferred the knee that received APTs over contralateral MBTs. In our cohort, TKA with an APT in one knee and an MBT in the contralateral knee recorded similar clinical results and perceived ranges of motion. Patients in general preferred the knee that received an APT over contralateral knee with an MBT.

Keywords: bilateral knee replacement; total knee arthroplasty; all-polyethylene tibia; metal-backed tibia; staged bilateral knee arthroplasty

1. Introduction

Total knee arthroplasty (TKA) is one of the most frequent orthopaedic procedures and the definitive treatment of knee arthritis. Even if promising new technologies have been developed in knee arthroplasty, implant selection is still discussed [1,2]. Most total knee replacements have been performed with metal-backed tibial components (MBTs). All-polyethylene tibial components (APTs) are primarily implanted in older and low-demand patients [3]. Numerous studies have compared MBTs and APTs, describing similar clinical outcomes and implant survivorship [4–6]. The first-generation APT designs often failed to aseptic loosening; thus, many orthopaedic surgeons are still reluctant to use APTs [7]. Nowadays, considering improvements in implant design, material quality, and the economic strain on health care, APT utility is regaining popularity [8,9].

Our institution has a long tradition in arthroplasty with APTs, choosing APTs not only in cases of elder patients. A previous study described excellent long-term clinical

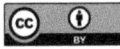

results and survivorship of APTs [10]. Moreover, in a clinical comparison of 812 patients with NexGen TKA APTs and MBTs, we suggest that APTs are equal or even superior to metal-backed components across the age categories [3]. Further examination of the topic in a biomechanical analysis on APTs showed a similar induced response in patients of the 60–70-year-old age groups as well as remodelling and modelling of the periprosthetic tibia, which is a beneficial factor in implant survivorship [11].

Despite numerous studies that have compared APTs with MBTs, none of them specifically analysed the clinical outcomes and the overall patient preference in patients who had undergone a staged bilateral knee replacement, having one knee with MBTs and the contralateral knee with APTs, implanted in a single orthopaedic department using the same surgical technique. The purpose of this retrospective study was to compare clinical results, perceived range of motion, and overall preference among patients who had undergone staged bilateral TKA with APTs and contralateral TKA with MBTs.

2. Materials and Methods

2.1. Sample Characteristics

For this retrospective comparative study, a dataset of 62 patients from a single centre who underwent staged bilateral TKA between 2009 and 2022 was selected. All of the patients had one knee with an MBT and an APT in the contralateral knee (Figure 1). In total, this represented 124 knee replacements, 34 of which had an APT on the right side, 28 with an APT on the left side, 34 with an MBT on the left side, and 28 with an MBT on the right side. There were 37 females and 25 males. The only indication for TKA was primary knee arthritis; patients with post-traumatic or other non-primary knee arthritis were excluded from this study (Table 1).

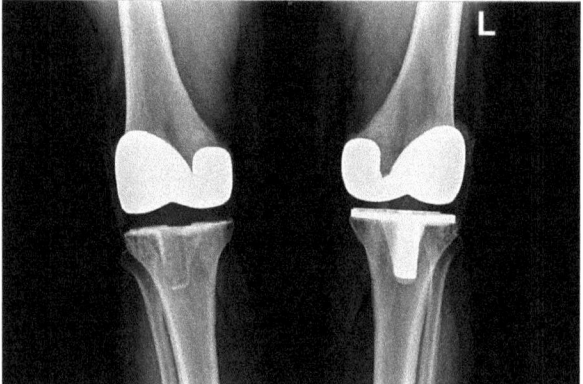

Figure 1. Radiological imaging of representative patient with staged bilateral TKA, right side with TKA APT implanted and left side with MBT.

Table 1. Sample characteristics.

Features	Bilateral TKA
Number of patients (knees)	62 (124)
Age at inclusion (years) APT MBT	74.1 ± 3.56 (66–82) 69.9 ± 3.69 (61–79) $p < 0.00001$
Sex Female Male	37 (59.7%) 25 (40.3%)

Table 1. Cont.

Features	Bilateral TKA
Average follow-up (years)	
APT	4.14 ± 3.19 (1–12)
MBT	7.45 ± 3.01 (1–12) $p < 0.00001$
Diagnosis	
Primary osteoarthritis	124 (100%)
Surgical approach	
Medial parapatellar	124 (100%)

Patients were followed up for at least 1 year, from 1 to 12 years postoperatively. The mean follow-up was 4.14 years for APTs and 7.45 years for MBTs (Figure 2). The mean age at the time of MBT implantation was 69.9 years and that at the time of APT implantation was 74.1 years. Exclusion criteria were a minimum 1-year follow-up and a maximum interval of 10 years between the first TKA and the TKA of the other side.

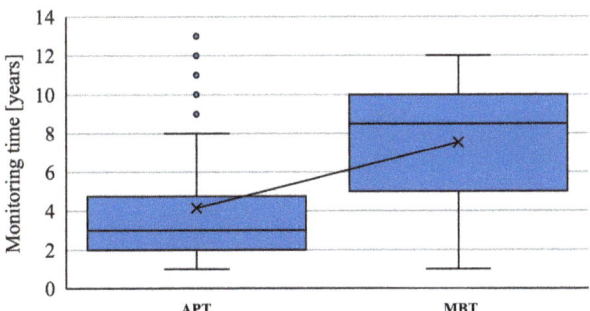

Figure 2. Follow-up patients with staged bilateral TKA in our institution from 2009 to 2022 for each implant type.

2.2. Evaluation

The primary efficacy endpoint compared was the clinical outcome of the implants as per the Knee Society Score before and after the procedure, which was assessed at a minimum of 1-year follow-up and eventually modified at the last examination, with both the knee-specific score (KS) and general functional score (FS) [12]. Both scores range from 0 to 100 (excellent) [12]. The secondary efficacy endpoint was the determination of the maximum range of motion in patients observed at a minimum of 1-year follow-up and eventually modified at the last examination. The range of motion was measured with a goniometer (universal goniometer) while the patient was lying on the exam table. The last efficacy point was an examination of the subjective implant preference of the patients between APTs and MBTs. Patients were asked directly to choose the knee they were satisfied with the most.

2.3. Implant Types

Four different systems of cemented TKA CR, two per type, were used (Figure 3). The all-polyethylene knee system variants included Sigma DePuy ($n = 16$) and NexGen Zimmer ($n = 46$). The metal-backed knee system variants included Search Evolution Aesculap ($n = 37$) and NexGen Zimmer ($n = 25$). The implant selection was based on current research evidence and advances in the field of orthopaedics to ensure the best outcomes for each patient.

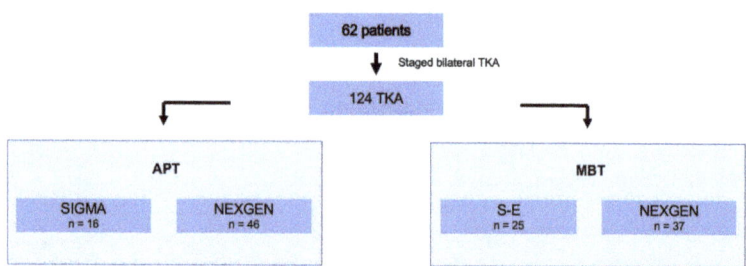

Figure 3. Sample distribution and TKA system variants used in staged bilateral TKA in our institution from 2009 to 2022.

2.4. Surgical Technique

In all cases, the same surgical technique was utilised, following the standard principles used in our institution. The mechanical alignment concept and medial parapatellar approach to the knee were employed using a tourniquet cuff inflated at 300 mmHg. Patellar resurfacing was performed in select cases, while patellar denervation with electrocautery and osteophyte removal were conducted in all cases. Bone cement was applied to the implants, with a small amount pressed into the cancellous bone. At the end of the procedure, two suction drains were inserted to capture the blood loss during the first 24 h, and 1 g of tranexamic acid was applied intra-articularly. All patients received a single preoperative dose of prophylactic antibiotics (cefazolin) before the inflation of the tourniquet and 3 doses postoperatively. All patients participated in the same postoperative course and physical therapy during their 7-day hospital stay.

2.5. Statistical Methods

The statistical analysis was carried out using R version 4.0.5 (Bell Laboratories, Murray Hill, NJ, USA) software. The Fischer exact test was conducted to compare categorical variables between the two groups. A significance level of $p < 0.05$ was used. A 95% confidence interval (95% CI) was calculated. The non-parametric Mann–Whitney test was used to compare the clinical outcomes between the implants.

3. Results

Tibial component removal was performed in three knees overall, all of which had an implanted MBT, and there was no statistically significant relationship between the survival rate and the type of implant ($p = 0.2439$). The cause of removal in two of the cases was due to aseptic loosening of the tibial component. The first occurred 4 years after the implantation and the second 10 years after the implantation. The last case of tibial component removal was because of arthrofibrosis, a reduced range of motion to 60 degrees of flexion, and an extension deficit of 5 degrees.

3.1. Functional Outcome

The mean measured KS of knees before the TKA with an APT was 47.11 and the mean KS of contralateral knees before the TKA with an MBT was 48.54 ($p = 0.01684$) (Figure 4). The mean measured FS of knees before the TKA with an APT was 44.35 and the mean FS of contralateral knees before the TKA with an MBT was 46.29 ($p = 0.01352$) (Figure 5). See Table 2.

Table 2. Preoperative KS and FS of patients with staged bilateral TKA in our institution from 2009 to 2022.

Overall	KS: APT	KS: MBT	FS: APT	FS: MBT
Mean	47.11	48.54	44.35	46.29
Std. Dev	4.00	3.56	4.09	3.83

Table 2. Cont.

Overall	KS: APT	KS: MBT	FS: APT	FS: MBT
Median	48	48	45	45
N.Valid	62	62	62	62

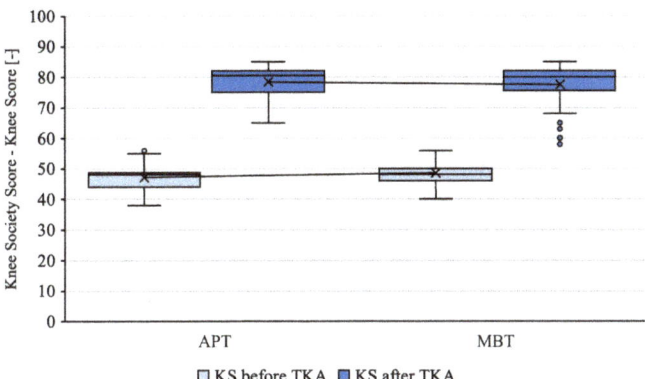

Figure 4. KS of implants in patients with staged bilateral TKA in our institution from 2009 to 2022.

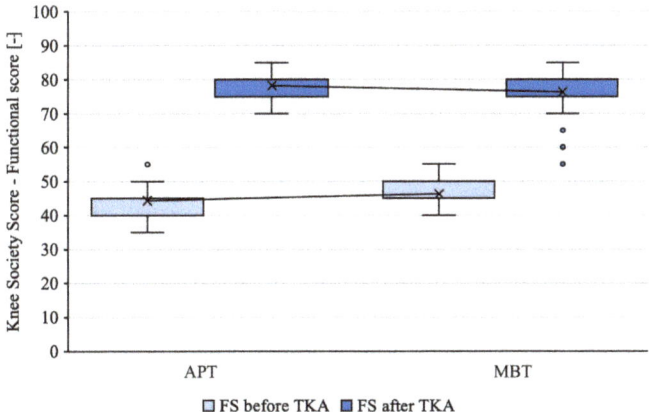

Figure 5. FS of implants in patients with staged bilateral TKA in our institution from 2009 to 2022.

The mean measured KS of knees with an APT was 78.37 and the mean KS of contralateral knees with an MBT was 77.4 ($p = 0.29372$) (Figure 4). The mean measured FS of knees with an APT was 78.22 and the mean FS of contralateral knees with an MBT was 76.29 ($p = 0.72786$) (Figure 5). See Table 3.

Table 3. Postoperative KS and FS at the last follow-up of patients with staged bilateral TKA in our institution from 2009 to 2022.

Overall	KS: APT	KS: MBT	FS: APT	FS: MBT
Mean	78.37	77.4	78.22	76.29
Std. Dev	5.11	6.87	4.44	7.06
Median	80.5	80	80	80
N.Valid	62	62	62	62

For both of the tibial components, there was a statistically significant improvement in FS and KS after the TKA ($p < 0.00001$).

3.2. Range of Motion

The mean knee flexion angle of knees with an APT was 103.8 ($\pm$8.21) degrees, and the mean flexion contracture was 6.25 degrees and occurred in eight knees. On the contrary, the mean knee flexion angle of contralateral knees with an MBT was 101.04 degrees ($\pm$14.29) ($p = 0.52218$), and the mean flexion contracture was 8 degrees and occurred only in five knees ($p = 0.5593$) (Figure 6). Manipulation under anaesthesia was necessary in one case because of stiffness in the APT. No cases were treated with arthroscopic or open lysis of adhesions.

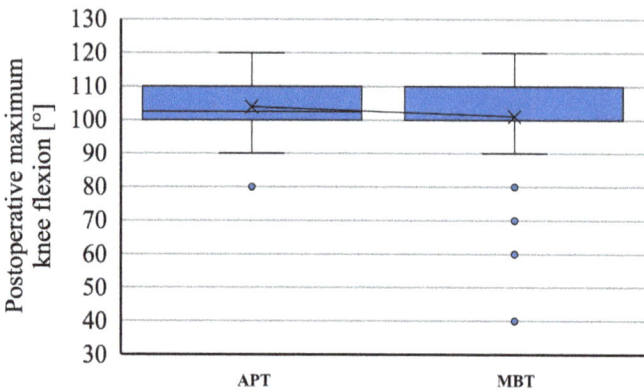

Figure 6. Maximum knee flexion in patients with staged bilateral TKA in our institution from 2009 to 2022.

3.3. Implant Preference

At the follow-up, patients were asked to directly compare their knees. A total of 54.8% of the patients preferred the knee that received an APT over the contralateral MBT. Meanwhile, 12.9% of the patients found no difference and 32.3% preferred the MBT (Figure 7).

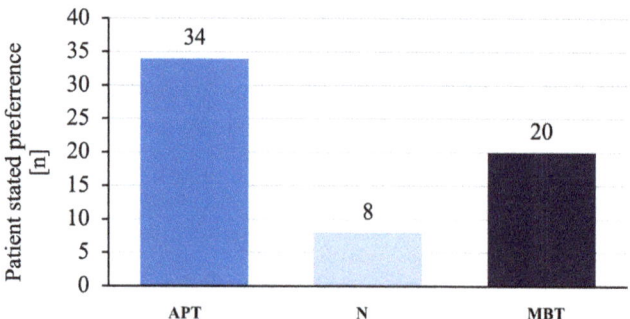

Figure 7. Patient-stated implant preference in staged bilateral TKA in our institution from 2009 to 2022.

4. Discussion

In modern orthopaedics, modular MBTs are preferred by the majority of orthopaedic surgeons over monoblock APTs [13]. The poor clinical results described in the 1980s notably lowered the utilisation rates of APTs [14]. Even though the design of these components and the polyethylene material used to make them have been significantly improved, APTs are still primarily recommended for older and low-demand patients [15]. Despite numerous papers comparing APTs and MBTs, there is no study specifically comparing these tibial components in bilateral TKA. This study compared the clinical outcomes of an APT in one knee and an MBT in the contralateral knee of the same patient in staged bilateral TKA.

Previous studies comparing these implants presented similar or even superior mid-term clinical survivorship of APTs [16,17]. In this study, out of a total of 124 TKAs, removal of the tibial component was necessary in three cases, and all of them were MBTs; removal of APTs was not necessary. There were no cases of polyethylene insert exchange, whereas modularity is considered to be a major advantage of MBTs [18]. Nouta et al., in meta-analysis comprising more than 12,500 TKAs, found no differences in clinical and functional outcomes between the two implants. The mean KS and FS for APTs and MBTs were found to be similar [19]. Another recent study comparing the two tibial components observed similar clinical results using the same evaluation method [20]. In the literature, there are only a few specific clinical comparisons between the components in bilateral staged TKA [21,22]. Our study recorded comparable clinical and functional outcomes using the Knee Society Score. The mean KS of APTs at the last follow-up (78.37) was similar to the mean KS of contralateral knees with MBTs (77.4). Analogously, the mean FS of APTs at the last follow-up (78.22) was comparable with the mean FS of contralateral knees with an MBT (76.29).

A recent study comparing the medium-term outcomes of the two implants described a similar range of motion in patients older than 70 years of age [20]. In this study, we recorded a similar maximal knee flexion when comparing the two tibial components. A slightly greater mean maximal flexion was measured in knees with APTs (103.8 degrees); on the contrary, the mean maximal flexion of knees with MBTs was 101.04 degrees. The difference in maximal knee flexion was not found to be significant. Flexion contracture was recorded in eight knees with APTs and five knees with MBTs. There was only a single patient with an APT undergoing manipulation under anaesthesia for stiffness.

Since APTs are primarily recommended for elderly patients, the implantation of the APTs was, in most cases, performed years after the implantation of MBTs. Additionally, we found excellent results of APTs in older patients [10]. Consequently, even if these older patients have previously received an MBT on the contralateral side during a previous surgery at a younger age, they still receive an APT. This explains the significant difference in the age at inclusion of the patients as well as the longer follow-up of patients with MBTs. Minimising the variation in follow-up durations was not feasible as we compared results for the same patient, and APTs were mostly implanted years later. Another issue we need to highlight is the lower KS and FS at the implantation of APTs. This could be probably explained by the age at implantation as the scoring system is associated with patient infirmity, especially in the case of the FS.

One crucial aspect following a TKA implantation is the overall satisfaction of the patient [23]. Therefore, we took into account the subjective preference of each patient by directly asking them to choose between the APT and the contralateral MBT. A similar method was used in a study comparing the overall preference among patients who had undergone staged bilateral TKA with a customised implant in one knee and an off-the-shelf implant in the contralateral knee [24]. In our query, 54.8% of the patients preferred the knee that received the APT over that with the contralateral MBT. Only 12.9% of the patients could not decide which of the knees they favoured.

The present study has several strengths that contribute to its reliability. Firstly, it possesses an appropriate sample size consisting of patients who underwent bilateral TKA. Additionally, the surgical technique employed was consistent across all patients, and the mean follow-up duration is notable. These strengths enabled us to effectively compare the performance of the two tibial component types. However, it is important to acknowledge the limitations of our study. Firstly, it had a retrospective design and varying follow-up durations for the studied knees. Additionally, some of the TKA cases only had a 1-year follow-up. Secondly, the sample consisted of four different systems of cemented TKA, with two variants for each type, which introduced some degree of variability. Considering these limitations, we believe that the obtained results are still meaningful and provide valuable insights into the comparison of the two tibial component types.

5. Conclusions

The present study provides evidence that TKA with an APT in one knee and an MBT in the contralateral knee exhibits comparable clinical and functional outcomes. Patients generally expressed a preference for the knee that received the APT over that with the contralateral MBT. Taking into account their limitations, our findings could influence implant selection, encouraging more frequent utilisation of TKAs with an APT.

Author Contributions: Conceptualisation, V.A. and L.N.; methodology, T.T. and L.P.; software, P.B. (Petr Boháč); validation, T.T. and L.N.; formal analysis, P.B. (Pavel Brančík); V.A.; investigation, V.A., M.M., and L.P.; resources, T.T. and L.N.; data curation, V.A. and L.N.; writing—original draft preparation, V.A. and L.N.; writing—review and editing, M.M., L.P., P.B. (Pavel Brančík), T.V., and V.A.; visualisation, P.B. (Petr Boháč) and P.B. (Pavel Brančík); supervision, T.T.; project administration, T.T.; funding acquisition, T.T. and T.V. All authors have read and agreed to the published version of the manuscript.

Funding: This research received no external funding.

Institutional Review Board Statement: This study was conducted according to the guidelines of the Declaration of Helsinki. Consent was not deemed necessary by the ethics committee due to study design, which was based on routine clinical data.

Informed Consent Statement: Informed consent was obtained from all subjects involved in this study.

Data Availability Statement: The data presented in this study are available on request from the corresponding author. The data are not publicly available for privacy reasons.

Conflicts of Interest: The authors declare no conflict of interest.

References

1. Batailler, C.; Swan, J.; Sappey Marinier, E.; Servien, E.; Lustig, S. New Technologies in Knee Arthroplasty: Current Concepts. *J. Clin. Med.* **2020**, *10*, 47. [CrossRef]
2. Palazzuolo, M.; Antoniadis, A.; Mahlouly, J.; Wegrzyn, J. Total Knee Arthroplasty Improves the Quality-Adjusted Life Years in Patients Who Exceeded Their Estimated Life Expectancy. *Int. Orthop.* **2021**, *45*, 635–641. [CrossRef]
3. Apostolopoulos, V.; Nachtnebl, L.; Mahdal, M.; Pazourek, L.; Boháč, P.; Janíček, P.; Tomáš, T. Clinical Outcomes and Survival Comparison between NexGen All-Poly and Its Metal-Backed Equivalent in Total Knee Arthroplasty. *Int. Orthop.* **2023**, *47*, 2207–2213. [CrossRef]
4. Longo, U.G.; Ciuffreda, M.; D'Andrea, V.; Mannering, N.; Locher, J.; Denaro, V. All-Polyethylene versus Metal-Backed Tibial Component in Total Knee Arthroplasty. *Knee Surg. Sports Traumatol. Arthrosc.* **2017**, *25*, 3620–3636. [CrossRef]
5. Yassin, M.; Garti, A.; Weissbrot, M.; Ashkenazi, U.; Khatib, M.; Robinson, D. All-Polyethylene Tibial Components Are Not Inferior to Metal-Backed Tibial Components in Long-Term Follow-up of Knee Arthroplasties. *Eur. J. Orthop. Surg. Traumatol.* **2015**, *25*, 1087–1091. [CrossRef]
6. Mohan, V.; Inacio, M.C.S.; Namba, R.S.; Sheth, D.; Paxton, E.W. Monoblock All-Polyethylene Tibial Components Have a Lower Risk of Early Revision than Metal-Backed Modular Components: A Registry Study of 27,657 Primary Total Knee Arthroplasties. *Acta Orthop.* **2013**, *84*, 530–536. [CrossRef]
7. Voss, B.; El-Othmani, M.M.; Schnur, A.-K.; Botchway, A.; Mihalko, W.M.; Saleh, K.J. A Meta-Analysis Comparing All-Polyethylene Tibial Component to Metal-Backed Tibial Component in Total Knee Arthroplasty: Assessing Survivorship and Functional Outcomes. *J. Arthroplast.* **2016**, *31*, 2628–2636. [CrossRef]
8. Ryan, S.P.; Steele, J.R.; Plate, J.F.; Attarian, D.E.; Seyler, T.M.; Bolognesi, M.P.; Wellman, S.S. All-Polyethylene Tibia: An Opportunity for Value-Based Care in Bundled Reimbursement Initiatives. *Orthopedics* **2021**, *44*, e114–e118. [CrossRef]
9. Kumar, V.; Hasan, O.; Umer, M.; Baloch, N. Cemented All-Poly Tibia in Resource Constrained Country, Affordable and Cost-Effective Care. Is It Applicable at This Era? Review Article. *Ann. Med. Surg.* **2019**, *47*, 36–40. [CrossRef]
10. Nachtnebl, L.; Tomáš, T.; Apostolopoulos, V.; Pazourek, L.; Mahdal, M. Long-Term Results of Total Knee Replacement Using P.F.C. Sigma System with an All-Polyethylene Tibial Component. *Acta Chir. Orthop. Traumatol. Cech.* **2021**, *88*, 412–417.
11. Apostolopoulos, V.; Tomáš, T.; Boháč, P.; Marcián, P.; Mahdal, M.; Valoušek, T.; Janíček, P.; Nachtnebl, L. Biomechanical Analysis of All-Polyethylene Total Knee Arthroplasty on Periprosthetic Tibia Using the Finite Element Method. *Comput. Methods Prog. Biomed.* **2022**, *220*, 106834. [CrossRef]

12. Insall, J.N.; Dorr, L.D.; Scott, R.D.; Scott, W.N. Rationale of the Knee Society Clinical Rating System. *Clin. Orthop. Relat. Res.* **1989**, *248*, 13–14.
13. Australian Orthopaedic Association National Joint Replacement Registry. Annual Report. Adelaide. AOA 2020: Table KT2 10 Most Used Femoral Prostheses in Primary Total Knee Replacement. Available online: https://aoanjrr.sahmri.com/documents/10180/689619/Hip%252C+Knee+%2526+Shoulder+Arthroplasty+New/6a07a3b8-8767-06cf-9069-d165dc9baca7 (accessed on 30 December 2022).
14. Doran, J.; Yu, S.; Smith, D.; Iorio, R. The Role of All-Polyethylene Tibial Components in Modern TKA. *J. Knee Surg.* **2015**, *28*, 382–389. [CrossRef]
15. Gustke, K.A.; Gelbke, M.K. All-Polyethylene Tibial Component Use for Elderly, Low-Demand Total Knee Arthroplasty Patients. *J. Arthrop.* **2017**, *32*, 2421–2426. [CrossRef]
16. Herschmiller, T.; Bradley, K.E.; Wellman, S.S.; Attarian, D.E. Early to Midterm Clinical and Radiographic Survivorship of the All-Polyethylene Versus Modular Metal-Backed Tibia Component in Primary Total Knee Replacement. *J. Surg. Orthop. Adv.* **2019**, *28*, 108–114.
17. Selvan, D.R.; Santini, A.J.A.; Davidson, J.S.; Pope, J.A. The Medium-Term Survival Analysis of an All-Polyethylene Tibia in a Single-Series Cohort of over 1000 Knees. *J. Arthrop.* **2020**, *35*, 2837–2842. [CrossRef]
18. Kelley, B.; Mullen, K.; De, A.; Sassoon, A. Modular Metal-Backed Tibial Components Provide Minimal Mid-Term Survivorship Benefits Despite Increased Cost and Frequency of Use: A Retrospective Review of the American Joint Replacement Registry Database. *J. Arthrop.* **2022**, *37*, 1570–1574.e1. [CrossRef]
19. Nouta, K.A.; Verra, W.C.; Pijls, B.G.; Schoones, J.W.; Nelissen, R.G.H.H. All-Polyethylene Tibial Components Are Equal to Metal-Backed Components: Systematic Review and Meta-Regression. *Clin. Orthop. Relat. Res.* **2012**, *470*, 3549–3559. [CrossRef]
20. Jabbal, M.; Clement, N.; Walmsley, P.J. All-Polyethylene Tibia Components Have the Same Functional Outcomes and Survival, and Are More Cost-Effective than Metal-Backed Components in Patients 70 Years and Older Undergoing Total Knee Arthroplasty: Propensity Match Study with a Minimum Five-Year Follow-Up. *Bone Jt. Open* **2022**, *3*, 969–976. [CrossRef]
21. Najfeld, M.; Kalteis, T.; Spiegler, C.; Ley, C.; Hube, R. The Safety of Bilateral Simultaneous Hip and Knee Arthroplasty versus Staged Arthroplasty in a High-Volume Center Comparing Blood Loss, Peri- and Postoperative Complications, and Early Functional Outcome. *J. Clin. Med.* **2021**, *10*, 4507. [CrossRef]
22. Cammisa, E.; Sassoli, I.; La Verde, M.; Fratini, S.; Rinaldi, V.G.; Lullini, G.; Vaccari, V.; Zaffagnini, S.; Marcheggiani Muccioli, G.M. Bilateral Knee Arthroplasty in Patients Affected by Windswept Deformity: A Systematic Review. *J. Clin. Med.* **2022**, *11*, 6580. [CrossRef]
23. Sugita, T.; Miyatake, N.; Aizawa, T.; Sasaki, A.; Kamimura, M.; Takahashi, A. Quality of Life after Staged Bilateral Total Knee Arthroplasty: A Minimum Five-Year Follow-up Study of Seventy-Eight Patients. *Int. Orthop.* **2019**, *43*, 2309–2314. [CrossRef]
24. Schroeder, L.; Dunaway, A.; Dunaway, D. A Comparison of Clinical Outcomes and Implant Preference of Patients with Bilateral TKA: One Knee with a Patient-Specific and One Knee with an Off-the-Shelf Implant. *JBJS Rev.* **2022**, *10*, e20.00182. [CrossRef]

Disclaimer/Publisher's Note: The statements, opinions and data contained in all publications are solely those of the individual author(s) and contributor(s) and not of MDPI and/or the editor(s). MDPI and/or the editor(s) disclaim responsibility for any injury to people or property resulting from any ideas, methods, instructions or products referred to in the content.

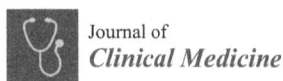

Article

Enhancing Precision and Efficiency in Knee Arthroplasty: A Comparative Analysis of Computer-Assisted Measurements with a Novel Software Tool versus Manual Measurements for Lower Leg Geometry

Ulrike Wittig [1,2], Amir Koutp [1,*], Patrick Reinbacher [1], Konstanze Hütter [1], Andreas Leithner [1] and Patrick Sadoghi [1]

[1] Department of Orthopaedics and Trauma, Medical University of Graz, 8036 Graz, Austria; ulrike.wittig@medunigraz.at (U.W.); patrick.reinbacher@medunigraz.at (P.R.); konstanze.huetter@medunigraz.at (K.H.); andreas.leithner@medunigraz.at (A.L.); patrick.sadoghi@medunigraz.at (P.S.)
[2] Department of Trauma Surgery, Landesklinikum Wiener Neustadt, 2700 Wiener Neustadt, Austria
* Correspondence: amir.koutp@medunigraz.at; Tel.: +43-316-385-81202

Abstract: (1) Background: The aim of this prospective study was to evaluate measurement software in comparison with manual measurements using inter-observer and intra-observer variability on radiographs in the preoperative planning of total knee arthroplasty. (2) Methods: Two independent observers retrospectively measured the mechanical lateral proximal femoral angle (mLPFA), the mechanical lateral distal femoral angle (mLDFA), the joint line convergence angle (JLCA), the mechanical medial proximal tibial angle (mMPTA), the mechanical lateral distal tibial angle (mLDTA), the hip–knee angle or mechanical tibial–femoral axis angle (HKA), and the anatomical–mechanical angle (AMA) on 55 long-leg anteroposterior radiographs manually twice, followed by measurements using dedicated software. Variability between manual and computer-aided planning was assessed, and all measurements were performed a second time after 14 days in order to assess intra-observer variability. (3) Results: Concerning intra-observer variability, no statistically significant difference was observed regarding the software-based measurements. However, significant differences were noted concerning intra-observer variability when measuring the mLDFA and AMA manually. Testing for statistical significance regarding variability between manual and software-based measurements showed that the values varied strongly between manual and computer-aided measurements. Statistically significant differences were detected for mLPFA, mLDFA, mMPTA, and mLPTA on day 1, and mLPFA, mMPTA, and mLPTA on day 15, respectively. (4) Conclusions: Preoperative planning of leg axis angles and alignment using planning software showed less inter- and intra-observer variability in contrast to manual measurements, and results differed with respect to manual planning. We believe that the planning software is more reliable and faster, and we would recommend its use in clinical settings.

Keywords: leg axis; leg axis angles; leg axis alignment; planning software

Citation: Wittig, U.; Koutp, A.; Reinbacher, P.; Hütter, K.; Leithner, A.; Sadoghi, P. Enhancing Precision and Efficiency in Knee Arthroplasty: A Comparative Analysis of Computer-Assisted Measurements with a Novel Software Tool versus Manual Measurements for Lower Leg Geometry. *J. Clin. Med.* 2023, *12*, 7581. https://doi.org/10.3390/jcm12247581

Academic Editor: Christian Carulli

Received: 22 October 2023
Revised: 4 December 2023
Accepted: 6 December 2023
Published: 8 December 2023

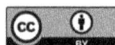

Copyright: © 2023 by the authors. Licensee MDPI, Basel, Switzerland. This article is an open access article distributed under the terms and conditions of the Creative Commons Attribution (CC BY) license (https://creativecommons.org/licenses/by/4.0/).

1. Introduction

While revision total knee arthroplasty (TKA) is not commonly associated with the surgical technique, it remains crucial to recognize its significance, as factors like inappropriate component size, malposition, and malalignment of the components can still contribute to the necessity for revision [1,2]. Therefore, thorough preoperative planning of relevant leg axis angles and, thus, varus/valgus alignment is an important factor in order to achieve optimal postoperative knee function [3].

Thus, preoperative planning is an important tool in total knee arthroplasty (TKA), especially concerning a reduction in intraoperative errors related to implant sizing, soft tissue balancing, and bony resections [4,5]. Consequently, many researchers have aimed to increase the reliability of preoperative planning [6–8].

The international gold standard in clinical preoperative planning is based on two-dimensional (2D) geometrical analysis of anterior–posterior (AP) standing long-leg radiographs by placing translucent templates on the radiographs [7,9]. Several studies have proposed that digital 2D planning might be more precise regarding the prediction of implant size [10,11]. Moreover, some studies have evaluated the accuracy of computed tomography (CT)-based three-dimensional (3D) planning and suggested that this might be more precise concerning the alignment and rotation of the components [12–14]. However, the accuracy of the novel measurement software Image Biopsy Lab (Vienna, Austria) has not been described on long-leg radiographs.

The aim of this prospective study was, therefore, to evaluate the above-mentioned measurement software in comparison with conventional manual measurements using inter-observer and intra-observer variability on 2D radiographs.

Our hypothesis is that the use of measurement software is more reliable and efficient in preoperative planning compared to manual measurements.

2. Materials and Methods

This study was approved by the institutional review board (blinded for review). Fifty-five pseudonymized standardized anteroposterior long-leg views were randomly selected from a patient collective consisting of surgical candidates for total knee arthroplasty between January 2021 and April 2021, as these radiographs were taken for preoperative planning [9,10]. The radiographs were independently reviewed by two observers, first manually and then using measurement software LAMA^{TM} (Image Biopsy Lab GmbH, Vienna, Austria). The measurement was carried out by two senior residents with experience and specialization in knee arthroplasty. In a second step, two independent reviewers were selected to evaluate the variability between manual and computer-aided planning, which was defined as inter-observer variability. Moreover, the angles were then measured a second time after a time interval of 14 days to assess intra-observer variability. Seven standardized angles were measured in degrees as follows: (1) the mechanical lateral proximal femoral angle (mLPFA); (2) the mechanical lateral distal femoral angle (mLDFA); (3) the joint line convergence angle (JLCA); (4) the mechanical medial proximal tibial angle (mMPTA); (5) the mechanical lateral distal tibial angle (mLDTA); (6) the hip–knee angle or mechanical tibial–femoral axis angle (HKA); and (7) the anatomical–mechanical angle as the angle between the anatomical and mechanical axis of the femur (AMA). A graphical depiction of these angles on a long-leg view is presented in Figure 1.

2.1. Manual Measurements

The manual measurements were performed on blinded prints of the radiographs by drawing the baselines through significant points of the proximal and distal femur and tibia, respectively. The first baseline was drawn through the central point of the femoral head and the tangent of the great trochanter. The second baseline runs through the most prominent protrusions of the medial and lateral femoral condyles. Analogously, the most prominent points of the proximal and distal tibia were connected with the third and fourth baseline. Next, the anatomical axis was drawn by connecting two central lines through the diaphyses of the femur and tibia. Additionally, the mechanical axis of the femur was drawn through the central point of the femoral head and the center of the femoral condyles. The mechanical axis of the tibia was drawn through the center of the tibial tubercles and the center of the previously marked distal tibial baseline. The mLPFA is the lateral angle between the femoral mechanical axis and the first baseline. The mLDFA is the lateral angle between the femoral mechanical axis and the second baseline. The JCLA, which has a positive value in case of varus deformity and a negative value in case of valgus deformity, constitutes the angle between the second and third baseline. The mMPTA is the medial angle between the third baseline and the mechanical axis of the tibia. The mLDTA is defined as the lateral angle between the fourth baseline and the mechanical axis of the tibia. The HKA, whose positive or negative value is determined analogously to the JLCA, constitutes the angle between the mechanical femoral and mechanical tibial axis. Finally, AMA is the angle between the anatomical and mechanical femoral axis.

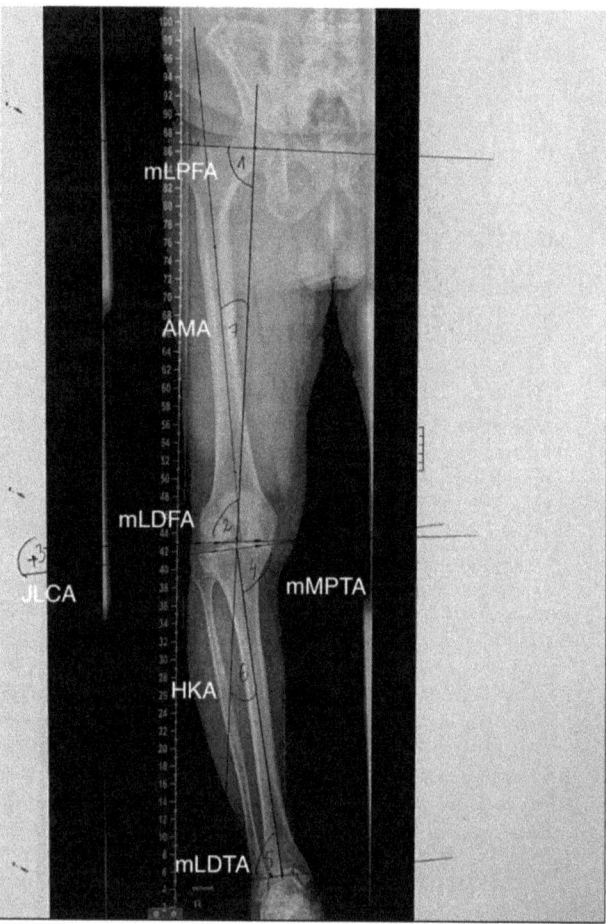

Figure 1. A graphical depiction of the angles measured on a long-leg radiographic view. (1) mLPFA; (2) mLDFA; (3) JLCA; (4) mMPTA; (5) mLDTA; (6) HKA; (7) AMA.

2.2. Software Measurements

The automatic localization of anatomical features of the femur, tibia, and calibration ball to assess all landmarks was needed to perform the required measurements. The AI-based software uses deep learning algorithms and multiple U-Net-based convolutional neural networks. A magnification factor was applied for length measurement based on the detection of a calibration ball. By segmenting a calibration ball and calculating a magnification factor based on the calibration ball size (25 mm) and the diameter of the segmentation (pixel units), the length calibration was performed. The measurement of the following angles was performed on each long-leg radiograph: hip–knee angle (HKA); anatomical–mechanical angle (AMA); joint line convergence angle (JLCA); mechanical lateral distal femoral angle (mLDFA); mechanical lateral distal tibial angle (mLDTA); mechanical lateral proximal femoral angle (mLPFA); mechanical medial proximal tibial angle (mMPTA); mechanical axis deviation (MAD); leg length; femur length; and tibia length. This is further illustrated in Figures 2 and 3.

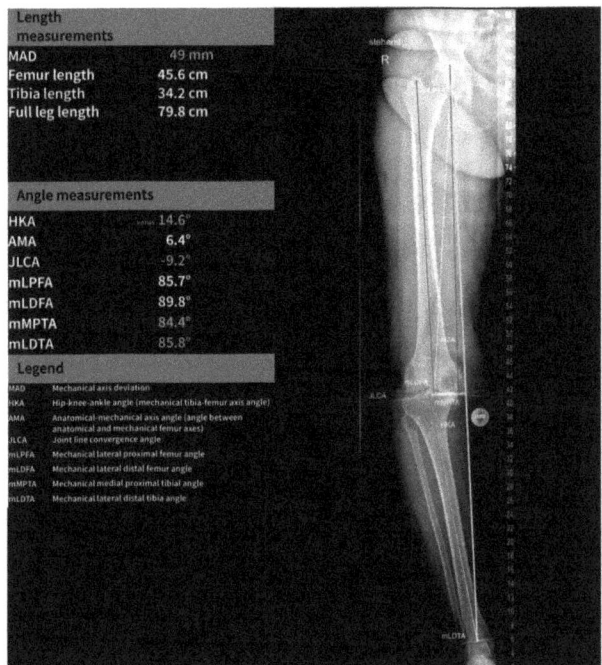

Figure 2. A graphical depiction of software-based measurements of standardized angles on a longleg view.

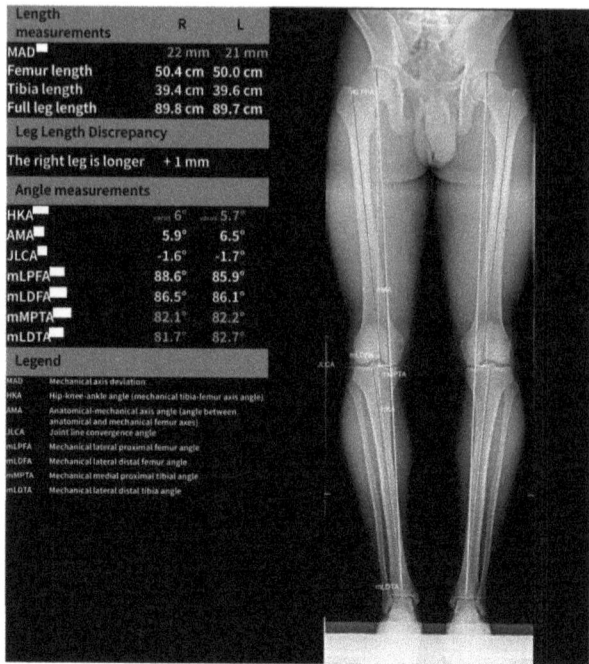

Figure 3. A graphical depiction of software-based measurements of standardized angles on long-leg views of both legs.

2.3. Statistical Analysis

Statistical analysis was performed using Statistical Package for the Social Sciences (SPSS) version 27.0 software (IBM Corp., Armonk, NY, USA). In order to quantify intra-observer variability as well as variability between manual and computer-aided planning (inter-observer variability), the t-test was used. Paired t-tests were used in order to assess intra-observer variability, while t-tests for independent samples were performed to check for variability regarding manual and computer-aided planning. A confidence interval of 95% was assumed, and a p-value < 0.05 was considered statistically significant. Moreover, a descriptive summary of the data was performed using summary tables.

The interrater reliability of measurements was assessed using intraclass correlation coefficients (ICCs) and the confidence interval.

3. Results

Axial deviation, femoral and tibial length, and full leg length were measured using the software. At day 1, the axial deviation was a mean of 12.1 cm (SD: 28.6), and the femoral and tibial length was on average 50.4 cm (SD: 3.1cm) and 39.3 cm (SD: 3.0 cm), and full leg length was a mean 89.5 cm (SD: 5.9 cm)At day 15, axial deviation was measured as a mean of 12.4 cm (SD: 28.7 cm), femoral and tibial length were at a mean of 50.4 cm (SD: 3.0 cm) and 39.3 cm (SD: 3.0 cm), and full leg length was measured as 89.6 cm (SD: 5.9 cm) on average.

A descriptive summary of the mean values and standard deviations of the manual and software-based measurements regarding the leg axis angles on days 1 and 15, respectively, is depicted in Table 1.

Table 1. Summary of mean values and standard deviation (SD) at day 1 and day 15.

	Manual d1	Manual d15	Software d1	Software d15
mLPFA	90.3 (SD: 4.7)	89.7 (SD: 3.9)	91.7 (SD: 4.8)	91.8 (SD: 4.8)
mLDFA	89.2 (SD: 4.1)	88.0 (SD: 3.9)	88.1 (SD: 2.9)	88.2 (SD: 2.9)
JLCA	3.3 (SD: 3.7)	3.3 (SD: 3.9)	2.4 (SD: 4.0)	2.5 (SD: 4.0)
mMPTA	89.5 (SD: 3.3)	88.9 (SD: 3.4)	87.8 (SD: 2.8)	87.8 (SD: 2.8)
mLPTA	88.5 (SD: 3.5)	87.9 (SD: 3.2)	86.2 (SD: 3.8)	86.1 (SD: 3.8)
HKA	2.6 (SD: 7.1)	2.8 (SD: 7.6)	2.6 (SD: 7.6)	2.7 (SD: 7.6)
AMA	6.7 (SD: 1.1)	7.0 (SD: 1.6)	6.9 (SD: 1.1)	6.9 (SD: 1.1)

Values are in degrees; SD = standard deviation; d1 = day 1; d15 = day 15; manual = manual measurements of both readers.

Concerning intra-observer variability, no statistically significant difference was observed regarding the software-based measurements. However, significant differences were noted concerning intra-observer variability when measuring the mLDFA and AMA manually. Moreover, the other manual measurements showed no statistical significance.

The test for statistical significance regarding the variability between manual and software-based measurements showed different results regarding the individual angles. For some angles, values varied strongly between manual and computer-aided measurements. Statistical significance was detected for mLPFA, mLDFA, mMPTA, and mLPTA on day 1, and mLPFA, mMPTA, and mLPTA on day 15, respectively. A summary of the p-values associated with the respective leg axis angles is outlined in Table 2.

Table 2. Summary of intra- and inter-observer variability.

Knee Angles	Intra-Observer Variability (Manual)	Intra-Observer Variability (Software)	Inter-Observer Variability d1	Inter-Observer Variability d15
mLPFA	$p = 0.285$	$p = 0.320$	$p = 0.026$	$p < 0.001$
mLDFA	$p = 0.012$	$p = 0.320$	$p = 0.035$	$p = 0.741$
JLCA	$p = 0.822$	$p = 0.435$	$p = 0.114$	$p = 0.103$
mMPTA	$p = 0.164$	$p = 0.320$	$p < 0.001$	$p = 0.010$
mLPTA	$p = 0.097$	$p = 0.276$	$p < 0.001$	$p < 0.001$
HKA	$p = 0.726$	$p = 0.320$	$p = 0.934$	$p = 0.943$
AMA	$p = 0.030$	$p = 0.320$	$p = 0.087$	$p = 0.594$

d1 = day 1, d15 = day 15.

The ICC revealed a value of 0.99 for the measurement of the interrater reliability, which, according to [15], corresponds to excellent agreement.

4. Discussion

The aim of this prospective study was, therefore, to evaluate the measurement software Image Biopsy Lab (Vienna, Austria) in comparison with conventional manual measurements using inter-observer and intra-observer variability on 2D radiographs.

One of the most important findings of the present study was that regarding four of the seven measured angles on day 1 (mLPFA: $p = 0.026$; mLDFA: $p = 0.035$; mMPTA: $p < 0.001$; mLPTA: $p < 0.001$) and three on day 15 (mLPFA: $p < 0.001$; mMPTA: $p = 0.010$; mLPTA: $p < 0.001$), statistically significant differences between manual and software-based measurements were detected, indicating that manual and software-based planning of leg axes leads to differential results. Additionally, the small difference in inter-observer variability between days 1 and 15 might indicate that the learning curve of performing manual measurements more precisely is quite small after only one repetition. Furthermore, intra-observer variability shows no significant results concerning software-based planning, possibly implying that this method might be more precise, and thus measurements may be more reliable and consistent between different time points. Testing for intra-observer variability of manual measurements revealed statistically significant differences regarding two angles (mLDFA: $p = 0.012$; AMA: $p = 0.030$), pointing towards poorer reliability of manual measurements with increased variability.

Potential explanations for reduced intra-observer variability during software-based analysis include the ability to zoom parts of the radiograph, enabling more exact determination of relevant landmarks for drawing. Moreover, transparent films may slide, which can consequently lead to inaccurate drawings and thus reduced reliability. Additionally, the goniometer has a 1° scale, and no further accuracy is possible.

In 2006, Hankemeier et al. [16] performed an analysis of intra-observer reliability regarding computer-assisted analysis of lower limb geometry and compared these findings to manual measurements on conventional radiographs. In this study, one single surgeon reviewed 59 long-leg radiographs five times and measured the mLPFA, mLDFA, mMPTA, mLDTA, JLCA, and AMA, respectively. The authors concluded that computer-assisted analysis increases intra-observer reliability, which is in accordance with the findings of this present study.

In a more recent study by Schröter et al. [17], the interrater reliability of two digital planning software for high tibial osteotomy was evaluated. In accordance with our results, high interrater reliability could be found using digital planning software.

A similar study reporting on the reliability of an imaging software in the preoperative planning of high tibial osteotomy detected high reliability and consistency between the conventional paper print method and the software-assisted method [18]. This further supports the hypothesis of our study regarding the reliability of measurement software in preoperative planning.

In this study, the anatomical axis was drawn by connecting two central lines through the diaphysis of the femur and tibia. The assessment of the anatomical axis is known to be difficult due to the bowing of the femoral shaft. Moreland [19] defined the anatomical axis as the connecting line between the midpoint of the medial-to-lateral width of the femoral diameter at half of the femoral length and 10 cm above the joint line. The literature showed varying definitions of the anatomical axis, but no significant differences were detected between them [20]. Another problem accompanied with planning on plain radiographs is rotational abnormality. It was shown that planning is rather precise when rotation is neutral, but that pathological rotation of the femur may lead to deviations, making estimated corrections proportional to the degree of malrotation necessary [21].

A further recent study by Pagano et al. [22], evaluating the role and efficiency of AI-powered software in total knee arthroplasty, showed excellent agreement with expert metrics in most knee angles and axial alignments assessed; however, it indicates limitations in the assessment of JLCA, the Mikulicz line, and in patients with a body mass index higher than 30 kg/m^2, which is comparable to our findings.

Several previous studies have reported on the inter-observer and intra-observer reliability of software-based 2D and 3D planning of component sizes for TKA [23]. It was reported that inter- and intra-observer reliability for component sizes was higher with CT-based 3D planning, comparing directly to two other published research articles that have performed preoperative 2D planning, supporting the fact that 3D planning using CT or MRI may lead to more precise measurements [24,25].

In addition to its use in preoperative planning, artificial intelligence is also used as a diagnostic tool for osteoarthritis of the knee, where studies have shown an increase in interrater reliability, which confirms our findings [26].

There were several limitations associated with the present study. First, measurements were only performed on standardized X-rays that are routinely performed in the preoperative setting. This comes with the advantage that no additional radiation is applied to the patient; however, planning might be more precise when performed on CT imaging, which is, on the other hand, associated with greatly increased radiation exposure compared to conventional radiographs. Second, measurements were only performed by two independent reviewers. The power of the findings might be increased by having the radiographs analyzed by more reviewers and including more experienced specialists or senior physicians. Furthermore, analysis of the radiographs at more than two time points may also enhance the validity and precision of the results. Scale, contrast, and brightness can affect the software evaluation of X-ray images. These factors can affect the software's ability to recognize landmarks or perform measurements, especially if the contrast quality of the X-ray images is not sufficient or the brightness is not set optimally. To minimize such effects, a standardized acquisition method is used when capturing X-ray images for analysis and to ensure that the image quality is sufficient. Paying attention to these factors and, if necessary, adjusting the settings can help to improve the reliability of software evaluation and the accuracy of manual measurements in orthopaedic imaging. As a university hospital, we are also subject to regular quality controls in order to be able to react accordingly. Additionally, no power analysis for the number of physicians, the number of patient cases, and repetitive measurements was performed. However, [15] postulated that, as a rule of thumb, at least 30 heterogeneous patient cases should be included.

5. Conclusions

Preoperative planning of leg axis angles and alignment using planning software showed less inter- and intra-observer variability in contrast to manual measurements, and results differed with respect to manual planning. We believe that the planning software is more reliable and would recommend its use in clinical settings.

Author Contributions: U.W.: Writing of the manuscript, data administration, approval of the final draft. A.K.: Data administration, revising manuscript, approval of the final draft. P.R.: Statistics, measurements of radiographs, revising manuscript, approval of the final draft. K.H.: measurements of radiographs, revising manuscript, approval of the final draft. A.L.: Revising the manuscript, approval of the final draft, study idea. P.S.: Revising manuscript, approval of the final draft, study idea. All authors have read and agreed to the published version of the manuscript.

Funding: This research received no external funding.

Institutional Review Board Statement: The study was conducted in accordance with the Declaration of Helsinki and approved by the Institutional Review Board The Ethics Committee of the Medical University of Graz, the study protocol (30-253 ex 17/18).

Informed Consent Statement: Not applicable.

Data Availability Statement: The data presented in this study are available on request from the corresponding author.

Conflicts of Interest: Andreas Leithner and Patrick Sadoghi received industrial grants from DePuySynthes, alphamed, and Medacta not related to the submitted manuscript. The remaining authors have no potential conflict of interest to declare.

References

1. Berend, M.E.; Small, S.R.; Ritter, M.A.; Buckley, C.A.; Merk, J.C.; Dierking, W.K. Effects of femoral component size on proximal tibial strain with anatomic graduated components total knee arthroplasty. *J. Arthroplast.* **2010**, *25*, 58–63. [CrossRef]
2. Ritter, M.A.; Faris, P.M.; Keating, E.M.; Meding, J.B. Postoperative alignment of total knee replacement. Its effect on survival. *Clin. Orthop. Relat. Res.* **1994**, *299*, 153–156. [CrossRef]
3. Kinzel, V.; Scaddan, M.; Bradley, B.; Shakespeare, D. Varus/valgus alignment of the femur in total knee arthroplasty. Can accuracy be improved by pre-operative CT scanning? *Knee* **2004**, *11*, 197–201. [CrossRef] [PubMed]
4. Kniesel, B.; Konstantinidis, L.; Hirschmüller, A.; Südkamp, N.; Helwig, P. Digital templating in total knee and hip replacement: An analysis of planning accuracy. *Int. Orthop.* **2014**, *38*, 733–739. [CrossRef] [PubMed]
5. Schroer, W.C.; Berend, K.R.; Lombardi, A.V.; Barnes, C.L.; Bolognesi, M.P.; Berend, M.E.; Ritter, M.A.; Nunley, R.M. Why are total knees failing today? Etiology of total knee revision in 2010 and 2011. *J. Arthroplast.* **2013**, *28*, 116–119. [CrossRef]
6. Goyal, N.; Stulberg, S.D. Evaluating the Precision of Preoperative Planning in Patient Specific Instrumentation: Can a Single MRI Yield Different Preoperative Plans? *J. Arthroplast.* **2015**, *30*, 1250–1253. [CrossRef]

7. Hirschmann, M.T.; Konala, P.; Amsler, F.; Iranpour, F.; Friederich, N.F.; Cobb, J.P. The position and orientation of total knee replacement components: A comparison of conventional radiographs, transverse 2D-CT slices and 3D-CT reconstruction. *J. Bone Jt. Surg. Br.* **2011**, *93*, 629–633. [CrossRef]
8. Tiefenboeck, S.; Sesselmann, S.; Taylor, D.; Forst, R.; Seehaus, F. Preoperative planning of total knee arthroplasty: Reliability of axial alignment using a three-dimensional planning approach. *Acta Radiol.* **2022**, *63*, 1051–1061. [CrossRef]
9. The, B.; Diercks, R.L.; van Ooijen, P.M.A.; van Horn, J.R. Comparison of analog and digital preoperative planning in total hip and knee arthroplasties. A prospective study of 173 hips and 65 total knees. *Acta Orthop.* **2005**, *76*, 78–84. [CrossRef]
10. Hsu, A.R.; Kim, J.D.; Bhatia, S.; Levine, B.R. Effect of training level on accuracy of digital templating in primary total hip and knee arthroplasty. *Orthopedics* **2012**, *35*, e179–e183. [CrossRef]
11. Kobayashi, A.; Ishii, Y.; Takeda, M.; Noguchi, H.; Higuchi, H.; Toyabe, S. Comparison of analog 2D and digital 3D preoperative templating for predicting implant size in total knee arthroplasty. *Comput. Aided Surg.* **2012**, *17*, 96–101. [CrossRef]
12. Ettinger, M.; Claassen, L.; Paes, P.; Calliess, T. 2D versus 3D templating in total knee arthroplasty. *Knee* **2016**, *23*, 149–151. [CrossRef] [PubMed]
13. Jazrawi, L.M.; Birdzell, L.; Kummer, F.J.; Di Cesare, P.E. The accuracy of computed tomography for determining femoral and tibial total knee arthroplasty component rotation. *J. Arthroplast.* **2000**, *15*, 761–766. [CrossRef] [PubMed]
14. Konigsberg, B.; Hess, R.; Hartman, C.; Smith, L.; Garvin, K.L. Inter- and intraobserver reliability of two-dimensional CT scan for total knee arthroplasty component malrotation. *Clin. Orthop. Relat. Res.* **2014**, *472*, 212–217. [CrossRef] [PubMed]
15. Koo, T.K.; Li, M.Y. A Guideline of Selecting and Reporting Intraclass Correlation Coefficients for Reliability Research. *J. Chiropr. Med.* **2016**, *15*, 155–163. [CrossRef] [PubMed]
16. Hankemeier, S.; Gosling, T.; Richter, M.; Hufner, T.; Hochhausen, C.; Krettek, C. Computer-assisted analysis of lower limb geometry: Higher intraobserver reliability compared to conventional method. *Comput. Aided Surg.* **2006**, *11*, 81–86. [CrossRef]
17. Schröter, S.; Ihle, C.; Mueller, J.; Lobenhoffer, P.; Stöckle, U.; van Heerwaarden, R. Digital planning of high tibial osteotomy. Interrater reliability by using two different software. *Knee Surg. Sports Traumatol. Arthrosc.* **2013**, *21*, 189–196. [CrossRef] [PubMed]
18. Lee, Y.S.; Kim, M.K.; Byun, H.W.; Kim, S.B.; Kim, J.G. Reliability of the imaging software in the preoperative planning of the open-wedge high tibial osteotomy. *Knee Surg. Sports Traumatol. Arthrosc.* **2015**, *23*, 846–851. [CrossRef]
19. Moreland, J.R. Mechanisms of failure in total knee arthroplasty. *Clin. Orthop. Relat. Res.* **1988**, *226*, 49–64. [CrossRef]
20. Gopurathingal, A.A.; Bhonsle, S. Inter-Observer and Intra-Observer Reliability of 2D Radiograph-Based Valgus Cut Angle Measurement in Preoperative Planning for Primary Total Knee Arthroplasty. *Cureus* **2021**, *13*, e12788. [CrossRef]
21. Swanson, K.E.; Stocks, G.W.; Warren, P.D.; Hazel, M.R.; Janssen, H.F. Does axial limb rotation affect the alignment measurements in deformed limbs? *Clin. Orthop. Relat. Res.* **2000**, *371*, 246–252. [CrossRef] [PubMed]
22. Pagano, S.; Müller, K.; Götz, J.; Reinhard, J.; Schindler, M.; Grifka, J.; Maderbacher, G. The Role and Efficiency of an AI-Powered Software in the Evaluation of Lower Limb Radiographs before and after Total Knee Arthroplasty. *J. Clin. Med.* **2023**, *12*, 5498. [CrossRef] [PubMed]
23. Miura, M.; Hagiwara, S.; Nakamura, J.; Wako, Y.; Kawarai, Y.; Ohtori, S. Interobserver and Intraobserver Reliability of Computed Tomography-Based Three-Dimensional Preoperative Planning for Primary Total Knee Arthroplasty. *J. Arthroplast.* **2018**, *33*, 1572–1578. [CrossRef] [PubMed]
24. Kastner, N.; Aigner, B.A.; Meikl, T.; Friesenbichler, J.; Wolf, M.; Glehr, M.; Gruber, G.; Leithner, A.; Sadoghi, P. Gender-specific outcome after implantation of low-contact-stress mobile-bearing total knee arthroplasty with a minimum follow-up of ten years. *Int. Orthop.* **2014**, *38*, 2489–2493. [CrossRef]
25. Kastner, N.; Sternbauer, S.; Friesenbichler, J.; Vielgut, I.; Wolf, M.; Glehr, M.; Leithner, A.; Sadoghi, P. Impact of the tibial slope on range of motion after low-contact-stress, mobile-bearing, total knee arthroplasty. *Int. Orthop.* **2014**, *38*, 291–295. [CrossRef]
26. Neubauer, M.; Moser, L.; Neugebauer, J.; Raudner, M.; Wondrasch, B.; Führer, M.; Emprechtinger, R.; Dammerer, D.; Ljuhar, R.; Salzlechner, C.; et al. Artificial-Intelligence-Aided Radiographic Diagnostic of Knee Osteoarthritis Leads to a Higher Association of Clinical Findings with Diagnostic Ratings. *J. Clin. Med.* **2023**, *12*, 744. [CrossRef]

Disclaimer/Publisher's Note: The statements, opinions and data contained in all publications are solely those of the individual author(s) and contributor(s) and not of MDPI and/or the editor(s). MDPI and/or the editor(s) disclaim responsibility for any injury to people or property resulting from any ideas, methods, instructions or products referred to in the content.

MDPI
St. Alban-Anlage 66
4052 Basel
Switzerland
www.mdpi.com

Journal of Clinical Medicine Editorial Office
E-mail: jcm@mdpi.com
www.mdpi.com/journal/jcm

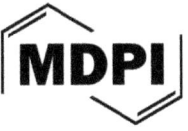

Disclaimer/Publisher's Note: The statements, opinions and data contained in all publications are solely those of the individual author(s) and contributor(s) and not of MDPI and/or the editor(s). MDPI and/or the editor(s) disclaim responsibility for any injury to people or property resulting from any ideas, methods, instructions or products referred to in the content.

www.ingramcontent.com/pod-product-compliance
Lightning Source LLC
LaVergne TN
LVHW070626100526
838202LV00012B/738